# Occupational Therapy:
# The First 30 Years

*1900 to 1930*

# Occupational Therapy: The First 30 Years
## *1900 to 1930*

❦ ❦ ❦

Virginia Anne Metaxas Quiroga, PhD

The American
Occupational Therapy Association, Inc.

Copyright © 1995 by the American Occupational Therapy Association, Inc.
All Rights Reserved.

*Occupational Therapy: The First 30 Years, 1900 to 1930* may not be reproduced in whole or in part, by any means, without permission.

For information address: The American Occupational Therapy Association, Inc., 4720 Montgomery Lane, PO Box 31220, Bethesda, MD 20854-1220.

*Disclaimers*

"This publication is designed to provide accurate and authoritative information in regard to the subject matter covered. It is sold or distributed with the understanding that the publisher is not engaged in rendering legal, accounting, or other professional service. If legal advice or other expert assistance is required, the services of a competent professional person should be sought."

> *From the Declaration of Principles jointly adopted by the*
> *American Bar Association and a Committee of Publishers and Associations.*

It is the objective of the American Occupational Therapy Association to be a forum for free expression and interchange of ideas. The opinions expressed by the contributors to this work are their own and not necessarily those of either the editors or the American Occupational Therapy Association.

Edited by Margo Johnson

Designed by Robert Sacheli

Printed in the United States of America

ISBN 1-56900-025-5

*To Beatrice Wade*
*1903–1994*

# Contents

Acknowledgments . . . . . . . . . . . . . . . . . . . . . . . . . . . . . xi

**Foreword**
by Robert K. Bing . . . . . . . . . . . . . . . . . . . . . . . . . . . . . 1

**Introduction.**
**The First Generation of Occupational Therapists:
A Study of Dual Authority** . . . . . . . . . . . . . . . . . . . . . 11

    A Brief Background on Activity Treatment
    Before the Twentieth Century . . . . . . . . . . . . . . . . 19

## Part I.
## The Rise of Occupational Therapy . . . . . . . . 29

**Chapter 1.**
**"The Jane Addams of Occupational Therapy":
Eleanor Clarke Slagle and
Women's Work in the Age of Reform** . . . . . . . . . . . . . 33

    The Importance of Hull House . . . . . . . . . . . . . . . . 37

    Aspiring Professional Eleanor Clarke Slagle . . . . . . . 42

**Chapter 2.**
**Psychiatry:
The Medical Birthplace of Occupational Therapy** . . . 51

    Young Dr. Dunton . . . . . . . . . . . . . . . . . . . . . . . . . . 53

    William Rush Dunton, Jr., at the
    Sheppard and Enoch Pratt Hospital . . . . . . . . . . . . . 55

    Spokesperson for the Neophyte Profession . . . . . . . . . 61

**Chapter 3.**
**Nurses for Invalid Occupations:
Susan E. Tracy and the
Expansion of Occupational Therapy** . . . . . . . . . . . . . 69

    Susan E. Tracy and the Adams Nervine Asylum . . . . . 73

    Founding of the Experiment Station
    for the Study of Invalid Occupations . . . . . . . . . . . . 79

    Altruistic Lady or Independent Professional? . . . . . . . 83

## Chapter 4.
### A Patient at Work is a Patient Half Cured: Herbert James Hall, the Arts and Crafts Movement, and Early Occupational Therapy Theory ........... 91

    The Devereux Workshops ..................... 96

    "O.T. Equivalents, Immunities, and Substitutions" .. 101

    The Influence of Emmanuelism ................. 103

## Chapter 5.
### Education of "the Handicapped": Occupational Therapy and Physical Rehabilitation Before World War I ........................ 113

    The Authentic Self: George Edward Barton at Consolation House ......116

    Philip King Brown and the Care of Patients With Tuberculosis .................. 125

    Susan Cox Johnson and Evelyn Lawrence Collins in New York City ........ 130

# Part II.
# World War I and Occupational Therapy ................ 143

## Chapter 6.
### "No More Cripples": The Reconstruction Movement ................. 149

    The Wartime Reconstruction Movement ......... 151

    The Reconstruction Aides ...................... 157

## Chapter 7.
### "Do Your Bit for the Boys": Occupational Therapy's Response to the Call for Service ................ 171

    The National Society for the Promotion of Occupational Therapy .......... 174

    The New York War Service Classes for Training Reconstruction Aides in Occupational Therapy ...................... 177

    Elizabeth Greene Upham and Milwaukee-Downer College ................ 182

Philanthropic Support
and the Service Ethic .................... 185

Typical Career Tracks of
the Reconstruction Aide Generation ............ 189

# PART III.
# STABILIZATION AND
# STANDARDIZATION IN THE 1920s ............ 203

## CHAPTER 8.
## Professional Culture and Education
## in Occupational Therapy in the 1920s ............ 209

Professional Culture:
Recruitment, Mentoring, and Networking ........ 212

The Beginnings of Education Reform ............ 218

Minimum Standards for
Courses of Training in Occupational Therapy ...... 223

## CHAPTER 9.
## Men, Medical Identity,
## and Survival in the 1920s ..................... 233

Herbert James Hall, Horatio M. Pollack,
and Record Keeping ....................... 238

Thomas B. Kidner,
Rehabilitation, and Tuberculosis ................ 242

Occupational Therapy and
the Problem of Commercialism ................ 244

William Rush Dunton, Jr., and the
Committee on Publicity and Publication ......... 245

Everett S. Elwood and
the Perils of Professional Growth ................ 250

# PART IV.
# SEEING IS BELIEVING:
# EXHIBITIONS AND PHOTOGRAPHS ............. 259

The Prewar Era (Photographs 11–14) ............ 264

Wartime (Photographs 15–19) .................. 270

The Postwar Period (Photographs 20–24) ......... 274

The Legacy of the First Generation .............. 278

# Acknowledgments

*Acknowledgments*

In the early 1980s, when I was a graduate student in the History Department at the State University of New York at Stony Brook, Professor Fred Weinstein made a comment that I appreciate only now. He said, "No one ever writes anything alone." During the several years that I worked on this book, I realized the wisdom of his words as I leaned on the expert advice and support of many historians, occupational therapists, librarians, archivists, editors, and friends. I owe these women and men much gratitude, for without their help, I would never have completed this work.

I must first thank the American Occupational Therapy Foundation for initiating the idea to write a history of the profession of occupational therapy, and for providing financial support. Martha Kirkland and especially Nedra Gillette contacted me regularly over the years, helping keep me and the project focused. Martha, Nedra, Mary Binderman, Robert Bing, Chester Burns, Marion Crampton, Kathlyn Reed, Susan Reverby, Ruth Levine Schemm, Mildred Schwagmeyer, Kay Barker Schwartz, Nancy Snyder, and Wilma West, all members of the ad hoc Critical Historical Issues Committee, met with me at the very beginning to identify significant people and topics to be included in the book. Several members of this committee collaborated with me as the project progressed.

So many occupational therapists, appreciative of the profession's fine tradition and history, were astoundingly supportive in helping me accomplish this work. Wilma West offered useful suggestions on drafts of several chapters, but more than that, as everyone knows, she was the vital spirit behind the project. Mildred Schwagmeyer saw that I would be able to conduct necessary research in St. Louis; she even opened her home to me so that I had a place to stay. Equally generous, Diane Gibson provided me with friendship, elegant accommodations, and access to research materials at the Sheppard-Pratt Hospital which historians can usually only dream about. Kitty Reed sent me many helpful materials, as well as editorial suggestions on early drafts. Terry Anne E. Litterst generously shared materials and ideas about the Boston School of Occupational Therapy. Cheryl Mattingly trustingly gave me the use of her apartment while I was in Chicago, even though she herself was not there. Over a cup of tea, Beatrice Wade graciously shared personal stories with me about the founding years of the profession. Also providing information and support were Carolyn Baum, Wendy Colman, Nadine Davis, Nancy Ellis, Norma Howat, Jacqueline Jones, Barbara Loomis, Caroline Morris, Frances Palmer, Lillian Parent, Sharon Schwartzberg, and numerous others whom I have not named. I am thankful to them all. Finally, for his untiring work in preserving occupational therapy's history, Robert K. Bing deserves the gratitude of the entire profession, but for now, I express only my thanks to him for his help with my work. Bob's enthusiasm, humor, gentle yet rigorous criticism, and insight into the minds of occupational therapists of long ago, was crucial to my interpretation of the history of occupational therapy. Bob is a consummate mentor and simultaneously a cooperative peer, a friend with whom I could enjoy sharing both my frustrations and my findings.

Since the inception of this work, my colleagues in women's history and in the social history of medicine have encouraged me countless times. Morris Vogel critically read and commented on early drafts of many chapters. Susan Reverby, whose work in the history of nursing has profoundly influenced me, helped me clarify many ideas in my work. Her input enabled me substantially to improve the final product. Other helpful colleagues were Rima Apple, Ruth Schwartz Cowan, Janet Golden, and Judith Walzer Leavitt, all of whom read parts of the manuscript at various points of its development. I owe my greatest debt to the members of my history writers' group: Polly Beals, Lucy Bowditch, C. Jane Covell, David McDonald, and Cynthia Ward, who gave freely of their time and attention. They challenged me intellectually, and also gave me much-needed emotional support when I faltered from time to time, as all authors do.

I thank the National Endowment for the Humanities for helping defray travel costs to Chicago and San Francisco (NEH Travel to Collections Grant, ID Number FE-24008-89, received during the period June to November, 1989).

I thank the archivists and the librarians of the following institutions, whose professional commitment and enthusiasm helped me uncover information not previously found: the Columbia County Historical Society, Kinderhawk, New York; the Delaware County Historical Association, Delhi, New York; the New York State Historical Association, Cooperstown; the National Archives, Washington, D.C.; the Library of the Health Sciences, University of Illinois at Chicago; the National Library of Medicine, Bethesda, Maryland; the Faulkner Hospital–Adams House, Boston, Massachusetts; the Library of Congress, Washington, D.C.; the Moody Library of the University of Texas Medical Branch, Galveston; the Philadelphia School of Occupational Therapy; the Medical Archives of the Hospital of the University of Pennsylvania, Philadelphia; the Sheppard-Pratt Hospital, Towson, Maryland; the New York Hospital–Cornell Medical Center Medical Archives, New York City; Teachers College Archives of Columbia University, New York City; Montefiore Hospital Archives, New York City; the Medical Library, University of California, San Francisco; the Francis A. Countway Library of Medicine, Harvard University, Cambridge, Massachusetts; the Alan Mason Chesney Medical Archive, Johns Hopkins Medical Institutions, Baltimore, Maryland; the Nils Yngve Wessell Library, Tufts University, Medford, Massachusetts; the New York Genealogical and Biographical Society, New York City; the Department of Occupational Therapy, College of Allied Health Sciences, Thomas Jefferson University, Philadelphia; the Newberry Library, Chicago; the State Historical Society of Wisconsin, Madison; the Wilma L. West Library, American Occupational Therapy Foundation, Bethesda, Maryland; the San Francisco Historical Society; the Archives and History of Medicine, School of Medicine, Washington University, St. Louis, Missouri; the Department of Occupational Therapy, Washington University, St. Louis, Missouri; McLean Hospital Archives, Belmont, Massachusetts; the New York Public Library; and the Buley Library, Southern Connecticut State University.

A special thanks to Inci Bowman for her masterful handling of the Official Archives of the American Occupational Therapy Association, and especially for showing me materials that were categorized as "unprocessed." Librarian Mary Binderman of the Wilma L. West Library, and the staff, never wavered in their commitment to seeing this work reach its potential. So often they sent me materials when I could not make the trip to Maryland.

I am very grateful to Margo Johnson, whose editorial skills have me in absolute awe. She kept me honest in more ways than I can possibly explain. Many thanks to Elizabeth Holcomb and all the staff of the Nonperiodical Publications Department of the American Occupational Therapy Association for seeing this project to its completion.

Friends and family, my most valued relationships, deserve the most thanks, of course. Thanks to my dear friends Sandy Morse and Tony Tommasi, both of whom have watched over me and my work since the 1970s when I was an undergraduate student at the State University of New York at Old Westbury.

Lorraine Edwards listened to me obsess over the writing of this book during hundreds of our exercise walks and telephone conversations; her steady encouragement kept me on track. My sisters Anne D. Metaxas and Victoria C. Metaxas and my brother Charles C. Metaxas have always been there for me. Only we know how much our loving parents, the late Stella and Dennis Metaxas, still guide and sustain us. Finally, thanks to the three men with whom I share a full life, my sons Paul and Alex and my husband Tony, for their patience, care, and willingness to share me with my other love, history.

*Virginia Anne Metaxas Quiroga*
*Norwalk, Connecticut*
*January 1995*

# Foreword

*by*
Robert K. Bing

*Foreword*

In the early years of this century, a woman emerged as this country's first management consultant. Mary Parker Follett had as a client a window-shade business that was about to fail. The company hired Follett to determine the causes of and the cure for the problem. After interviewing customers, employees, and management, she recommended that the company reconceptualize its enterprise; rather than be in the window-shade business, it should be in the light-control business. Once this expanded view took hold, the company flourished beyond expectations.

Follett coined the term and the concept, the Law of the Situation. It asks the questions, "What is the business you *really* are in?" and "What is the business you think it would be *useful* for you to be in?"

In these waning years of the twentieth century, nearly all of us are taking inventories and determining to one extent or another what business we are in or ought to be in. Seemingly we are preparing for some marked, possibly dramatic changes, some type of new enterprise. More than a few people are predicting that the coming of the next millennium will usher in a quite different way of thinking and behaving. At present, everything seems to be in flux. No two days are quite alike. We can be surprised at a moment's notice. The gravitational pull of the millennium seems to signal that we have a lot of stuff to deal with and to straighten out. We need to get right with ourselves and others. There is a distinct feeling that something is about to happen.

This phenomenon is not troubling to historians. They realize that there is something curiously special about the last decade of each century, an unusual surge of energy to clear the old century's agenda and make ready for the new century. The syndrome of the '90s focuses on both the past and the future.

For instance, during the 1490s, the King and Queen of Spain were clearing their country's agenda by defeating the Moors and expelling the Jews. At the same time they were financially underwriting the initial voyages of Columbus, which took him westward in search of the Orient's riches. Spain needed these riches to realize its desire to dominate the next century. Thus began the Age of Discovery.

Another important decade of the '90s occurred in the eighteenth century. The Age of Enlightenment in Europe was at full power. From this fervor came the antecedents of occupational therapy. The French were attending a revolution over past injustices and new social and political ideals, clearing away an outworn agenda. The English were similarly involved in reconceptualizing attitudes and principles that governed humanity and society. Philippe Pinel, a physician and a reformer, was a product of the French Revolution. He initiated moral treatment in the care of people considered insane. William Tuke, a deeply religious Quaker and an English philanthropist, founded the York Retreat and ushered in an era of reforms emphasizing the humane care of persons with mental illness. By the beginning of the nineteenth century, many of these ideals and practices had been transported to the newly established United States and had become important building blocks in the American cultural experiment.

The 1890s was a decade of 1,000 movements. Everything was "modern": unions, art, drama, economics, politics, industry. The modern women's movement ultimately became the twentieth century's feminist movement. It was a time of changing manners, roles, styles, and fashions—an age of anticipation and transition. There was a distinct feeling that something was coming to an end and something new was about to happen. Indeed, the American Century was about to dawn.

The 1990s have come to be known by some as a "New Age." In contrast to the 1890s, the present decade is taking shape in 10,000 movements and 100,000 opinions. Everyone has an opinion on nearly every subject; everyone is stridently offering advice. Social, political, economic, technological, and philosophical issues and debates abound, crowding our everyday lives. Most of these debates are about issues left over from previous decades. At times the din is deafening, and more than a few of us long for a period of silence and contemplation. We are constantly pushed and pulled by change, to the point that some of us are beginning to agree with the wit who declared, "Progress is just fine, so long as it does not go on too long."

Meanwhile, the push is on to complete this century's agenda and to prepare for the next century and the new millennium. An odd assortment of activities has appeared. Some people have taken up reading and interpreting Nostradamus's prophetic verse from the 1550s; they hope to find out how the century will end. Others are investing time, effort, and resources in the paraphernalia and the practices of the New Age. This cultural phenomenon has also given rise to "alternative medicine," which is now a nearly $30-billion-a-year industry. Many of the alternatives have an ancient lineage.

The dramatic resurgence of fundamentalism is ever present. Historians believe it to be a reaction to modernism and abrupt change. In times of turbulence we tend to turn to structure, rather than to debatable ambiguities. As a society, we have been through this before. With the onset of the Industrial Revolution some 200 years ago, Protestant revivalism emerged to counteract the unprecedented changes of people moving from cottage industries to factories and replacing hand tools with machinery. Contemporary observers believe that as long as we experience cultural turbulence related to great change, revivalism and fundamentalism will remain. Once we no longer require so much structure to cope with change, fundamentalism will recede in importance.

Socially we are reexamining a founding construct of the American culture. Until very recently we nearly all subscribed to the belief that we were a multiethnic country with the capabilities of creating a new American culture. This was thought to be a brilliant solution, not possible anywhere else in the world. "*E pluribus unum*"—"one out of many"—which appears on the United States seal and coinage, means precisely that: a cultural synthesis. Because of past insensitivities, multiculturalism and political correctness have appeared and given rise, as the historian Arthur Schlesinger states, "to the conception of the U.S. as a nation composed not of individuals making their own choices but of inviolable ethnic and racial groups. It rejects the historic American goals of assimilation and integration . . . The balance is shifting from *unum* to *pluribus*" (from "one" to "many"). Should this separatist trend be allowed to continue, Schlesinger adds, "the result can only be the fragmentation, resegregation and tribalization of American life."[1]

The melting pot would be melted down and made into a monument to our new, quaint ways.

Daniel Boorstin, Pulitzer Prize–winning historian, writer, and former Librarian of Congress, recently lamented as "un-American" the emergence of hyphenated Americans, a distinct symbol of the 1990s: "I believe there are only *Americans* [emphasis in original] . . . There has been so much emphasis recently on the diversity of our peoples. I think it's time that we reaffirmed the fact that what has built our country is community and that community is not dependent on government. It's dependent on the willingness of people to build together." American community building, Boorstin continued, stands in stark contrast to "the fanaticisms and miseries of much of the rest of the world, . . . the terrors of ethnic cleansing in Europe, the horrors of tribal warfare in Africa and the oppressions of totalitarianism, which by no means has entirely disappeared."[2]

Health care, with all its social, political, economic, technological, and philosophical ramifications, has been elaborately laid out for everyone's scrutiny and comment. Rarely in our history has a topic been so thoroughly examined, debated, and brought into our homes and business places with such detail. Since the Kennedy and Johnson eras of the 1960s and the passage of Medicare and Medicaid, government involvement in medical practice and health care has been unprecedented. With the many-faceted enterprises of medicine and health care becoming the conjoint business of industry, insurance and drug companies, public and private institutions, and federal and state governments, it is little wonder that we are experiencing a medical arms race as intensely competitive as any military arms race. The politics of resentment is everywhere, and we are in the midst of a revolution and a reformation whose outcomes are still very much in doubt.

The occupational therapy profession is caught up in the whirlwind of change. In addition to wondering where we will wind up, on whose side we should be in the revolution, and what positions we should take in the reformation, we are attempting to determine what business we really are in or what business it would be useful for us to be in. We are in the midst of our own twentieth-century "fin de siècle," and we suspect that some dramatic things are about to happen.

No less than any other health profession, occupational therapy is coming to realize in this last decade of the twentieth century that we have a lot of stuff to deal with and to straighten out. We need to get right with ourselves and with all others. Witness some of the issues currently under consideration: (1) our current squabbles with similar professions, such as nursing and physical therapy; (2) our experimental endeavors to establish some kinds of alliances with like-minded professions; (3) our continuing attempts to gain political recognition through licensure; (4) the reexamination of the name and the ultimate roles of the occupational therapy assistant and aide; (5) our present review of appropriate relationships with medicine and social services; (6) the ongoing discourse about the proper educational preparation for entry-level practice; (7) our emerging notions about different behaviors that occupational therapy practitioners should employ with patients and clients; (8) the appropriateness of clinical and academic research in fulfilling the promise of occupational therapy; (9) our current reexamination of long-standing concepts of occupation, function, independence, and the psychosocial core of occupational therapy; (10) the splitting of practice into discrete, medically determined entities, thereby creating hyphenated occupational therapists, as it were; all of which has resulted in a *conspiracy of disunity*, replacing professional *unum* with *pluribus* and potentially setting the stage for fragmentation, segregation, and tribalization of the profession; and (11) the mechanical bias that has crept into practice, at the expense of spiritualism, a long-standing, dearly held belief.

A treatment that holds the promise of an early cure for many of our ills lies in a fresh look at where we came from and where we have been. This must be as vigorously pursued as our endeavors to prepare for our future. If a touchstone is needed, it might well be William James's dictum, "We live forward; we understand backwards," or if we prefer, Kierkegaard's observation, "Life must be lived forwards, but can only be understood backwards."

We should approach this activity with a few basic suppositions. Almost any way we might turn, any route we might follow, someone, sometime, has traveled it. From this supposition we ought to gain assurance that much of what troubles us today troubled our founders and professional ancestors; nevertheless, with uncommon perseverance and fortitude, they succeeded well beyond their original intentions or expectations.

A second assumption is that the fundamental belief system that drove those in the past propels us today. Occupational therapy is an ideal born in a philosophical movement, that became activated through the good works of women and men who unalterably believed that those who were sick and disabled could *regain*, *retain*, and *attain* some semblance of function within the limitations imposed by the human organism and the expectations of society; and that this might occur by the most obvious means of all—reorganization through occupation, through activity, through leisure, and through rest.[3]

Still another supposition is this: as Hugh Sidey has noted, "History is a marvelous collection of stories about men and women who refuse to accept the common verdict that certain achievements [are] impossible."[4] Travels to our professional archives and diggings confirm that occupational therapy's early history in this century is replete with stories of the ideals, the deeds, the hopes, and the works of *individuals*, rather than groups or organizations. All of them were infused with unusual zeal and an unwillingness to accept compromise or defeat. They advanced changes in attitudes and practices that reduced or eliminated outmoded inhumanity toward people who were sick and disabled. These same men and women assumed the responsibilities of caring about and for persons who were not highly valued by society, most particularly those who were considered nonproducing and economically burdensome to their families and the community.

We should come back from excursions to our archives with a profound appreciation that the original, single purpose of preparing occupational therapy practitioners was to create individuals who could care for patients, their families, and the community. The primary idea was for practitioners to perform a service, not to establish economic enterprises that would guarantee a profit. Nor was it ever intended that occupational therapy practitioners would become indentured servants to physicians, or sycophants to the business people running institutions. Neither was there an intention to transform occupational therapy practitioners into researchers, adding more responsibilities to an already burdened practice, thereby putting at potential risk the original purpose—to care for patients.

By learning, perhaps for the first time, about the problems that our founders and their immediate successors faced, and the ways in which they resolved these vexing difficulties, we can gain assurance that problems ultimately are solved or go away. How these remarkable individuals coexisted and collaborated with both friends and adversaries offers us encouragement that we can do the same, with measurable success.

The stories about the founders, particularly those about Eleanor Clarke Slagle and William Rush Dunton, Jr., provide us with a rich lode of information on how we can reverse the disturbing trend of splitting our practice into seemingly unrelated entities. We need to reaffirm that what built our profession was a communal spirit, a oneness of purpose, an intent *to build together*, in spite of the realization that occupational therapy practitioners would ultimately scatter liberally over the medical and health-related landscapes. A common language and a common culture, pieced together by these outstanding individuals, have brought us through to today, with all the empowerment we currently enjoy. If the founders had permitted practitioners of that time to segment themselves into media-based or medically related entities, we would not have a profession today. At best we might be a loosely fashioned confederation of far-distant professional relatives, residing in a many-roomed mansion of indistinct architecture.

Reading our history should be of particular value to a younger generation of shakers and movers who fervently believe that their world is new, that all their problems are freshly minted, and that they need only employ reason and emotion to come to some resolutions. A legacy of experience, acquired from understanding the past, whether remote or recent, provides invaluable assistive information in deciding what to do, or not to do, today about the future.

Finally, a knowledge and an appreciation of the pathways that our progenitors traveled offer us substantial knowledge that enhances our competence, understanding, and courage. Unlike the ancient mariners who had to use incomplete maps and fear those unknown regions marked as "Here Be Dragons," our professional ancestors left behind well-drawn charts of their progress and practice. Often they had to make do with very few resources; yet they were proud of their accomplishments and wrote copiously about their work. Their creativeness, frequently under dire conditions, is today a source of marvel and imagination, full of concepts and ideas that can serve us well and stiffen our backbones.

I commend to readers this very well documented history of the first decades of twentieth-century occupational therapy, so ably recounted by Professor Virginia Quiroga. I sincerely hope that readers will experience an array of insights and emotions as our profession's past is unrolled for our enlightenment and understanding.

*Robert K. Bing, EdD, OTR, FAOTA*
*Professor Emeritus*
*University of Texas Medical Branch, Galveston*

## NOTES

1. Arthur Schlesinger, "The Cult of Ethnicity, Good and Bad," *Time*, 8 July 1991, 21.
2. As quoted in T. Szulc, "The Greatest Danger," *Parade*, 25 July 1993, 4, 5–6.
3. Paraphrased from Robert K. Bing, "Occupational Therapy Revisited: A Paraphrastic Journey," *American Journal of Occupational Therapy* 35 (1981): 500.
4. Hugh Sidey, "The Presidency," *Time*, 1 December 1980, 18.

# Introduction

## The First Generation *of* Occupational Therapists

### A Study of Dual Authority

## Introduction

> Occupational therapy is defined as any activity, mental or physical, definitely prescribed and guided for the distinct purpose of contributing to and hastening recovery from disease or injury.
> H. A. Pattison, *physician, National Tuberculosis Association*

> Occupational therapy is directed activity which differs from all other forms of therapy in that it is given in increasing doses as the patient improves.
> Eleanor Clarke Slagle, *occupational therapist,*
> *New York State Department of Mental Hygiene*

> Occupational therapy is the science of organized work for invalids.
> Herbert James Hall, *physician, Devereux Workshops, Marblehead, Massachusetts*

Ever since the health profession of occupational therapy emerged in the early 1910s, it has had to explain itself to the world of medicine and to the public. The word "therapy" seems to have been understood easily: most Americans then and now would agree that therapy is some kind of treatment for either a physical or a mental disorder. The word "occupational" has been the troublesome one. During the 1910s many interpreted it to denote "vocational." The first generation of occupational therapists, however, meant much more than that by the word. They took a holistic approach to health care, believing that to achieve good health, a patient had to engage body, mind, and spirit in the process of healing. Healing, they argued, came about when patients were "occupied" with work, in particular, with craft activity. By interacting with individual patients and by observing with their own eyes, the early occupational therapists learned that occupational therapy restored physical function, improved mental attitude, and in general, lessened suffering, thus quickening convalescence.

In the early part of the twentieth century, such thinking offered Americans a critique of mainstream scientific medicine, which by that time had enthusiastically adopted the methods, the philosophy, and the tools of laboratory science, medical reductionism, and high technology. Occupational therapists and their supporters, many of whom were physicians, challenged the powerful leaders of scientific medicine. Scientific medicine had made significant gains in the fight against acute and infectious diseases, the advocates of occupational therapy acknowledged, but humanistic as well as scientific methods and values had to remain central in American medicine. Occupational therapy, they asserted, provided a necessary corrective to scientific medicine's overly objective approach. Patients were not merely diseased organs or tissues to be seen through the lens of the microscope or the image of a radiograph. They were whole persons needing care beyond the acute stages of illness. Furthermore, occupational therapists argued, complex social, economic, and biological reasons caused disease, not single microbes.

On the other hand, occupational therapy fit perfectly into the medical mainstream of the early twentieth century. Medical leadership was turning its attention from acute to chronic diseases. New medical specialties were proliferating to care for patients with psychiatric disorders, tuberculosis, heart disease, arthritis, and other degenerative and disabling conditions. Hospitals and clinics were springing up to support the growth of chronic care and medical specialization. Occupational therapy was yet another new profession to provide services during this period.

As occupational therapy created its professional boundaries during the 1910s, it wove the threads of its fabric from a variety of disciplines and social movements. Leaders took principles and practices from nursing, teaching, medicine, psychiatry, arts and crafts, rehabilitation, self-help, orthopedics, mental hygiene, social work, and more, enriching occupational therapy's professional depth and breadth.

Yet these varied perspectives caused problems as well. The first generation of occupational therapists found it difficult to create a concise body of knowledge, authority, and identity in the early twentieth century's evolving culture of professionalism and medical hierarchy.[1] In a time when scientific medicine seemed nearly obsessed with measurement—what health care professionals might today call "patient outcomes"—occupational therapists focused on process. The dilemmas of balancing the scientific and humanistic trends inherent in occupational therapy, of finding occupational therapy's place in American medicine, and of meeting the aims of scientific medicine still plague the profession today.

Occupational therapy was on the defensive at its emergence in the early twentieth century for at least two reasons: (1) occupational therapists believed that they had to fight the powerful world of scientific medicine and (2) occupational therapy was a new profession for *women*. Thus occupational therapy not only challenged early-twentieth-century mainstream medicine, but also contemporary, socially constructed gender roles. Most

Americans still assumed that a woman's place was in the private domestic sphere, or, if she entered health care, in nursing, as an assistant to a physician.

This book, a study of the early history of occupational therapy, shows how the profession chose to legitimize its authority in the world of medicine and with the general public by drawing on the dual authority of men in medicine and women in charity networks. Occupational therapy's male and female founders instituted a gender-defined division of labor. The men essentially built the necessary bridges to the largely male medical world. They made sure that occupational therapy took on the expected trappings of a profession, such as a theoretical base and a journal of research findings. Further, they assumed positions of authority in the American Occupational Therapy Association. From its founding in 1917 as the National Society for the Promotion of Occupational Therapy until after World War II, with the exception of one year, male physicians or men closely related to mainstream medicine served as president of the association. Often too, male physicians held conspicuous positions on boards of training schools and practice clinics.

This does not mean that the women played passive roles in the building of the profession, however. Most schools and clinics that have trained and provided workplaces for occupational therapists since 1917 have been founded, underwritten, and managed by a cooperating community of female practitioners and charity workers, often members of women's clubs or philanthropic organizations such as the Junior League or the Red Cross. As a result, these institutions have held a generous degree of autonomy and freedom from male-dominated medical and educational organizations, resting instead on a rich tradition of volunteer and charity activities among nineteenth-century American women.[2]

How important were women's values in molding occupational therapy's professional identity? Was occupational therapy's multidisciplinary nature the most formative characteristic in shaping its relationship to modern American health care? Examining the years 1900–1930, this study analyzes occupational therapy's first generation of practitioners and the institutions that they created. During those years the founders defined the profession's boundaries, developed theories of practice, increased the number of practitioners, strategized to convince the American public and the medical world of the value of occupational therapy, built many institutions in which to train practitioners and treat patients, and established standards for training and practice.

This all became possible in the context of women's entrance into professional work, which began in the late nineteenth century.[3] As women born in the last quarter of that century earned college degrees, they pursued in unprecedented numbers a variety of professions, mainly social work, education, medicine, nursing, and law. The body of literature in this subfield of women's history is growing. Other than studies of the history of American nursing, however, little attention has been paid to the growth and development of the many female-dominated health professions that emerged in the early twentieth century.[4] The stories of physical therapy, dietetics, and dental hygiene, for example, are yet to be told. This study serves as a partial corrective to such oversights.

Many studies of women's professional work have analyzed the cultural and ideological context in which middle- and upper-class women actively sought to establish a place for themselves outside the traditional sphere of marriage and family. Aspiring female professionals expanded the limits of nineteenth-century separate-sphere ideology by arguing that women's moral superiority, natural nurturing qualities, and altruism could and should be applied beyond the private family for the good of society. In a world rapidly changing from a rural to an urban context and from an agricultural to an industrial base, socially conscious women with professional aspirations fought to share in addressing the problems of modern society by improving conditions in the nation's schools, slums, hospitals, and social settlements. Fraught with conflict between traditional and modern female roles, many professional women of this transitional generation found that they could advance their influence on society by drawing on the strengths of women's networks as well as by aligning themselves with men in positions of authority. The women of Hull House in the 1890s, for example, expanded their political power and, by extension, their programs of social conscience, by affiliating with male reformers and male-dominated institutions.[5] The founding generation of occupational therapists adopted this strategy as well. Eleanor Clarke Slagle, who was part of the Hull House community in the first decade of this century, spearheaded the effort.

This study of the first generation of occupational therapists attempts to analyze the values that drew women to the field and to explain the personal and professional conflicts that they experienced. Unfortunately the primary sources available for examination were limited. Only a few founding-generation members born in the last decades of the nineteenth century have survived for interviews.[6] Worse, the leadership of the founding generation of occupational therapists left no personal papers. This gap is particularly striking considering that many female physicians, nurses, social workers, and educators of the early twentieth century left private papers such as diaries and letters for historians to examine; perhaps they understood their crucial role in the history of women's professional work. Even more puzzling is the fact that first-generation occupational therapists left few autobiographies or detailed records of their life work, as did social workers Jane Addams and Julia Lathrop or nurse Lillian Wald of the same generation.[7]

The dearth of published and unpublished primary sources has left later generations of occupational therapists with many questions concerning the origins of the founding generation. For example, little is known about the personal lives of three of occupational therapy's most prominent founders. A simple fact such as the true birth date of Eleanor Clarke Slagle, who was considered the mother of the profession and was often called by her contemporaries "the Jane Addams of occupational therapy," is unknown.[8] The early life of Susan E. Tracy, a nurse who wrote the field's first and for many years its most important textbook, is at best sketchy.[9] No one knows where Susan Cox Johnson received her training in arts and crafts, even though she held prestigious positions in that field at the Montefiore Home and Hospital for Chronic Diseases and at Teachers College, Columbia University, in the 1910s and 1920s.[10] What childhood influences led these women to lives of service? Who were their mentors? Why did Slagle marry, and why did she divorce? Did Tracy and Johnson consciously choose not to marry in order to pursue meaningful work outside traditional marriage and family? What were their opinions of the men with whom they worked to promote the field of occupational therapy?

Were these omissions in the record part of an effort—deliberate or otherwise—to cover what might have been considered inadequate credentials? Slagle, Tracy, and Johnson held no college degrees. Did they or following generations obscure the record because of a fear of negative consequences for their beloved occupational therapy? Did Slagle, Tracy, and Johnson project a self-effacing public image because they simply fell back on socially acceptable personality traits for women of the late Victorian era?

*Introduction*

The limited resources suggest that they shared at least some ambivalence about asserting powerful public images. They often deferred to medical authority, but only when necessary; they took charge in the female circles of their own institutions.

Fortunately, and ironically, men associated with occupational therapy have contributed to collecting, saving, and publishing historical materials. Psychiatrist William Rush Dunton, Jr., fondly known as the father of occupational therapy, first conceived of it in a professional medical model during the 1910s. Later he founded the profession's national journal and then edited it for many years. This journal has been an extremely valuable source of information.[11] In 1948 physician Sidney Licht published a collection of original writings establishing that occupational therapy's history predated the Christian era.[12] Occupational therapist Robert K. Bing, one of the few men to enter the field since it attained professional status in this century, and a recent president of the American Occupational Therapy Association, made sure that the extant papers of Dunton were saved, along with the records of the American Occupational Therapy Association.[13] Moreover, because Dunton lived a long life, Bing had the opportunity to interview him during the 1960s. Later Bing wrote a thorough and very useful biography as a doctoral dissertation.[14]

Recently many authors interested in establishing the profession's philosophical and historical antecedents have written papers and dissertations chronicling the American Occupational Therapy Association and various leaders and institutions.[15] Fortunately too, many of the schools founded during World War I saved historical materials, as did many private and public hospitals and clinics.[16] The resources surveyed for this study included the records of many training institutions and hospitals; the professional writings of occupational therapists, physicians, and psychiatrists; World War I records of the Office of the Surgeon General and other government agencies; newspaper articles; and the personal testimonials of practitioners. There were artifacts and photographs for examination as well, occupational therapy being a profession of many tools, prosthetic devices, and patient-made craft products. At the Pennsylvania Hospital in Philadelphia, a model of the occupational therapy department building, made by patients, stands in the office of the director of occupational therapy today. One can tip the roof back for a closer view. At the Sheppard and Enoch Pratt Hospital in Towson, Maryland, huge looms used for weaving during the 1910s by patients who were mentally ill are stored in the attic of the

Casino Building. Also, the audiovisual department is preserving a photograph collection of the history of the hospital, which includes many images of practitioners using occupational therapy to treat patients.[17] In many other places, photographs illustrating the enthusiasm with which patients engaged in arts and crafts and the dedication with which practitioners undertook their work still exist to serve as documents for the historian.[18]

Photographs 1 and 2 (following pages), taken in 1918 of World War I occupational therapy reconstruction aides at Fort McPherson, Georgia—photograph 2 including Surgeon General William C. Gorgas—reflect the internal dilemma experienced by the first generation of occupational therapists in the United States. A spirit of sisterhood and public service first drew them to occupational therapy; yet to ensure permanence for what Herbert James Hall would later call a "new profession for women," they had to show the public a facade of crisp professionalism. This study illuminates the ways in which the first generation of occupational therapists actively tried to integrate their traditional values as women into the ideology of professional medicine.

## A Brief Background on Activity Treatment Before the Twentieth Century

According to Sidney Licht, the earliest evidence of occupational therapy can be found in ancient times, in physicians' treatment of persons considered insane. One hundred years before the birth of Christ, the Greek physician Asclepiades initiated humane treatment of patients with mental illness using activity, including therapeutic baths, massage, exercises, and music. In doing so, he challenged the more common, somatic approach advocated by Hippocrates, who employed the severe methods of bloodletting, emetics, and purges to free patients of the evil spirits causing their illness. A century later, the Roman Celsus rejected the somatic approach, prescribing music, travel, conversation, light, and exhausting exercise for his suffering patients. Galen, who influenced physicians for the next fourteen centuries, completely "disregarded the psychological approach to mental illness," recommending somatic remedies considered harsh by modern standards.[19]

In medieval Europe, humane treatment of persons considered insane was rare. Persons who were mentally ill were associated with demons. Most of them were executed as witches. Others found themselves in hospitals, chained by the ankles and the wrists, and at times by the neck as well. Licht argues that the establishment of hospitals radically changed the care of these people. In hospitals, he writes, "physicians were able to see large numbers of psychotics under one roof and finally realize the mass inhumanity with which they were managed."[20]

As late as the eighteenth century in Europe, hospital superintendents relied on restraints, torture, and punishment in their treatment of persons considered insane, until the commencement of a reform movement, often attributed to the work of Philippe Pinel and Johann Christian Reil on the Continent and William Tuke in England.[21] In the French hospital Bicêtre, Pinel replaced metal chains with moral restraint. "Continuous work," he argued, "interrupts the chain of morbid thoughts, fixes the attention on more pleasant subjects and by means of exercise maintains order in any group of patients."[22] He instituted rigorous work and leisure activities in 1786. Reil improved on Pinel's ideas by including handcrafts and fine arts in his patients' regimens.[23] Tuke, a Quaker, created similar moral therapy regimens at the York Retreat in 1796.[24]

**Photograph 1:** Reconstruction aides, "Spirit of Sisterhood and Service." (AOTA Archives)

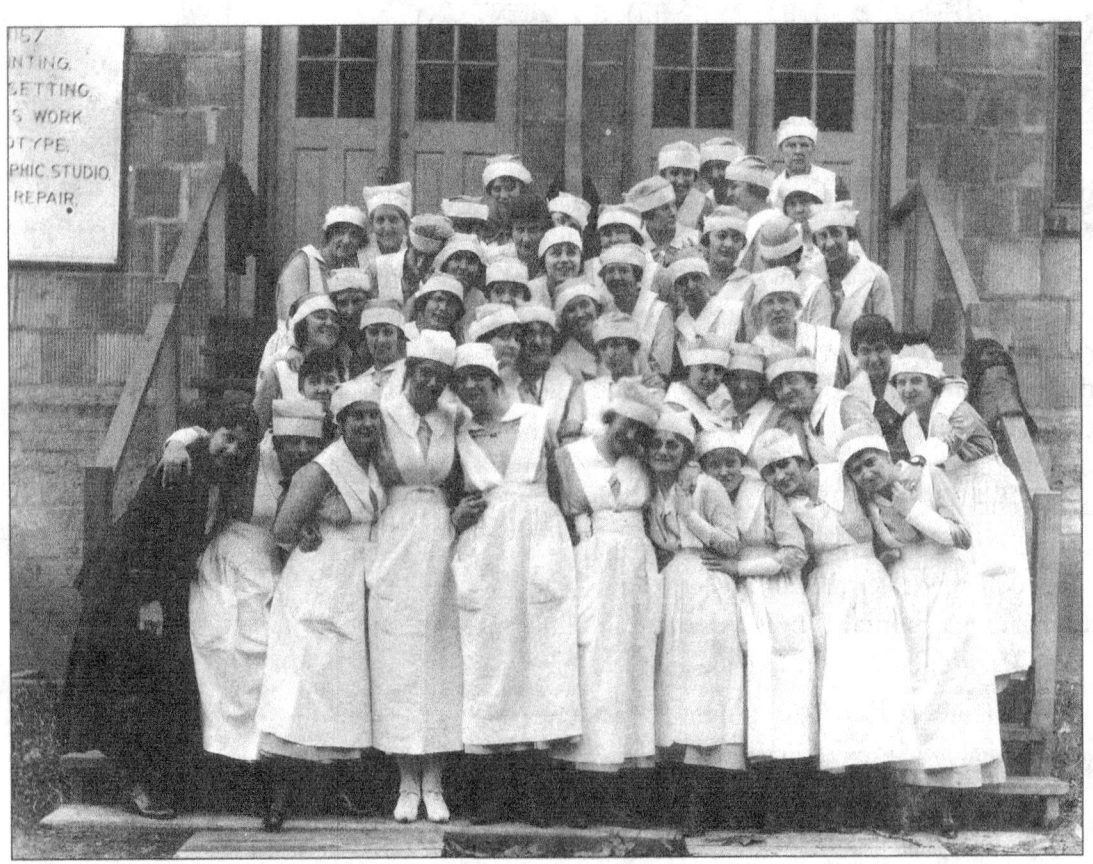

In the early nineteenth century, as several Americans traveled to Europe and visited these hospitals, a movement to reform the care of persons considered insane took root on this side of the Atlantic. Thomas Scattergood, a Quaker minister, helped found the Friends' Asylum for the Insane near Philadelphia in 1817, after his visit to the York Retreat.[25] Rufus Wyman, a physician well versed in Tuke's ideas, established the Connecticut Retreat for the Insane in Hartford in 1821.[26] Thomas Story Kirkbride, a physician at the Pennsylvania Hospital for the Insane, in the Philadelphia area, wrote extensively on moral therapy and organized the first national association of hospital superintendents, the American Medico-Psychological Association.[27]

During the middle decades of the nineteenth century, interest in activities for patients considered insane waned. In spite of all the hope for the efficacy of moral therapy, patients largely remained ill. As the generation of hospital superintendents led by Kirkbride died, so did many moral therapy programs, and hospitals for persons considered insane became custodial, at least temporarily.[28]

*Introduction*

**Photograph 2:** Reconstruction aides with Gen. Gorgas, "Crisp Professionalism." (AOTA Archives)

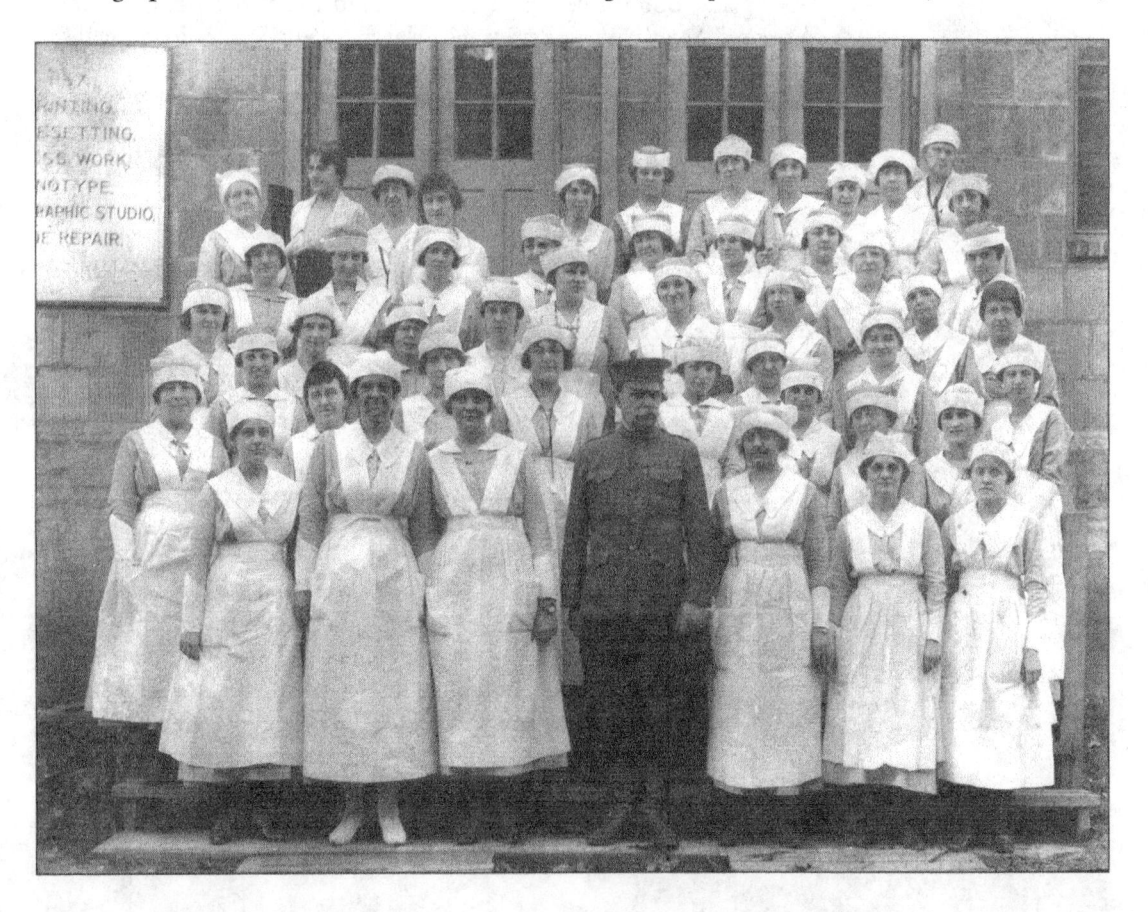

At the turn of the twentieth century, however, with the rebirth of the reform impulse, the notion of work as a therapeutic measure in the care of persons considered insane revived. Moreover, as physicians and reformers became interested in chronic diseases other than mental illness, such as tuberculosis and disability caused by congenital factors, environment, or injury, work therapy found other arenas of application. Part I examines this reawakening of interest in work as therapy. ❦

## Notes

1. Burton J. Bledstein, *The Culture of Professionalism: The Middle Class and the Development of Higher Education in America* (New York: W. W. Norton and Company, 1976). For a description of American medicine's gradual evolution toward science and technology, see Paul Starr, *The Social Transformation of American Medicine: The Rise of a Sovereign Profession and the Making of a Vast Industry* (New York: Basic Books, 1982).

2. The following studies describe women's charity and volunteer work in the nineteenth century and the transformation of that tradition into professional work in the early twentieth century: LeRoy Ashby, *Saving the Waifs: Reformers and Dependent Children, 1890–1917* (Philadelphia: Temple University Press, 1984); Dorothy G. Becker, "Exit Lady Bountiful: The Volunteer and the Professional Social Worker," *Social Service Review* 34 (March 1964): 57–72; Joan Jacobs Brumberg, " 'Ruined' Girls: Changing Community Responses to Illegitimacy in Upstate New York, 1890–1920," *Journal of Social History* 18 (Winter 1984): 247–63; Allen F. Davis, *Spearheads for Reform: The Social Settlement and the Progressive Movement, 1890–1914* (New York: Oxford University Press, 1967); Virginia Drachman, *Hospital with a Heart: Women Doctors and the Paradox of Separatism at the New England Hospital, 1862–1969* (Ithaca, N.Y.: Cornell University Press, 1984); Lori D. Ginzberg, *Women and the Work of Benevolence: Morality, Politics, and Class in the Nineteenth Century United States* (New Haven, Conn.: Yale University Press, 1990); Donna L. Franklin, "Mary Richmond and Jane Addams: From Moral Certainty to Rational Inquiry in Social Work Practice," *Social Service Review* 60 (December 1986): 504–25; Nancy A. Hewitt, *Women's Activism and Social Change: Rochester, New York, 1822–1872* (Ithaca, N.Y.: Cornell University Press, 1984); Wendy Kaminer, *Women Volunteering: The Pleasure, Pain, and Politics of Unpaid Work from 1830 to the Present* (Garden City, N.Y.: Anchor Press, 1984); Roy Lubove, *The Professional Altruist: The Emergence of Social Work as a Career, 1880–1930* (Cambridge: Harvard University Press, 1965); Robyn Muncy, *Creating a Female Dominion in American Reform, 1890–1935* (New York: Oxford University Press, 1991); Peggy Pascoe, *Relations of Rescue: The Search for Female Moral Authority in the American West, 1874–1939* (New York: Oxford University Press, 1990); Julia B. Rauch, "Women in Social Work: Friendly Visitors in Philadelphia, 1880," *Social Service Review* 49 (June 1975): 241–59; and Kathleen

Woodroofe, *From Charity to Social Work in England and the United States* (Toronto, Canada: University of Toronto Press, 1962).

3. Some examples of the history of women's professional work are Penina G. Abir-Am and Dorinda Outram, eds., *Uneasy Careers and Intimate Lives: Women in Science, 1789–1979* (New Brunswick, N.J.: Rutgers University Press, 1987); Joan Jacobs Brumberg and Nancy Tomes, "Women in the Professions: A Research Agenda for American Historians," *Reviews in American History* 10 (June 1982): 276–96; Lela B. Costin, *Two Sisters for Social Justice: A Biography of Grace and Edith Abbott* (Chicago: University of Illinois Press, 1983); Dee Garrison, *Apostles of Culture: The Public Librarian and American Society, 1876–1920* (New York: Free Press, 1979); Penina Migdal Glazer and Miriam Slater, *Unequal Colleagues: The Entrance of Women into the Professions, 1890–1940* (New Brunswick, N.J.: Rutgers University Press, 1987); C. Jane Gover, *The Positive Image: Women Photographers in Turn of the Century America* (Albany: State University of New York Press, 1986); James W. Grimm, "Women in the Female-Dominated Professions," in *Women Working: Theories and Facts in Perspective*, ed. Ann H. Stromberg and Shirley Harkness (Palo Alto, Calif.: Mayfield Publishing Company, 1978); Barbara J. Harris, *Beyond Her Sphere: Women and the Professions in American History* (Westport, Conn.: Greenwood Press, 1978); Patricia M. Hummer, *The Decade of Elusive Promise: Professional Women in the United States, 1920–1930* (Ann Arbor, Mich.: UMI Research, 1979); Daniel J. Walkowitz, "The Making of a Feminine Professional Identity: Social Workers in the 1920s," *American Historical Review* 95 (October 1990): 1051–75; and Ronald G. Walton, *Women in Social Work* (London: Routledge and Kegan Paul, 1975).

4. Some studies of the history of American nursing are JoAnn Ashley, *Hospitals, Paternalism, and the Role of the Nurse* (New York: Teachers College Press, 1976); Barbara Melosh, *"The Physician's Hand": Work, Culture, and Conflict in American Nursing* (Philadelphia: Temple University Press, 1982); Susan M. Reverby, *Ordered to Care: The Dilemma of American Nursing, 1850–1945* (Cambridge: Cambridge University Press, 1987); and Nancy Tomes, "Little World of Our Own: The Pennsylvania Hospital Training School for Nurses, 1895–1907," in *Women and Health in America*, ed. Judith Walzer Leavitt (Madison: University of Wisconsin Press, 1984), 467–81.

5. Katherine Kish Sklar, "Hull House in the 1890s: A Community of Women Reformers," *SIGNS* 10 (1985): 658–77. In this article Sklar discusses the work of Jane Addams, Julia Lathrop, and Florence Kelley, all of whom lived at Hull House in the 1890s. The three women had similar socioeconomic and educational backgrounds, but as Sklar reveals, along with others such as Grace and Edith Abbott and Sophonisba Breckinridge, they also shared a family political tradition. All had fathers or brothers who were very active in politics, and this socialized them to promote using political solutions for social problems. At least two important founders of the profession of occupational therapy had close male relatives who were active in politics. Eleanor Clarke Slagle's brother was a United States congress-

man from New York, and Elizabeth Upham Davis's father was the attorney for a United States senator from Wisconsin.

6. The American Occupational Therapy Foundation began an oral history project in the 1980s. Project personnel have completed interviews of thirty-five occupational therapists, most of whom were born after 1900.

7. Jane Addams, *Twenty Years at Hull House* (1910; reprint, New York: New American Library, 1960); Addams, *My Friend Julia Lathrop* (New York: Macmillan, 1935); Lillian Wald, *The House on Henry Street* (New York: Henry Holt and Company, 1915).

8. Eleanor Clarke Slagle was born circa 1871 in Hobart, New York, and died in 1942, according to Edward T. James, Janet W. James, and Paul S. Boyer, eds., *Notable American Women, 1607-1950* (Cambridge: Belknap Press of Harvard University Press, 1971), 3:296-98. Other sources give 1876 as her year of birth. Her tombstone is dated 1868.

9. Much of the available information about Susan E. Tracy (1864-1928) is very superficial. Basic biographical information can be found in sources on the history of nursing, such as Martin Kaufman, ed., *The Dictionary of American Nursing Biography* (Westport, Conn.: Greenwood Press, 1988), 370-71, and in sources on the history of occupational therapy, such as articles in the *Maryland Psychiatric Quarterly* and the *American Journal of Occupational Therapy* that are cited in chapter 3, note 2.

10. According to Kathlyn L. Reed and Sharon R. Sanderson, *Concepts of Occupational Therapy* (Baltimore: Williams and Wilkins Company, 1983), Susan Cox Johnson (1876-1928) was born in Corsicana, Texas. She later taught high school in Berkeley, California, and wrote a textbook called *Textile Studies* (Berkeley, Calif.: W. R. Morris, 1912). Once she arrived in New York City in 1916, her career is better documented. See chapters 5, 7, and 8 for discussions of Johnson's significance.

11. For a brief history of occupational therapy's official journals, see Myra L. McDaniel, "Forerunners of the *American Journal of Occupational Therapy*," *American Journal of Occupational Therapy* 25 (1971): 41-52.

12. Sidney Licht, ed., *Occupational Therapy Source Book* (Baltimore: Williams and Wilkins Company, 1948).

13. The collection is amply described in Inci A. Bowman, *Guide to the Archives of the American Occupational Therapy Association* (Galveston: University of Texas Medical Branch, n.d.).

14. Robert K. Bing, "William Rush Dunton, Junior—American Psychiatrist: A Study in Self" (Ed.D. diss., University of Maryland, 1961).

15. Just a few histories written by occupational therapy practitioners and supporters are Robert K. Bing, "Occupational Therapy Revisited: A Paraphrastic Journey," *American Journal of Occupational Therapy* 35 (1981): 365-402; Bing, "William Rush Dunton, Junior"; Wendy

Colman, "A Study of Educational Policy Setting in Occupational Therapy, 1918–1981" (Ph.D. diss., New York University, 1984); Ruth E. Levine, "The British Origins of the Use of Arts and Crafts in Occupational Therapy" (Paper presented at the Written History Seminar, Sixty-third Annual Meeting of the American Occupational Therapy Association, Portland, Ore., April 1983); Levine, "The Influence of the Arts-and-Crafts Movement on the Professional Status of Occupational Therapy," *American Journal of Occupational Therapy* 41 (1987): 248–53; Sidney Licht, "The Founding and Founders of the American Occupational Therapy Association," *American Journal of Occupational Therapy* 21 (1967): 269–77; Licht, *Source Book*; Terry Anne E. Litterst, "Boston School of Occupational Therapy, 1918–1930: The Formation of a Professional Educational Institution" (Paper presented at the Written History Seminar, Sixty-third Annual Meeting of the American Occupational Therapy Association, Portland, Ore., April 1983); Litterst, "Occupational Therapy: The Role of Ideology in the Development of a Profession for Women," *American Journal of Occupational Therapy* 46 (1992): 20–27; Barbara Loomis, "The Henry B. Favill School of Occupations and Eleanor Clarke Slagle," *American Journal of Occupational Therapy* 46 (1992): 34–38; Barbara Loomis and Beatrice Wade, *Chicago: Occupational Therapy Beginnings: Hull House* (Chicago: University of Illinois at Chicago, Henry B. Favill School of Occupations, Eleanor Clarke Slagle Department of Occupational Therapy, 1973); "Presidents of the American Occupational Therapy Association (1917–1967)," *American Journal of Occupational Therapy* 21 (1967): 290–98; and Special 75th Anniversary Issue, *American Journal of Occupational Therapy* 46 (1992): 9–85.

16. For this study I examined the records of the Boston School of Occupational Therapy, the Milwaukee-Downer College School of Occupational Therapy, the New York War Service Classes for Training Reconstruction Aides in Occupational Therapy, the Philadelphia School of Occupational Therapy, and the St. Louis School of Occupational Therapy, all founded in 1917 or 1918. Some of the hospitals that I visited were the Sheppard and Enoch Pratt Hospital in Towson, Maryland; the Faulkner Hospital in Jamaica Plain, Massachusetts; the Rush-Presbyterian Hospital in Chicago; the New York Hospital in New York City; the Montefiore Hospital and Medical Center (known in the 1920s as the Montefiore Home and Hospital for Chronic Diseases) in New York City; and the McLean Hospital in Boston.

17. A special thanks to Diane Gibson, occupational therapist in charge of patients' activities at the Sheppard-Pratt Hospital, for taking me to see the weaving room in the Casino Building and for finding the photographs hidden in a closet in the old laundry building on the hospital grounds.

18. See the list of photographs held at the Official Archives of the American Occupational Therapy Association, in Bowman, *Guide to the Archives*. Taking photographs of patients involved in craft work and showing displays of finished products were very common between 1910 and 1930. The purpose of these photographs, I believe, was to quantify patients' productivity.

19. Licht, *Source Book*, 1–4.

20. Ibid., 5–6.

21. Ibid., 6–8; Bing, "Occupational Therapy Revisited," 503–4; letter, Bing to the author, 2 February 1995. Samuel Tuke is often credited with founding the York Retreat and introducing moral therapy regimens there, but according to Bing, the credit should go to Samuel's grandfather William Tuke (1732–1822), a Quaker and a wealthy merchant, and to Samuel's father Henry (1755–1814), who is often considered a cofounder with William. Samuel (1784–1857) was the family member who wrote about the York Retreat, in *Description of the Retreat: An Institution near York for Insane Persons of the Society of Friends: Containing an Account of Its Origins and Progress, the Modes of Treatment, and a Statement of Cases* (York, England: Alexander, 1813; reprint, London: Dawsons of Pall Mall, 1964).

22. Licht, *Source Book*, 19.

23. Ibid., 25–30.

24. Ibid., 40–56.

25. Ibid., 8; Bing, "William Rush Dunton, Junior," 60.

26. Licht, *Source Book*, 8–9.

27. Ibid., 73–80.

28. Nancy Tomes, *A Generous Confidence: Thomas Story Kirkbride and the Art of Asylum-keeping, 1840–1883* (Cambridge: Cambridge University Press, 1984), passim.

# PART I

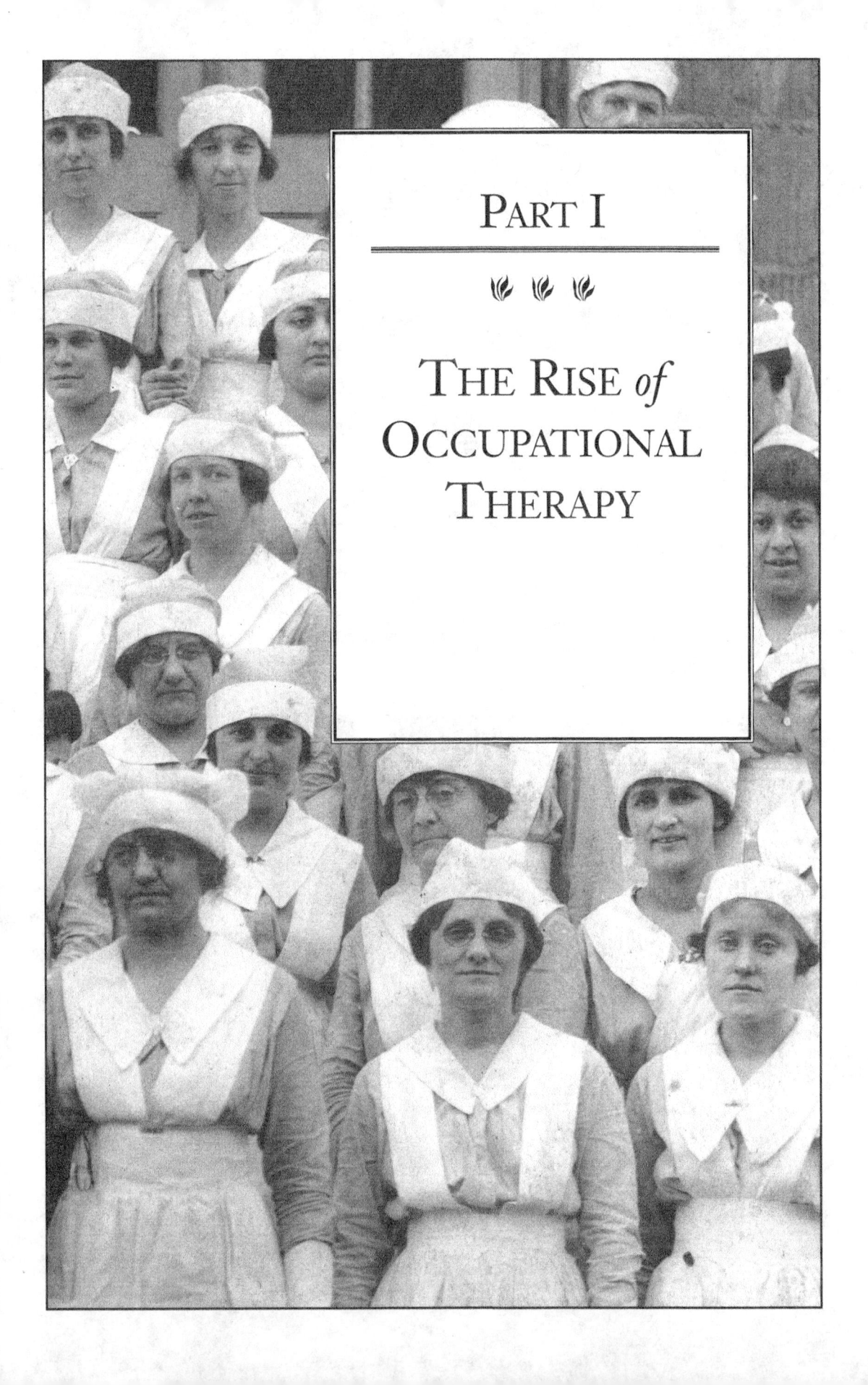

## THE RISE *of* OCCUPATIONAL THERAPY

During the 1910s in locations all over the United States, reformers promoted the idea that work restored the health of "invalids" victimized by the deleterious effects of industrialization and urbanization. Tuberculosis, arthritis, neurasthenia, and industrial injuries, they argued, could be treated by individualized programs of supervised arts and crafts. Coming from a decidedly middle-class "therapeutic world view," as many Progressive Era reformers did, these creators of occupational therapy directly addressed the health problems associated with modern life by combining the traditional values of the work ethic and crafts with scientific and medical principles.[1]

Why did the idea of "occupying" patients receive so much attention at this particular time in American history, and why was there an emphasis on crafts? Was not an obsession with handcrafts ironic, given that America was undergoing vast industrialization and machine-made products were becoming the norm? If the apparent defensiveness of occupational therapy proponents is an indicator, contemporary critics sneeringly viewed craft work by patients as anachronistic if not frivolous. Yet proponents of occupational therapy saw the introduction of arts and crafts into the lives of patients as the path to health. They believed that the development of occupational therapy was one answer to what they perceived as myriad medical and social ills plaguing American society in a time of vast change. Women in particular saw working in occupational therapy as part of a long-standing tradition of ameliorating the plight of downtrodden victims of industrial society.

Part I explains occupational therapy's multidisciplinary and holistic approaches to the care of patients by analyzing the values and the motivations of several important founders of the profession. It also shows how the founding years set the stage for a division of labor by gender within the profession. The five chapters in Part I feature the work of important founders at their respective institutions: Eleanor Clarke Slagle, mental hygiene advocate, at the Chicago School of Civics and Philanthropy; William Rush Dunton, Jr., psychiatrist, at the Sheppard and Enoch Pratt Hospital in Towson, Maryland; Adolph Meyer, psychiatrist, at the Henry Phipps Psychiatric Clinic, Johns Hopkins Hospital, in Baltimore; Susan E. Tracy, nurse, at the Adams Nervine Asylum and at the Experiment Station for the Study of Invalid Occupations, both in Jamaica Plain, Massachusetts; Herbert James Hall, physician, at the Devereux Workshops, then at the Devereux Mansion, a sanatorium for neurasthenics, in Marblehead, Massachusetts; George

Edward Barton, patient with tuberculosis, arts and crafts advocate, and organizer and first president of the National Society for the Promotion of Occupational Therapy, at Consolation House in Clifton Springs, New York; Philip King Brown, physician, at the San Francisco Polyclinic Hospital and at the Arequipa Sanatorium for women with tuberculosis, in Marin County, California; and Susan Cox Johnson, educator and craftswoman, at Teachers College, Columbia University, and at the Montefiore Home and Hospital for Chronic Diseases, both in New York City.

These founders came from backgrounds in social work, medicine, psychiatry, nursing, architecture, and teaching, and they were profoundly influenced by the arts and crafts, efficiency, mental hygiene, antituberculosis, and women's philanthropy and reform movements of the early twentieth century. They held connections to hospitals, schools, and social organizations based in Baltimore, Boston, Chicago, and New York, but even before World War I, their influence had spread to locations as far as upstate New York and the West Coast. They identified themselves as pioneers of a new therapeutic method within medical science, but they believed that their work had important implications for American society at large. Their task was to convince others of the important relationship between creative work and health.

## Note

1. For a discussion of the concept of a therapeutic world view, see T. J. Jackson Lears, *No Place of Grace: Antimodernism and the Transformation of American Culture, 1880–1920* (New York: Pantheon Books, 1981), 47–59.

# Chapter 1

## "The Jane Addams *of* Occupational Therapy"

Eleanor Clarke Slagle
and Women's Work
in the Age of Reform

*"The Jane Addams of Occupational Therapy"*

In summer 1911, Eleanor Clarke Slagle inaugurated a lifelong labor of love. She set out as a reformer interested in mental hygiene, but quickly her efforts evolved into building a new profession for women, to be called occupational therapy. For this contribution she came to be known by her contemporaries as "the Jane Addams of occupational therapy." Slagle (see photograph 3) began her work by taking a course in "curative occupations and recreations" at the Chicago School of Civics and Philanthropy.[1] The course, an outgrowth of the mental hygiene movement, used the latest educational methods by providing students with theoretical lectures, craft training, and practical clinical experience. The school itself, supported by Chicago settlement women Jane Addams and Julia Lathrop, served as a major recruiting and socializing agency, bringing aspiring young professional women into what historian Robyn Muncy calls "the female dominion in American reform."[2] This chapter explains the rise of occupational therapy by placing it in the context of women's reform and professional activities in the decades surrounding the turn of the twentieth century. Further, the chapter places Slagle in a peer group of women such as Addams and Lathrop who were part of a transitional generation that transformed volunteer reform work into professionalism.

Women's work in reform movements began long before this transitional generation of women. Since the middle of the nineteenth century, American middle-class women had actively organized all-female public activities by extending the traditional role known as "true womanhood." The so-called cult of true womanhood emerged during the first decades of the nineteenth century, when a competitive and acquisitive industrialized America seemed to be replacing the earlier ideal of a rural

Christian republic. In this period most American women internalized an ideology that assigned them to embody the Christian virtues of piety, purity, domesticity, and submissiveness. Home, family, and church, not politics and the marketplace, were to be the main centers of women's attention and activity.[3]

Almost immediately, women seemed unsatisfied with concentrating their nurturing qualities and their perceived moral superiority on the circumscribed sphere of home and family. Without rejecting the notion of self-sacrificing service to others, or a Christian focus, but chafing against the limitations of domesticity, they carved a place for themselves in the public sphere. They argued that their values as Christians and as females had an important place in reforming the world beyond the private sphere. They worked in numerous settings, including churches, missionaries, moral reform societies, and various charity institutions, which most often served women and children. These many organizations were frequently founded, supported, and completely run by women, with little, if any, participation by men. Tirelessly they enlarged women's sphere by ameliorating the plight of the poor and the suffering and by uplifting the fallen in an ever-evolving, seemingly heartless and sinful urban and industrial society.[4]

During the nineteenth century, along with the widening sphere for women came new educational opportunities. As early as the 1830s and the 1840s, women such as Catharine Beecher, Mary Lyon, and Emma Willard, crusaders for the education of American women in seminaries, successfully argued that women's crucial role in influencing their own children to be responsible citizens and virtuous Christians required formal education. Seminaries turned out hundreds of women who would be part of the first women's profession in America, teaching. After all, leaders in education asserted, if women were the appropriate

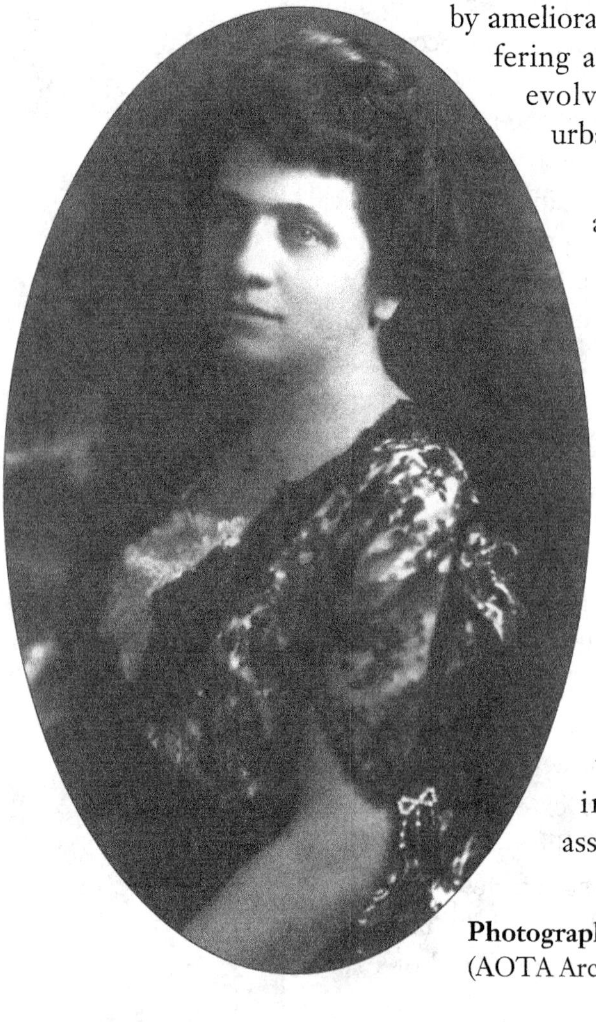

**Photograph 3:** Portrait of Eleanor Clarke Slagle. (AOTA Archives)

ones to foster the nation's conscience, then they could have even more influence by becoming teachers and subsequently reaching even larger numbers of future citizens. Between 1860 and 1890, American women advanced on the education continuum by entering colleges, where they were further imbued with values such as service and altruism.

As a result, the first generation of college-educated women built new professions that bridged the gap between women's and men's worlds at the turn of the century. Earnest in their internalized responsibility to serve others, many chose never to marry; they dedicated their entire adult lives to fields such as nursing, social work, and teaching. Others who lived more traditionally as wives and mothers nonetheless continued their reform work by joining the legions of American women who founded secular reform organizations: the Children's Aid Society, the General Federation of Women's Clubs, the National Association of Colored Women, the National Consumers' League, the Young Women's Christian Association, and hundreds of other national and local groups. At no other time in American history have women been better organized to conduct reform work than they were around the turn of the twentieth century.[5]

## The Importance of Hull House

When Eleanor Clarke Slagle went to Chicago in 1911, she entered one of the most dynamic centers of women's reform in America. The institutional heart of women's reform in Chicago pulsated in the Hull House Settlement. In 1889, several years after graduating from the Rockford (Illinois) Female Seminary, Jane Addams and Ellen Gates Starr founded Hull House; later it became an important training ground for women's political and professional work. An innovative institution modeled after Toynbee Hall in London, Hull House was dedicated to bridging the gulf between middle-class reformers and the hordes of poor and immigrant residents of the industrialized city of Chicago. Different from Toynbee Hall, which drew many male residents, most of whom were studying for the ministry, Hull House was an all-female secular community providing middle-class educated American women with a respectable alternative to marriage and family life, and viable opportunities to become involved in public reform.

Hull House and Jane Addams led what became a widespread settlement movement in the United States. By 1900, over 100 settlements had been founded in the United States. In 1911, Addams became the head of the National Federation of Settlements, a post she held until 1935. By 1911, at least 215 settlements existed in cities all over the United States, 53 percent of which were female-only institutions. This level of involvement attests to the enthusiasm with which women fulfilled public, and eventually professional, roles in American reform.[6]

Building on, but differing from, women's previous philanthropic traditions, the practice of Hull House was for residents actually to live in the working-class neighborhoods of Chicago. There they studied the conditions under which their impoverished neighbors lived, seeking not only to provide immediate aid, but to address the root causes of poverty. They thought, as good Progressives should, that by using scientific methods to analyze the city's social, health, educational, and economic conditions, and then by educating the public on these issues, they could rouse interest in reform and make changes for the better.

Many of the projects that Hull House sponsored were particularly geared to aiding women and children, an area in which philanthropic women had long felt authorized to work. During Hull House's first decade it founded day-care services for the children of working mothers, playgrounds, cooperative living quarters for working women, a public kitchen for working families, and individualized aid to women in crisis.[7]

Eventually Hull House residents realized that the problems they faced required more than local amelioration; they soon engaged in city politics, calling on men in prominent political positions to help improve labor and housing conditions. In time they turned to state and national politics for more permanent solutions to problems, again using well-developed connections with men in power.[8] One example of Hull House's success in developing a national focus was the creation of the Children's Bureau in 1912, an agency described by Muncy as "the first female stronghold in the federal government."[9]

Strong political ties between Hull House's leadership and powerful men were important, but equally integral to the success of its aims were networks existing between Hull House residents and individual female patrons. Well-to-do women generously supported the settlement's projects and thereby provided opportunities for young women with professional aspirations. According to Muncy, Jane Addams initiated a "fellowship system" whereby she solicited the aid of wealthy women to support given projects. A variety of women's clubs and organizations also financed Hull House undertakings. For example, the Chicago Kindergarten Organization, founded by wealthy women to provide education for poor young children, paid the salaries of two Hull House kindergarten teachers. Thus the coalition not only accomplished helping impoverished youngsters, a good work well within the confines of women's charity sphere, but also provided aspiring female professionals with jobs.[10]

Hull House also served as a meeting place for proponents of contemporary social movements that directly influenced the later development of occupational therapy. For example, in 1897 the Chicago Arts and Crafts Society organized at Hull House. There many middle- and upper-class Chicagoans participated in this larger American and British movement by studying a variety of arts and crafts processes and thus resisting what they perceived to be the tyranny of the machine. At twice-monthly meetings the society aimed to revitalize and ennoble the meaning of work by re-creating the ideal of the crafts person, in spite of the fact that society members lived in the machine age. Under the auspices of the society, for example, Ellen Gates Starr held bookbinding classes in which "design and workmanship, beauty and thoroughness [were] taught to a small number of apprentices."[11] At various times, workshops were held in pottery, metal, wood, and textiles.

Craft work, as society members saw it, provided opportunities for them as non-working-class people to capture what they perceived to be a productive and meaningful life experience. By actually using their hands, creating specimens of pottery, wood, glass, metal, or cloth, the members hoped to gain insight into the problem with which they struggled incessantly—alienation in modern life. In discussions, members analyzed and critiqued America's rapid and seemingly complete capitulation to "industrial organization and the machine," which had created a world in which they felt lost and aimless.[12]

Reflecting a sense of stewardship toward the working-class and immigrant population of Chicago, and harboring fears about the potential restlessness of that population, they talked about "the present state of the factories and the workmen therein." Realizing the inevitability of industrialization, they justified the moderate use of the machine because of its potential to relieve "workmen from drudgery." By insisting that "the machine no longer be allowed to dominate the workman and reduce his production to a mechanical distortion," they projected their own interpretation of the experience of workers in modern life.[13]

Jane Addams and Ellen Gates Starr certainly believed, on the basis of their observations of women workers, that alienation existed among their less-fortunate female neighbors. "At Hull House," Addams said, "we constantly see immigrant girls who enter factory life so . . . [poorly] . . . prepared for industry that they not only receive low wages but become quickly discouraged with American life."[14] In 1900, in response to their concerns about workers' alienation and immigrants' problems with assimilation, and after obtaining the financial backing of some wealthy Chicago women, Addams and Starr created an educational institution called the Hull House Labor Museum. At the museum, which primarily examined the history of textile production, Addams tried to instill pride in immigrant women's traditional textile-producing skills. She recruited Syrian, Greek, Italian, Russian, and Irish women to demonstrate spinning and weaving. Charts displayed on the wall illustrated the long history of hand labor in the making of threads, comparing the years of primacy of the stick spindle with the very brief period when the spinning wheel was used, and then with the era of steam-driven machines. At times Addams displayed textile implements and tools, raw materials, and finished products.

To Addams, educational activities such as those offered by the Hull House Labor Museum helped alleviate tensions that workers experienced. Influenced by the philosophy of contemporary Chicago educator John Dewey, an advocate of learning by doing or by actual experience, Addams believed that if workers learned the "history and growth of industrial processes," they would feel more connected to and less hostile toward factory processes of labor.[15] Succinctly she said, "If a child goes into a sewing factory with a knowledge of the work she is doing in relation to the finished product; if she is informed concerning the material she is manipulating and the processes to which it is subjected; if she understands the design she is elaborating in its historic relation to art and decoration, her daily life is lifted from drudgery to one of self-conscious activity, and her pleasure and intelligence is [sic] registered in her product."[16]

During the winter of 1901–2, in a typical schedule of events, the department of textiles of the Hull House Labor Museum correlated its history lessons with practical classes in weaving and design, thus bringing participants from the abstract to the actual creation of a finished product. Members of the Chicago

Arts and Crafts Society cooperated in the venture by serving as instructors. In short, Hull House invited workers from the nearby factories to join residents in tracing the "primitive methods to the factories of the vicinity," where the "enlarged and developed tool [would] be rediscovered."[17] Addams wanted workers to come to the museum to be "entertained, to work with the tools with which they are already familiar, to study charts and diagrams which are simple and graphic, to attend lectures which may illustrate their daily work, and give them some clew [sic] to the development of the machine and the materials which they constantly handle."[18] Such a program, Addams claimed, conceived of education in terms that John Dewey would call "a continuing reconstruction of experience."[19]

Occupational therapy had not yet taken root in the first decade of the twentieth century, yet as it began to bud after 1910, it would graft many ideas and practices from the arts and crafts and education reform movements. Occupational therapists, for example, vigorously adopted craft work and experiential learning as central practices in their field, mainly because they shared a world view with arts and crafts advocates and education reformers. As the next few chapters illustrate, occupational therapists also valued authentic experience, productivity, and civic action in their lives. More important, they believed that it was their duty to convince others of the virtues of such activity. Occupational therapists and reformers came from similar segments of American society: the vast majority were middle or upper class, educated, white, Protestant, and urban. Because many of the tasks inherent in arts and crafts and education, such as weaving, and teaching young children, were extensions of traditional women's work, women were well represented in these reform movements. Occupational therapy combined the skills of craft work and teaching with those of caring for society's ill or needy—all of which were defined as proper women's work. Thus occupational therapy too would be a field highly dominated by women.

By the 1910s, arts and crafts ideology, education reform, and women's assumed natural capacity to help so-called invalids had merged, creating the basis of the new profession of occupational therapy. This does not explain why the field was defined as a "therapy," however. Distancing itself from education, occupational therapy took on medical trappings when arts and crafts ideology and education reform coupled with mental health care. Julia Lathrop linked them as she became involved in the mental hygiene movement. After Lathrop read Clifford Beers's autobiography, *A Mind That Found Itself*,[20] which described the contemporary plight of persons with mental illness and the need for reform in mental health care, and particularly after she attended the founding meeting of the Mental Hygiene Association in New Haven, Connecticut, in 1908, during which she was moved to tears, she returned to Chicago determined to begin work in mental health reform.[21]

Collaborating with Graham Taylor, a leader of the settlement movement and the director of the Chicago School of Civics and Philanthropy, Lathrop immediately started experimental classes at the school. As Taylor phrased it, the course was to train "institution attendants in occupations for the insane." Taylor convinced state hospital authorities to subsidize the course and give paid leaves of absence for attendants so that they could take it.[22] The "special course in curative occupations and recreations for attendants and nurses in institutions for the insane" emphasized "the *educational* as opposed to the *custodial* idea in the daily care of the mentally unsound [emphasis in original]."[23] A report that Taylor gave at the National Conference of Charities and Correction on the success of the first course helped attract hospital attendants from Indiana, New York, and other states during the next few years.[24] Eleanor Clarke Slagle later praised the six-week course for stimulating national interest in what she called "the normalizing effect of occupational work."[25]

## Aspiring Professional Eleanor Clarke Slagle

Eleanor Clarke Slagle took the course in curative occupations when she was about forty years old, but she had been imbued with the values of reform since childhood. Her character was shaped by an early life in rural upstate New York, where she discovered the importance of hard work and civic responsibility simply by observing her own immediate and extended family. Born circa 1871 in Hobart, New York, Ella May Clark, as she was then known, was the younger of two children, and the only daughter, of William John Clark, a cooper and later a sheriff of Delaware County, and Emmaline J. (Davenport) Clark.[26] The Clark and Davenport families had settled in Delaware County in the early nineteenth century and were well-known. Emmaline was related to John Davenport, one of the founders of Yale University. Many Clarks and Davenports were active abolitionists, and several of the men in both families served in the Union Army during the Civil War. The marriage between William Clark and Emmaline Davenport took place shortly after William returned from serving as a second lieutenant in the New York Infantry during the Civil War. William was thirty-six years old when he married, Emmaline only sixteen. She gave birth first to a son, John Davenport Clark, in 1869, and then to Ella May two years later, bearing both before she reached the age of twenty.[27]

The members of Eleanor Clarke Slagle's family in her early childhood followed traditional late-nineteenth-century gender roles. Father William was reportedly a "strict disciplinarian with a rigid adherence to a firm sense of right and wrong," mother Emmaline a "soft and frivolous woman" who spoiled her son and daughter.[28] In certain ways John and Ella May were treated equally: they were baptized together at St. Peter's Episcopal Church in Hobart on New Year's Eve, 1876, and they both attended private school at the Delaware Academy in nearby Delhi, New York. John had many more educational opportunities than his sister, however. He finished high school at Phillips Academy in Andover, Massachusetts, in 1894, and then went on to college in Colorado and to law school in Brooklyn, New York.[29] Ella May attended Hudson River Institute, Claverack College's high school program located near Hudson, New York, in 1885 and 1886, where she studied music, but she never attended college in a degree-granting program. The school nonetheless instilled in Ella May an urge to be civically responsible: it aimed to inculcate "refined manners, elevated social character, cultivated taste, and Christian morals" in its students.[30] A coeducational institution, Hudson River Institute may also have helped prepare Ella May to work comfortably with men, which she later did with seeming ease and grace.

Eleanor Clarke Slagle left no personal papers; thus many gaps in her personal history cannot be filled. Historians know little of the period between her school days and her appearance in Chicago, for example. They do know that she married Robert E. Slagle, the son of the Reverend Peter and Mrs. Cordelia (Beam) Slagle of Chicago, at St. Peter's Episcopal Church in Hobart on April 19, 1894, and that the couple planned to make their home in Chicago.[31] Historians do not know, however, what Robert did for a living, where and how Ella May and Robert met, whether or not the marriage was a happy one, whether there were ever any children, why the couple lived in St. Louis for some years, and whether the couple divorced. In 1937, Eleanor Clarke Slagle described herself as a "long time widow," but a grandniece later contradicted that statement, saying that Slagle was divorced.[32]

Slagle apparently never spoke of the seventeen years between her wedding and her appearance at the Chicago School of Civics and Philanthropy in 1911, so it is difficult to say precisely why she pursued a professional life in occupational therapy. There is evidence that she was involved in some way in reform work. In the early 1920s she wrote a resumé that was headed by the following statement: "Covering a period of years of interest in the unfair social attitude toward the dependency of mentally and physically handicapped, followed by lectures on Social Economics by Professor Henderson, Chicago University, Jane Adams [sic], Hull House, Julia Lathrop, now of the Children's Bureau, I took up: . . . [the special course in 1911 and continued on in occupational therapy]."[33]

The health history of Slagle's family provides grounds for speculation on why she became interested in occupational therapy. She was surrounded by disability and chronic illness from childhood to adulthood. In several instances she found it her duty to be the family caretaker, and this experience oddly enough prepared her for a career in working with persons who were sickly or disabled. Her father was probably ill throughout her life: he returned from the Civil War partially disabled, having been wounded by a gunshot to the neck.[34] No evidence exists of the injury's effect on his ability to function, and whether Eleanor had to tend to him as a child or as a young woman is not known. She definitely assumed a caretaking role when he became ill in his later life, however. William Clark spent his final years with his married daughter Eleanor in St. Louis, leaving his wife and his upstate New York home behind. The marriage apparently dissolved, Emmaline returning to her father's home with John.[35]

Slagle's brother and her nephew, two other significant men in her life, suffered various ailments as well. John contracted tuberculosis in the 1890s, which led him to go to college in Colorado, where the climate and the altitude were believed to help relieve his chronic condition.[36] Estranged from his mother, who remarried after her husband William's death, John leaned on his sister for emotional support. He called her "Aunt Peggie," and she became in some ways his dearest friend and confidante, even closer to him than his wife Marian, whom he had met in college. Later he struggled with alcohol abuse, writing often to his teetotaling sister Eleanor of his troubles, including an unhappy marriage.[37] She supported him unhesitatingly until his death in an automobile accident in 1933. Eleanor's only nephew Jack, John's son, contracted polio in 1908 at two years of age; as a result of the disease, his right arm was severely incapacitated throughout his life.[38] Eleanor played the role of a loving and indulgent aunt to Jack in his childhood. In the 1920s she and her nephew both lived in New York City. Jack was in law school, but he spent much of his time rebelling against the rules, carousing with women, and consuming alcohol. John, who was in Washington, D.C., serving in Congress, put Eleanor in charge of getting control of Jack's finances and behavior. Never wavering in her duty to the family, Eleanor saw her nephew through his New York City years until he finally passed the bar examination in 1933.[39]

Seeing her father, brother, and nephew struggle with disabling injuries and debilitating illnesses may have been the personal experience that drove Eleanor Clarke Slagle to the Chicago School of Civics and Philanthropy in 1911. Practically speaking, Slagle as a single woman needed to find a means to earn a living. Immediately on completion of the course, which included both an academic focus and a field experience in which she studied Illinois hospitals and charitable institutions, Slagle procured employment in state hospitals in Michigan and New York, where she studied and organized "re-educational classes."[40]

Already gaining a name for herself in the fledgling field of occupational therapy and having made connections with Chicago leaders of the mental hygiene movement, in 1912, Slagle went to Baltimore to direct a new department of occupational therapy in the Henry Phipps Psychiatric Clinic of Johns Hopkins Hospital, which was headed by psychiatrist Adolph Meyer, formerly of Illinois. Slagle learned much while working with Meyer, including a method of occupational therapy treatment for patients with mental illness that she called "habit training," which she believed "re-educated" patients in "decent habits of living." "Broadly speaking," she once wrote, "re-education is substituting better habits (for bad habits) or the building of new habits to replace those which have been lost."[41] More to the point, she explained that occupational therapy "conserves the work habit and prevents invalid habits."[42]

In late 1913, Slagle attended the Maryland State Conference on Mental Hygiene, at which she met with her former colleague Graham Taylor of the Chicago School of Civics and Philanthropy. Taylor visited the Phipps Clinic, which he described in a letter to Julia Lathrop as "a wonderful place" that "impressively combined . . . work, science, and sympathy." Slagle, he told Lathrop, "besought" him to "renew . . . efforts to train others for the work she is so masterfully accomplishing and for which she thinks an increasing demand is sure to develop." Taylor not only saw the importance of occupational therapy in mental health care, but found that it could be well applied in tuberculosis prevention and care. Taylor pressed Lathrop to continue working with him to educate occupational therapy workers in more than just mental hygiene.[43]

Slagle's lobbying of Taylor apparently paid off: by early 1914 she had resigned her position at the Phipps Clinic to return to Chicago, the hotbed of reform. Back at the Chicago School of Civics and Philanthropy, she gave lectures on occupations. More significant, under the auspices of the Illinois Society for Mental Hygiene, she started a workshop for the chronically unemployed, called the Experimental Station. Although the program was organized primarily for patients with mental illness, "the demand was so great," Slagle later wrote, "that all types . . . of borderline mental cases and orthopedic cripples . . . were admitted."[44] Soon she headed a school of occupational therapy named after a recently deceased Chicago physician, Henry B. Favill, who was one of the founders of the Chicago Anti-Tuberculosis Society and a leader in national mental hygiene as well.[45]

Slagle stayed in Chicago for the next few years, but she made it her business to contact people in other cities who were beginning to see, as she did, that her work had the potential to become its own professional field. She nurtured the relationships that she forged with women and men involved in the mental hygiene and antituberculosis movements, and with female philanthropists who would finance her projects, and she made new allies among hospital physicians, psychiatrists, and nurses who worked directly with patients. The next chapter chronicles the work of the "father of occupational therapy," William Rush Dunton, Jr., a hospital psychiatrist who would be one of Slagle's closest colleagues.

# NOTES

1. Eleanor Clarke Slagle's attendance at the Chicago School of Civics and Philanthropy in summer 1911 is recorded in "Alumni Register, Chicago School of Civics and Philanthropy, 1903–1913," p. 64, Graham Taylor Papers, Chicago School of Civics and Philanthropy, Newberry Library, Chicago (hereafter Graham Taylor Papers). Slagle herself reported the year as 1910 ["Experience of Eleanor Clarke Slagle," resume, 1922, Papers of the American Occupational Therapy Association, Official Archives of the American Occupational Therapy Association, Wilma L. West Library, American Occupational Therapy Foundation, Bethesda, Maryland (hereafter AOTA Archives)]. I have used the school's date throughout this book.

2. Robyn Muncy, *Creating a Female Dominion in American Reform, 1890–1935* (New York: Oxford University Press, 1991).

3. Barbara Welter, "The Cult of True Womanhood: 1820–1860," *American Quarterly* 18 (Summer 1966): 151–74.

4. Barbara Berg, *The Remembered Gate: The Origins of American Feminism* (Oxford: Oxford University Press, 1978); Carroll Smith-Rosenberg, *Religion and the Rise of the American City: The New York City Mission Movement, 1812–1870* (Ithaca, N.Y.: Cornell University Press, 1978).

5. A few examples of important books on the history of women's education in the United States are Linda D. Gordon, *Gender and Higher Education in the Progressive Era* (New Haven, Conn.: Yale University Press, 1990); Kathryn Kish Sklar, *Catharine Beecher: A Study in American Domesticity* (New Haven, Conn.: Yale University Press, 1973); and Barbara Miller Solomon, *In the Company of Educated Women: A History of Women and Higher Education in America* (New Haven, Conn.: Yale University Press, 1985).

6. G. J. Barker-Benfield, "Jane Addams," in *Portraits of American Women from Settlement to the Present*, G. J. Barker-Benfield and Catherine Clinton (New York: St. Martin's Press, 1991), 341; Muncy, *Creating a Female Dominion*, 8–11.

7. Muncy, *Creating a Female Dominion*, 13.

8. Katherine Kish Sklar, "Hull House in the 1890s: A Community of Women Reformers," *SIGNS* 10 (1985): 658–77.

9. Muncy, *Creating a Female Dominion*, 38.

10. Ibid., 17.

11. Jane Addams, *Twenty Years at Hull House* (1910; reprint, New York: New American Library, 1960), 261.

12. *Hull House Bulletin* 2 (1897): 9.

13. Direct quotations regarding the Hull House Chicago Arts and Crafts Society, ibid. For a discussion of American arts and crafts ideology and its manifestations at Hull House, see T. J. Jackson Lears, *No Place of Grace: Antimodernism and the Transformation of American Culture, 1880–1920* (New York: Pantheon Books, 1981), 74–83.

14. Letter, signed President of Hull House, 18 May 1908, Hull House Association Records, Special Collections, Main Library, University of Illinois at Chicago.

15. *Hull House Bulletin* 6 (1903–4): 12.

16. As quoted in Lears, *No Place of Grace*, 80.

17. "First Report of the Labor Museum at Hull House," ca. 1898, p. 15, Jane Addams Papers, microfilm ed., Special Collections, Main Library, University of Illinois at Chicago.

18. Ibid.

19. Ibid.; Lears, *No Place of Grace*, 80.

20. Clifford W. Beers, *A Mind That Found Itself: An Autobiography* (New York: Longmans, Green, and Company, 1908).

21. Jane Addams, *My Friend Julia Lathrop* (New York: Macmillan, 1935), 162.

22. Letter, Graham Taylor to Governor Charles S. Deneen, 22 June 1909, Graham Taylor Papers.

23. Barbara Loomis, "Professional Occupational Therapy Education in Chicago, 1908–1920" (Paper presented at the Written History Seminar, Sixty-third Annual Meeting of the American Occupational Therapy Association, Portland, Ore., April 1983).

24. Letter, Graham Taylor to B. R. Burroughs (Secretary, Board of Administration, Springfield, Illinois), 11 March 1910, Graham Taylor Papers.

25. Loomis, "Professional Occupational Therapy Education," 2.

26. Eleanor Clarke Slagle left a remarkable professional record through her work with the American Occupational Therapy Association. Finding accurate data about her personal life, however, has been a true adventure. Some information about her early years appears in an entry in Edward T. James, Janet W. James, and Paul S. Boyer, eds., *Notable American Women, 1607–1950* (Cambridge: Belknap Press of Harvard University Press, 1971), 3:296–98. The author of the entry describes some of the inconsistencies in the record, even in such basic information as Slagle's correct birth date. For example, Slagle's death record in the New York State Department of Health gives her year of birth as 1876; her tombstone shows the year as 1868; and the census records list her age in 1875 as four and in 1880 as nine, which would make her birth year 1871. The 1880 census record for Delhi, First District, contains the following information about the Clark household: "William J. Clark, age 37, ex-sheriff; Emma J. Clark, age 32, wife, keeps house; John D., age 11, son, goes to school; Ella May, age 9, daughter, goes to school; McNett, Belle, servant, age 19; and Murray, John B., boarder, surrogate clerk." No information in any of the sources that I consulted explained when or why Ella May Clark began to use "Eleanor" as her first name and to spell her last name with a terminal "e". Information in note 31 suggests that she was using "Eleanor Mai" at the time of her wedding. Her brother John also changed the spelling of his last name from "Clark" to "Clarke."

27. That there was a twenty-year difference in age between William and Emma, or Emmaline, is described in Marian W. Clarke, "Memories of a Congressman's Widow," typescript, Marian W. Clarke Papers, New York State Historical Association, Cooperstown. The 1880 census record indicates that there was a five-year difference in age between them.

28. Paul T. DuVivier, "A Congressman during Hard Times" (M.A. thesis, State University of New York College at Oneonta, 1976), 1, Delaware County Historical Association, Delhi, New York.

29. Ibid., 3.

30. Randall N. Saunders, *Remembering Claverack College* (Hudson, N.Y.: Hudson Evening Register, 1944), 5. Information about Claverack College is taken from Saunders, *Remembering Claverack College*; and "Annual Circular of Claverack College and Hudson River Institute, Claverack, Columbia Co., New York," 1881, 1885, 1886, Claverack College Collection, Columbia County Museum, Kinderhook, New York. Ella May Clark is listed in the 1885 and 1886 circulars. Thanks to Helen M. McLallen, curator of the Columbia County Museum, for this information.

31. *The Delaware Gazette*, 25 April 1894, microfilm, New York State Historical Association, Cooperstown. The entire article reads: "A Fashionable Wedding: The social event at Hobart, last week was the marriage of Eleanor Mai Clark daughter of ex-sheriff Clark to Mr. Robert E. Slagle of Chicago on Thursday noon. The ceremony was at St. Peter's Episcopal Church, Reverend Thomas Burrows, the rector officiating. Miss Gage presiding at the organ. The ushers were Mr. F. D. Merritt of Chicago, Mr. J. D. Clark the brother of the bride; hon. Jason R. Cowan of Hobart and J. Gould Barlow of Grand Gorge. Miss Mary C. Hanford was the bridesmaid and Miss Lavina E. Griffin the maid of honor. The bride and groom will make their home in Chicago." Slagle's marriage and baptism records are listed in R. W. Vosburgh, ed., *Records of St. Peter's Episcopal Church in Village of Hobart, Town of Stamford, Delaware County, New York*, vol. 3, transcribed by the New York Genealogical and Biographical Society (New York City, 1921).

32. "Slagle, Eleanor Clarke (Mrs.)," resumé, ca. 1937, John Davenport Clarke Papers, New York State Historical Association, Cooperstown (hereafter John Davenport Clarke Papers); James et al., *Notable American Women*, 3:296–98. Slagle's grandniece, Catherine Clarke Colby of Newcastle, Maine, said in an interview for the entry in *Notable American Women*, "There were whole periods of her life she never mentioned" (p. 296).

33. Slagle's early career is well described in her resume, "Experience of Eleanor Clarke Slagle," 1922, Papers of the American Occupational Therapy Association, AOTA Archives.

34. New York Census, 1890, Special Schedules for Union Veterans of Civil War, microfilm, New York State Historical Association, Cooperstown. Information follows: "Clark, Wm. J.; 2nd lieutenant; Company J; 144 New York Infantry Regiment; August 9, 1862, date of enlistment; July 14, 1865, date of discharge. Gun Shot in Neck

(Disability Incurred)." In "A Congressman," biographer DuVivier reports that William Clark accompanied John Brown on the Harper's Ferry Arsenal raid.

35. DuVivier, "A Congressman," 1.

36. Ibid., 88.

37. Letters between John D. Clarke and Eleanor Clarke Slagle, 1928–31, John Davenport Clarke Papers. Many family photographs and scrapbooks attest to a close relationship between Eleanor and her brother and nephew.

38. DuVivier, "A Congressman," 104.

39. Letters between Clarke and Slagle, 1928–31, John Davenport Clarke Papers.

40. Eleanor Clarke Slagle, *State of New York Department of Mental Hygiene, Syllabus for Training of Nurses in Occupational Therapy*, 2d ed. (New York, 1944), 33.

41. Ibid.

42. Ibid., 19.

43. Letter, Graham Taylor to Julia Lathrop, 24 November 1913, Graham Taylor Papers.

44. "Experience of Eleanor Clarke Slagle," resume, 1922, Papers of the American Occupational Therapy Association, AOTA Archives.

45. John Favill, *Henry Baird Favill, 1860–1916: A Memorial Volume* (Chicago: privately printed, 1917), xiii; *History of Medicine and Surgery and Physicians and Surgeons of Chicago* (Chicago: Biographical Publishing Corporation, 1922), 175–76.

# Chapter 2

## Psychiatry

### The Medical Birthplace of Occupational Therapy

In 1914 the prestigious Sheppard-Pratt Hospital in Towson, Maryland, put together a series of photographs to be presented at a meeting of the American Medico-Psychological Association.[1] One of them, reproduced in this book as photograph 4, portrayed psychiatrist William Rush Dunton, Jr., later called the "father of occupational therapy," in a woodworking shop, leaning over a table working on a craft project. The photograph suggested that Dunton felt comfortable being shown doing carpentry at a time when most other physicians would be photographed only in the laboratory, at a desk, or at a patient's side.[2] Although psychiatry increasingly emphasized scientific routines, Dunton gave a clear message that work in the form of arts and crafts was an important component of therapy for patients.

In the first decades of the twentieth century, Dunton participated in a nationwide struggle to raise the status of psychiatry in American medicine.[3] Professionalizing occupational therapy, he thought, was an important step in that direction, for he believed that the new profession held the promise of combining humanitarian values with scientific routines. This chapter analyzes Dunton's role in building the new profession of occupational therapy in an age of increasing emphasis on science and efficiency in mental health care.

## Young Dr. Dunton

William Rush Dunton, Jr., grew up in a comfortable, middle-class, Gilded Age home in Philadelphia. His choice of medicine as a career and his lifelong interest in arts and crafts reflected familial traditions and his educational background. He was born near Philadelphia on July 24, 1868, the son of Jacob

Dunton, a drug manufacturer and an inventor, and Annie (Gordon Gemmill) Dunton. Jacob's mother, Mary (Rush) Dunton, was a second cousin of the famous physician Benjamin Rush, and she gave her maiden name to Jacob's brother, William Rush Dunton. Jacob and Annie named their third child William Rush Dunton after his uncle, a physician. Young William Rush Dunton received his early education from private tutors and at the Lauderbach and Germantown academies in Philadelphia. In 1888 he graduated from Haverford College with a Bachelor of Science; because he was so interested in theater, music, literature, and the arts, he stayed one more year to earn a Master of Arts. He then entered medical school at the University of Pennsylvania, graduating in June 1893. Young Dr. Dunton added "Junior" to his name so that Philadelphians could distinguish between him and his physician uncle.[4]

An interest in laboratory science, to which Dunton had been introduced while in medical school, took the graduate to Baltimore's Johns Hopkins Hospital, which was linked to Johns

**Photograph 4:** Dr. Dunton "doing a bit of woodworking in the occupational therapy shop." (Sheppard-Pratt Archives)

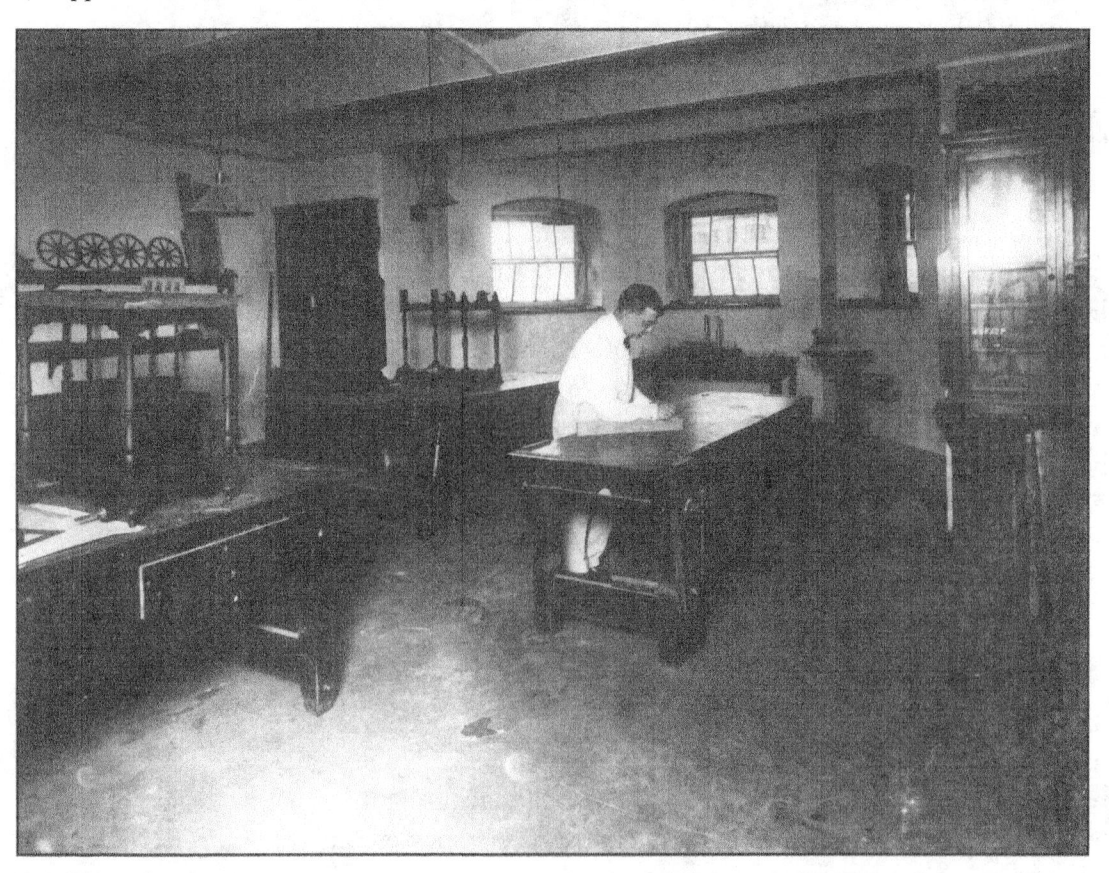

Hopkins Medical School, one of the most important centers of change in American medicine at the turn of the twentieth century.[5] At Johns Hopkins, Dunton was impressed by the emphasis on research; later he would pursue research at the Sheppard-Pratt Hospital. He was also impressed by the modern methods of asepsis, which he introduced at Philadelphia's Germantown Hospital during his service as a resident physician in late 1893. Dunton's time at Germantown Hospital gave him experience in general medicine. He gained experience in obstetrics and pediatrics at Children's Hospital, where he went in early 1895. There he met Nursing Superintendent Edna D. Hogan, whom he would later marry.[6]

Dunton's eventual decision to accept a position at the Sheppard Asylum (as the Sheppard and Enoch Pratt Hospital was then named) in Towson, Maryland, was part professional and part personal. Typically, young physicians of Dunton's day either joined the practices of older physicians or, if they had financial resources, opened their own private practices.[7] After Dunton's father experienced some financial difficulties, Dunton assumed that he would practice with his uncle. Dunton's interest in Hogan, however, met the strong opposition of the elder Dr. Dunton, who thought that his nephew ought to marry someone from as socially prominent a Philadelphia family as the Duntons. Young Dunton disagreed, thus risking any future association with his uncle. When he became engaged to Hogan in 1895, his professional relationship with his uncle ended.[8]

## WILLIAM RUSH DUNTON, JR., AT THE SHEPPARD AND ENOCH PRATT HOSPITAL

That same year Sheppard Asylum Superintendent Edward N. Brush hired William Rush Dunton, Jr., as assistant physician. The hospital had just opened in 1891, and Brush was building his staff. He placed Dunton in charge of a clinical and pathological laboratory. Brush and Dunton were part of a larger movement to raise the status of psychiatry by aligning it with other fields of medicine that were increasingly emphasizing the importance of laboratory science. Brush embodied the values of a generation of psychiatrists in America who tried to maintain traditional nineteenth-century charitable and humanitarian aims amid the advance of modern science. He hoped to offer patients "at once a hospital and an asylum" because he thought the role of the institution was twofold. Brush's goals, in other words, were either to restore the patient to health by using the best methods that medical science could offer, or to give the patient "an asylum and refuge, a protection from himself and the world."[9]

Dunton took on his new responsibilities with trepidation. Like many physicians of his time treating patients with mental illness, he felt inadequate and ill prepared.[10] Believing that psychiatry lagged behind other medical sciences in understanding the etiology, the diagnosis, and the treatment of mental illness, Dunton began his twenty-nine-year career at the Sheppard-Pratt Hospital in the laboratory. He looked into acid-alkali balances of urine in patients with manic-depressive illness, trying to show that the urine of patients in a manic state contained a high acid balance whereas the urine of patients in a depressed state had an elevated alkali balance. Dunton failed to prove this hypothesis. After several months of frustration, he realized that the laboratory would not furnish him with the help that he needed to care for patients. Brush reassigned Dunton to the clinical care of female patients.[11]

Medical school and postgraduate work had certainly prepared Dunton to give basic medical care to his patients, yet his lack of knowledge about the diagnosis and the treatment of his patients' mental problems led him to spend his first years at the hospital in study. After completing his daily duties, which included visiting the wards twice daily to check the condition of his patients and write entries in their medical charts, Dunton read various journals and books from Brush's library, among them the *American Journal of Insanity*. He was intrigued by the theories of many contemporary psychiatrists, especially those of Emil Kraepelin, whose work at a clinic in Heidelberg was having an important influence on American psychiatry in its struggle to develop modern diagnostic techniques. Kraepelin had combined a clinical-descriptive approach (taking of life histories) and a somatic approach (examination of body tissues) in studies of thousands of patients, resulting in the development of diagnosing mental illness by understanding its course and outcome. Dunton was also fascinated by the work of moral therapy advocates, such as the famous nineteenth-century Quaker William Tuke, of the York Retreat in England.[12]

His reading acquainted him with many of the basic controversies in American psychiatry of his time: among others, the somatic versus the environmental approach to determining etiology; the complexities of classifying mental illness; and the difficulties of ascertaining the efficacy of a variety of treatments. In the next several years Dunton threw himself into the pursuits of many of his contemporaries, publishing articles in such periodicals as the *American Journal of Insanity*, the *Journal of the American Medical Association*, the *Maryland Psychiatric Quarterly*, and the *Proceedings of the American Medico-Psychological Association* on subjects ranging from the diagnosis of dementia praecox (schizophrenia), to experiences with chloretone, to observations on blood pressure, to the *Packard* commitment case, which dealt with the rights of patients.[13]

Dunton's close reading of Samuel Tuke's report on the Tuke family's work at the York Retreat, which detailed the employment and amusement activities of patients, made him realize that this was one area in which the Sheppard Asylum needed improvement. Patients at the York Retreat regularly participated in "a judicious regimen of activity." Dunton decided to set up such a program at the hospital. Yet Dunton's approach differed from that of Tuke: he determined to bring activities for patients under the purview of scientific investigation. He could not begin this work, however, until the hospital was in a position to provide funding.[14]

Beginning in the later 1890s, Dunton and Brush had the financial backing that they needed. In 1896, Enoch Pratt, a wealthy merchant and philanthropist, gave the trustees a bequest of over $1.5 million dollars, with relatively few qualifications. He asked that certain building projects be completed, and that the hospital continue its commitment to caring for indigent patients as well as those able to pay. Finally, he asked that the traditional name of the institution—the Sheppard Asylum—be changed to the Sheppard and Enoch Pratt Hospital.[15]

To these requests the trustees gladly agreed. Brush welcomed the name change because it publicly declared the scientific aims of the institution.[16] Benjamin Pope, president of the Board of Trustees, also leaned toward a mission of not only offering curative treatment, but seeking an understanding of ways to prevent mental illness in the first place. He hoped that the science of psychiatry, that "most hidden and difficult branch of the curative art," would catch up to "the wonderful advances in other departments" of medicine.[17]

Brush made sure that the hospital took on the trappings of a research institution. He brought in Stewart Paton, a well-known neurologist, as director of the new clinical and pathological laboratory. He expanded the library to include fifty-two medical and psychiatric journals. He hired Clarence B. Farrar, a recent graduate of Johns Hopkins University, as clinical assistant, and sent Farrar to Heidelberg to study. On his return Farrar conducted pathological analyses of tissues from recently deceased patients. Staff members established contacts with other hospitals, institutions, and professional organizations. Brush lectured at the College of Physicians and Surgeons in Baltimore and was active in the Maryland State Mental Hygiene Association. Paton and Dunton gave a clinical course in psychiatry at Johns Hopkins, and Farrar lectured in the Department of Psychology at Johns Hopkins after his visit to Europe. Physicians from the Sheppard-Pratt Hospital joined the American Medico-Psychological Association, an elite group of hospital physicians (earlier called "hospital superintendents") interested in the study of mental disease.[18]

Further, hospital staff developed formal connections to the newly established Henry Phipps Psychiatric Clinic at nearby Johns Hopkins, headed by Adolph Meyer, probably one of the most influential psychiatrists in America from 1890 to 1940. One of Meyer's many contributions to American psychiatry was the development of the approach that he called "psychobiology." Meyer had initially trained in neurology, but by the 1890s he had broadened his scope to believe that psychiatry had to be based on both a somatic and a psychological approach. Thus in diagnosis and treatment he combined the life experience of patients with physiological and biological data. He urged that detailed life histories of patients be taken, bringing about a virtual revolution in the form and the content of patients' case records in America.[19]

Meyer has always been seen as a friend and a supporter of occupational therapy. Certainly his ideas about mental illness laid the ground for much interest in work therapy on the part of American psychiatrists in the first decades of the twentieth century. Influenced by Darwinian biology, Meyer saw healthy individuals holistically, as organisms that successfully interacted with and adapted to their environment.[20] In a paper on the philosophy of "occupation therapy," he wrote, "Our body is not merely so many pounds of flesh and bone . . . with an abstract mind or soul added to it. It is . . . a live organism pulsating with its rhythm of rest and activity." A mentally healthy individual, he elaborated, is "an organism that maintains and balances itself in the world of reality and actuality by being in active life and active use, i.e., using and living and acting its *time* in harmony with its own nature and the nature about it [emphasis in original]."[21] Those who cannot function well in their environment, he reasoned, are mentally ill, debilitated by certain defective habits learned early in life that prevent them from adapting to adulthood. For example, in a thesis that he developed about dementia praecox, Meyer argued that the condition was caused by a lack of adaptation, resulting in habit deterioration.[22] He believed that patients with such a condition could be cured by being involved in "habit training" regimens that would restore them to a balanced, healthful life.

Meyer's influence can be seen in the Sheppard-Pratt Hospital's commitment to upgrading the training of attendants and nurses, giving them the skills to be more active in the care of patients, rather than being merely custodial. In 1905 the Sheppard-Pratt Hospital established a training school for nurses, a common program in many other hospitals around the turn of the century. According to a later article by Dunton, certain classes emphasized teaching the nurses and the attendants various handcrafts believed to be ideal activities for habit training. Actually, work in handcrafts had begun in 1903, when a nurse from the hospital had learned raffia basketry so that she could introduce the arts and crafts to hospital patients. By 1908, Grace Fields, probably a craftswoman, was regularly instructing patients in a variety of crafts, including weaving, woodworking, metalworking, basketry, leather craft, and bookbinding. By 1915, two full-time and nine part-time teachers were conducting regular classes in handcrafts.[23]

Certainly the Sheppard-Pratt Hospital's commitment to both humanitarian and scientific aims and its proximity to Meyer's clinic in Baltimore directly affected Dunton's care of patients. By the early 1910s, detailed histories taken from patients on their entry into the hospital were being included in meticulously kept files. The files were far more comprehensive than the records for the 1890s, which were bound in large volumes by year and held much less information about the patients' lives both before and during their hospital stay.[24]

There was an obvious drive to regulate and rationalize the care of patients at the Sheppard-Pratt Hospital. Actual records show that clinical measurements such as blood pressure, temperature, and pulse were recorded twice daily. Nurses paid close attention to patients, monitoring the amount and the characteristics of urine, the frequency of bowel movements, and the number of hours of sleep. Moreover, Dunton used these observations in an attempt to correlate constitutional factors with mental condition.[25]

Hospital staff actively intervened in patients' daily routines, moving themselves beyond custodialism. Some patients received hydrotherapy treatments; others were encouraged to participate in outdoor leisure activities. The Casino Building, built in 1901 with money from the Pratt bequest, became the setting for many indoor activities. There patients participated daily in bowling, billiards, gymnastics, weaving, art work, sewing, and reading.

A subtle shift in thinking about the care of patients also occurred at the Sheppard-Pratt Hospital during these years. The caretakers assumed that patients should take some responsibility for their ultimate cure. In other words, although hospital staff acted on patients by performing medical procedures and by providing a highly structured environment, staff expected patients to participate in overcoming their illness by cooperating on the ward and working in the workshop. Nurses and occupational therapists regularly recorded patients' behavior and compliance, making these assessments on grid charts along with routine medical observations, such as "nourishment," "sleep," "excretions," and "special symptoms" like headaches and seizures. Staff commented on whether the patients were resistive, passive, or cooperative; whether they were happy, sad, or indifferent; and whether or not they participated in some form of occupation, such as reading, games, basketry, or sewing. These observations of mood and behavior, along with the standard medical observations, helped the staff judge the condition of individual patients.

The Sheppard-Pratt Hospital may have been a leader in the psychiatric community, but it was not the only hospital to introduce a regimen of craft work for patients in the early 1910s. Contemporary reports show that crafts were also regularly and successfully used in public mental hospitals that catered to lower-class patients. Between 1911 and 1915, occupations programs for patients increased in many large state hospitals.[26] Private hospitals also developed occupations programs during this period. The McLean Hospital in Boston and the Bloomingdale Hospital in New York are just two examples. Smaller private asylums such as the Adams Nervine Asylum in Jamaica Plain, Massachusetts, and the Devereux Mansion in Marblehead, Massachusetts, followed the trend.[27]

Indeed, all mental hospitals were under considerable pressure to establish an occupations program if they did not already have one. It was the criterion by which the prestige of individual institutions was measured. One report stated, "Diversional occupation, scientifically and systematically applied, marks the standing of a hospital, and if [it is] neglected or omitted, the patients are not receiving the most modern care and treatment to which they are entitled."[28]

In other words, a consensus among practicing psychiatrists held that occupying patients with work was a necessary component of successful therapy. C. Floyd Haviland, of the Kings Park Hospital on Long Island, New York, argued, "It seems almost trite to discuss the therapeutic value of occupation for the insane, so thoroughly has practical experience demonstrated that it is the most powerful single means at our command in curative treatment."[29] Dunton agreed: "Occupation is regarded as one of the most valued therapeutic measures."[30] T. J. Moher, of the Hospital for the Insane in Ontario, Canada, stated, "There is no other remedy known at the present time that is more productive of good results than occupation."[31]

By the early 1910s, then, there was broad interest in the use of occupations for patients, mainly because it seemed to help patients reach a healthier state. Yet many questions would also be raised because although practitioners widely agreed that occupational therapy worked, no one knew exactly why it did. Nor could practitioners explain why occupational therapy did not help seriously ill patients. Dunton and other leaders called for the development of a theory to underlie the treatment variously called "diversional occupation," "moral therapy," "reeducation," "ergotherapy," "work therapy," "industrial occupations," or just plain "occupations." Dunton wanted the soon-to-be-separate profession of occupational therapy "accorded the attention and respect" that he felt it deserved, presumably from the world of medicine. He, among others, lamented that the developing profession of occupational therapy was not considered "an exact science." He called for fellow practitioners to devise "instruments or methods" by which outcomes could be measured so that the work could be brought into accordance with the current scientific and systematic values of medicine.[32]

## Spokesperson for the Neophyte Profession

In Baltimore, William Rush Dunton, Jr., and Eleanor Clarke Slagle began a decades-long personal and professional relationship through which they tirelessly promoted occupational therapy. Between 1913 and 1915, when Slagle worked under Adolph Meyer in the newly established Occupations Department at the Phipps Clinic, she frequently visited the Dunton home.[33] During this time Dunton and Slagle planned the establishment of a national association. Dunton especially had an affinity for organizing such a group: he had organized the Maryland Psychiatric Society in 1908 and a Haverford College alumni group before that.[34]

Dunton took on the role of spokesperson for the neophyte profession, addressing important questions in several articles and books. In *Occupation Therapy: A Manual for Nurses* (1915), a book based on the occupations course for nurses offered at the Sheppard-Pratt Hospital beginning in fall 1911, Dunton attempted to explain how occupational therapy fit into current psychiatric theory. In a chapter titled "The Mechanism of Recovery by Occupation," Dunton displayed the influence of Adolph Meyer: He argued for diverting a patient's "attention" away from "brooding over the fancied sin he believes he has committed" and toward "other interests." Then, he said, a patient "regains better control of . . . attention and can voluntarily drive out the depressive thoughts." Using a schema developed by his colleague Clarence B. Farrar, Dunton went on to offer a mechanistic explanation of mental illness: "We are especially interested in the circle A which represents the focus of the attention or the conscious idea. In cases of depression this circle becomes small, owing to the inability to voluntarily fix the attention. In cases of excitement the circle becomes enlarged and ideas slip through it with great rapidity. In cases of dementia the circle is ragged and ideas are not clearly formed." In an unsatisfactory summary, he simplistically stated, "A little study, thought and observation will prove these statements" and make it "easily understood how occupation helps the patient by training the attention."[35]

Dunton and his colleagues Brush and Meyer struggled to find a place in which occupational therapy would fit amid the theoretical outlines of contemporary psychiatric thinking, yet new developments in the field frustrated their efforts. Sigmund Freud's psychoanalytic ideas, which concentrated more on individual analysis and less on broader social contexts, gained popularity in the American psychiatric community. Thus psychiatry entered a new period of transformation. This time the ideas of a generation of psychiatrists such as Brush, Dunton, and Meyer came under criticism.

Such criticism occurred at the Sheppard-Pratt Hospital, where first Brush and then Dunton left under pressure. On April 1, 1920, after nearly thirty years of service as physician-in-chief and superintendent of the hospital, Brush resigned, to be replaced by the luminary Harry Stack Sullivan, a strong advocate of Freudianism. Within two years Dunton too had departed.[36]

Both Brush and Dunton spent their final years at the hospital moving in directions that failed to coincide with the thinking of converts to Freudianism. They did not believe that the causes of mental illness, and possible cures, could be found within the individual patient. Although in "complete sympathy with scientific research," Dunton once said, "we should not despise empiricism." He was more than willing to attack mental illness from many sides and with colleagues from more than one field. Knowing that he could not prove on a purely scientific basis that occupational therapy worked, for example, he called for analyzing it from a broad perspective, one including "its relationship to social science, mental hygiene, vocational education, recreation, and other subjects."[37]

Dunton chose to support the growth of a new profession *allied* with psychiatry and medicine. The new profession, in order to survive, still had to convince the medical world and the general public of its value. This problem and other issues, including creating a workforce to ensure the continued growth of occupational therapy and expanding the settings in which occupational therapy would be practiced, would be foremost on the minds of the founding generation.

The next three chapters describe the work of several other founders, most of whom were centered in Boston, another important locus of activity in the early years of occupational therapy. They were Susan E. Tracy, an educator of nurses for "invalid occupations"; Herbert James Hall, a Harvard-trained physician and the founder of the Devereux Workshops in Marblehead, Massachusetts; George Edward Barton, an arts and crafts enthusiast and the first president of the National Society for the Promotion of Occupational Therapy; Philip King Brown, a Harvard Medical School graduate and the founder of the Arequipa Sanatorium for women with tuberculosis, in Marin County, California; and Susan Cox Johnson, the director of patients' activities at Blackwell's Island Hospital in New York City and later a faculty member at Teachers College, Columbia University.

*Part I:*
*The Rise of Occupational Therapy*

1. Dunton's photograph is part of a series titled "The Life of the Patient," found among several hundred photographs now being cataloged at the Sheppard-Pratt Hospital. I thank Diane Gibson, head of patients' activities, for making me aware of the existence of these photographs. She and Robert Gibson, executive president of the Sheppard-Pratt Hospital, are also cataloging and storing other artifacts from the hospital's history. Sources for the history of Sheppard-Pratt Hospital include Bliss Forbush and Byron Forbush, *Gatehouse: The Evolution of the Sheppard and Enoch Pratt Hospital, 1853–1986* (Baltimore: Sheppard and Enoch Pratt Hospital, 1986); and Bliss Forbush, *The Sheppard and Enoch Pratt Hospital, 1853–1970* (Philadelphia: J. B. Lippincott Company, 1970). A representative sample of the photographs from the series is published in Forbush and Forbush, *Gatehouse*.

2. For studies on the use of photographs in medical history, see Rima Apple, "Pictorial Essay," in *Women's Health and Medicine in America: A Historical Handbook*, ed. Rima Apple (New York: Garland, 1990), 271–81; Daniel M. Fox and Christopher Lawrence, *Photographing Medicine: Images and Power in Britain and America since 1840* (Westport, Conn.: Greenwood Press, 1988); and Daniel M. Fox and James Terry, "Photography and the Self-image of American Physicians, 1880–1920," *Bulletin of the History of Medicine* 52 (Spring 1978): 435–57.

3. For background on the history of the care of persons considered insane, see Ellen Dwyer, *Homes for the Mad: Life inside Two Nineteenth-Century Asylums* (New Brunswick, N.J.: Rutgers University Press, 1987); Gerald N. Grob, *Mental Illness and American Society, 1875–1940* (Princeton, N.J.: Princeton University Press, 1983); and Nancy Tomes, *A Generous Confidence: Thomas Story Kirkbride and the Art of Asylum-keeping, 1840–1883* (Cambridge: Cambridge University Press, 1984). On the transformation of American hospitals at the turn of the twentieth century, see Charles E. Rosenberg, *The Care of Strangers: The Rise of America's Hospital System* (New York: Basic Books, 1987); David Rosner, *A Once Charitable Enterprise: Hospitals and Health Care in Brooklyn and New York, 1885–1915* (Cambridge: Cambridge University Press, 1982); Paul Starr, *The Social Transformation of American Medicine: The Rise of a Sovereign Profession and the Making of a Vast Industry* (New York: Basic Books, 1982); and Morris Vogel, *The Invention of the Modern Hospital: Boston, 1870–1930* (Chicago: University of Chicago Press, 1980).

4. The biographical information on Dunton and the descriptions of Dunton's early years at the Sheppard-Pratt Hospital are from the thorough biography by Robert K. Bing, "William Rush Dunton, Junior—American Psychiatrist: A Study in Self" (Ed.D. diss., University of Maryland, 1961).

5. Kenneth Ludmerer discusses Johns Hopkins University and its prominence in American medical education in *Learning to Heal: The Development of American Medical Education* (New York: Basic Books, 1985).

6. Bing, "William Rush Dunton, Junior," 101–2.

7. Grob, *Mental Illness*, 31–32.

8. Bing, "William Rush Dunton, Junior," 102.

9. Forbush, *The Sheppard and Enoch Pratt Hospital*, 39–40.

10. Grob, *Mental Illness*, 30–45.

11. Bing, "William Rush Dunton, Junior."

12. Ibid., 110. See also the introduction to this book, note 21.

13. William R. Dunton, "Experience with Chloretone," *American Journal of Insanity* 58 (July 1901): 133; Dunton, "Some Points in the Diagnosis of Dementia Praecox," *American Journal of Insanity* 59 (July 1902): 53–61; Dunton, "Some Observations upon Blood Pressure in the Insane," *American Journal of Insanity* 61 (July 1904): 41–53; Dunton, "Mrs. Packard and Her Influence upon Laws for the Commitment of the Insane," *Johns Hopkins Hospital Bulletin* 18 (October 1907): 419–24. A book on Mrs. Packard (Mrs. Theophilus Packard, Jr., nee Elizabeth Parsons Ware) is Barbara Sapinsley, *The Private War of Mrs. Packard* (New York: Paragon Press, 1989).

14. Grob, *Mental Illness*, 31–32.

15. Bing, "William Rush Dunton, Junior," 110–16.

16. Ibid., 111–12; Forbush, *The Sheppard and Enoch Pratt Hospital*, 38–63.

17. Forbush, *The Sheppard and Enoch Pratt Hospital*, 39.

18. Ibid., 40–41.

19. According to Grob, *Mental Illness*, 112–18, Meyer was born in Switzerland in 1866 and received his M.D. from the University of Zurich in 1892. He then went to the United States. After holding a brief appointment at the University of Chicago and then spending three years at the Kankakee State Hospital in Illinois as a pathologist, Meyer went to Massachusetts, where he held a similar appointment at the Worcester Hospital from 1896 to 1901. He was director of the Pathological Institute of New York State from 1901 to 1908, when he took his positions as director of the Phipps Clinic and professor of psychiatry at Johns Hopkins Medical School.

20. Adolph Meyer, "The Philosophy of Occupation Therapy," *Archives of Occupational Therapy* 1 (1922): 1–10.

21. Forbush, *The Sheppard and Enoch Pratt Hospital*, 63.

22. Ibid., 41–50; William R. Dunton, "A Nurse's Occupation Course," in *Proceedings of the American Medico-Psychological Association* 19 (1912): 269–78.

23. Forbush, *The Sheppard and Enoch Pratt Hospital*, 41–50; Dunton, "A Nurse's Occupation Course," 269–78.

24. There are several hundred case records of patients available to scholars on request. The records from the 1890s are spotty, and are bound in volumes by year. The records from approximately 1897 to 1911 are missing. After 1911, each patient has an individual file,

including records of the patient's initial entrance into the hospital, physician's notes, medical records, photographs of the patient, results of various tests, and descriptions of the course of illness. Unfortunately for historians of nursing and occupational therapy, a large proportion of the nursing and occupational therapy notes were removed from the charts and discarded during the 1960s.

25. Grob, *Mental Illness*, 36–41.

26. See the *Proceedings of the American Medico-Psychological Association* in the years 1912–15, for example, for reports on occupations programs at the following hospitals: the Kankakee State Hospital, Illinois; the Laurel Sanitarium, Maryland; the Boston State Hospital in Dorchester, and the Taunton State Hospital, Massachusetts; the New Jersey State Hospital in Morris Plains; the Kings Park Hospital on Long Island, New York; the Massillon State Hospital, Ohio; and the Homeopathic State Hospital in Allentown, and the Norristown State Hospital, Pennsylvania.

27. S. B. Sutton, *Crossroads in Psychiatry: A History of the McLean Hospital* (Washington, D.C.: American Psychiatric Press, 1986). Information about occupational therapy and Bloomingdale Hospital can be found in Louis J. Haas, *Occupational Therapy for the Mentally and Nervously Ill* (New York: n.p., 1925); about occupational therapy and the Adams Nervine Asylum, in Susan E. Tracy, *Studies in Invalid Occupation* (Boston: Whitcomb and Barrows, 1910); and about occupational therapy and the Devereux Mansion, in Herbert J. Hall and Mertice M. C. Buck, *The Work of Our Hands: A Study of Occupations for Invalids* (New York: Moffat, Yard and Company, 1915).

28. "Report of the Committee on Diversional Occupation," in *Proceedings of the American Medico-Psychological Association* 21 (1914): 138; also in *American Journal of Insanity* 71 (July 1914): 214.

29. C. Floyd Haviland, "Occupation for the Insane," in *Proceedings of the American Medico-Psychological Association* 19 (1912): 249–61.

30. William R. Dunton, "Occupation as a Therapeutic Measure," *Medical Record* 83 (1913): 388–89.

31. As quoted in Arthur P. Herring, "Diversional Occupation of the Insane," in *Proceedings of the American Medico-Psychological Association* 19 (1912): 245–48.

32. William R. Dunton, "The Principles of Occupational Therapy," in *Proceedings of the First Annual Meeting of the National Society for the Promotion of Occupational Therapy* (Towson, Md.: NSPOT, 1918), 26–34.

33. The biographical material on Slagle is taken from Edward T. James, Janet W. James, and Paul S. Boyer, eds., *Notable American Women, 1607–1950* (Cambridge: Belknap Press of Harvard University Press, 1971), 3:296–98. Information on the course and its relationship to mental hygiene is drawn from Jane Addams, *My Friend Julia Lathrop* (New York: Macmillan, 1935), 151–52; and Barbara Loomis, "Professional Occupational Therapy Education in Chicago, 1908–1920" (Paper presented at the Written History Seminar, Sixty-third Annual Meeting of the American Occupational Therapy Association, Portland, Ore., April 1983). Career information about

Slagle appears in her resume, "Experience of Eleanor Clarke Slagle," 1922, Papers of the American Occupational Therapy Association, Official Archives of the American Occupational Therapy Association, Wilma L. West Library, American Occupational Therapy Foundation, Bethesda, Maryland (hereafter AOTA Archives); and in a letter, Slagle to Adolph Meyer, 9 October 1912, AOTA Archives.

34. Bing, "William Rush Dunton, Junior," 150–52.

35. William R. Dunton, *Occupation Therapy: A Manual for Nurses* (Philadelphia: W. B. Saunders Company, 1915), 27–33.

36. Bing, "William Rush Dunton, Junior," 177–79.

37. Dunton, "The Principles," 27.

# Chapter 3

## Nurses *for* Invalid Occupations

### Susan E. Tracy and the Expansion of Occupational Therapy

*Nurses for Invalid Occupations*

In 1910 when the American Society of Superintendents of Training Schools for Nurses met in New York City, Adelaide Nutting of Teachers College, Columbia University, arranged for a special exhibition. This "Educational Museum," as she labeled it, displayed experimental work in the new field of "occupations for invalids." One of the participants, Boston-based physician Herbert James Hall, showed handcrafts made by patients treated for "nervous exhaustion" at his small mental asylum in Marblehead, Massachusetts. The Chicago School of Civics and Philanthropy exhibited work by patients from Illinois mental hospitals. Susan E. Tracy's exhibit, "The Testing of Invalid Occupations in the Adams Nervine Asylum, Jamaica Plain, Massachusetts," showed handcrafts made by patients and ways to instruct nurses in this new field.[1]

Susan E. Tracy was an important figure in the movement to create the new profession of occupational therapy in the first decades of the twentieth century. Born in 1878 and graduated from the Massachusetts Homeopathic Hospital Nursing School in 1898, she, like Slagle, was a member of the first generation of professional women in the United States.[2] In 1906 she organized occupational therapy classes in her training school for nurses at the Adams Nervine Asylum. She trained practitioners not only in the Boston area, but in Chicago and New York, as she tried to establish occupational therapy as a subspecialty of nursing. In 1910 she published a textbook that was widely used in the field until at least 1940 (see photograph 5).[3] Another important contribution that Tracy made was to take occupational therapy from its limited place in psychiatric institutions to the homes of patients, an important locus of care in the early twentieth century. Her contemporaries in nursing and occupational therapy considered her a pioneer in advancing women's professional work.[4]

Yet Tracy did not always behave as a pioneer should; she balked at certain norms of professional behavior. For example, in 1917 she opted not to attend the much-publicized founding meeting of the National Society for the Promotion of Occupational Therapy, later called the American Occupational Therapy Association. Training newcomers to the field seems to have been more important to Tracy than establishing a national association. While the founders met in upstate New York, she stayed in Chicago to run occupations courses for nurses in the Rush-Presbyterian and Michael Reese hospitals. Did Tracy not concur that a national organization was vital to the development of the profession? Did she not agree that the public and the medical world had to be convinced of the value of occupational therapy?[5]

This chapter analyzes the profession-building strategies and the professional self-identity of Tracy not because they were unique but because the career tracks of many first-generation occupational therapists paralleled that of Tracy. Tracy and numerous other female occupational therapists between 1910

**Photograph 5:** Examples of craft work in Susan Tracy's book, *Invalid Occupations*.

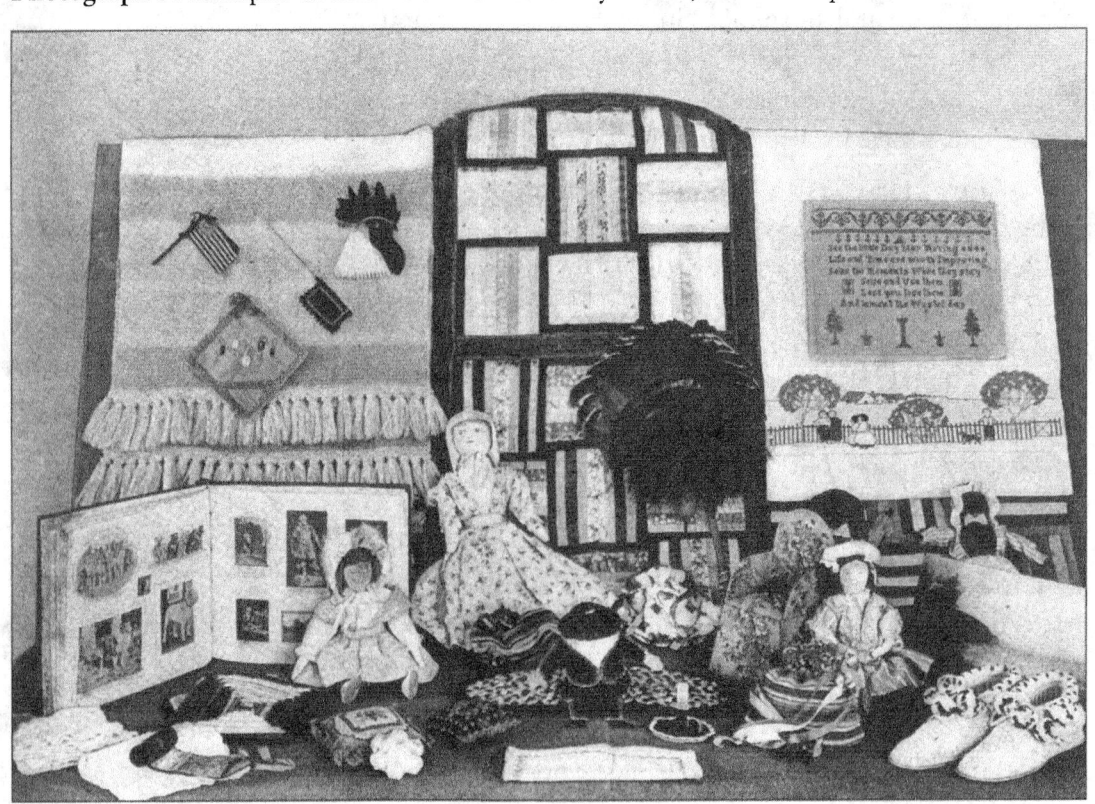

and 1930 seemed ambivalent about the field's taking on the typical trappings of professionalism—establishing a strong national association, coalescing a precise body of knowledge based on scientific theory, and so forth.[6] Many did not share the priorities of the male founders of this new profession. Had Tracy and other female occupational therapists internalized an ideology that encouraged subjectivity and passivity in women, and discouraged objectivity and leadership,[7] or was the adoption of a division of labor based on gender a deliberate strategy to help legitimize the field?

The chapter describes a gender-defined framework of organization that occupational therapy embraced in its founding years. From the 1910s until at least World War II, men strongly associated with mainstream medicine concentrated on building theory, dominating the profession's journal, and holding the presidency of the national association.[8] Women, by contrast, concentrated on establishing local institutions for practice and training, and developing experience-based practice. This analysis of Tracy's career illuminates occupational therapy's gender-defined division of labor, the role of occupational therapy in eliminating the rest cure, the short-lived link between nursing and occupational therapy, and the struggle within occupational therapy to define its professional boundaries.

## Susan E. Tracy and the Adams Nervine Asylum

Susan E. Tracy formally began her work in "invalid occupations" at the Adams Nervine Asylum in Jamaica Plain, Massachusetts, a small mental institution founded in the late nineteenth century. The Adams Nervine Asylum catered to "nervous invalids" rather than to persons who were seriously mentally ill, according to the resident physician, Daniel H. Fuller.[9] Indeed, patients had to be declared "not insane" to gain entry to the institution. Prospective patients presented Fuller with a certificate signed by their own physician stating that they could "be cured" by a stay at the asylum.[10]

Specifically, most of the patients at the Adams Nervine Asylum suffered from "neurasthenia," a newly identified illness. According to neurologist George M. Beard, then America's expert on neurasthenia, patients suffered from several symptoms, including "morbid anxiety, unaccountable [mental and physical] fatigue, irrational fears, and compulsive or inadequate sexual behavior."[11] Patients also complained of headaches, sleep and appetite disturbances, pains and aches, and depression.[12]

Late-nineteenth-century physicians declared that the illness was caused by the stresses of modern life. People had limited energy; when they were taxed by overwork, stress, or strain, in the marketplace or at home, one or more of their bodily systems broke down, provoking neurasthenia. Complete bed rest and a bland diet, to the point of infantilization, offered the only hope of restoring the exhausted patient to health. This so-called rest cure was popularized by elite Philadelphia physician S. Weir Mitchell.[13]

At the Adams Nervine Asylum around the turn of the century, the rest cure dominated the therapy program. Prescribed by the resident physician, the rest cure was actually delivered by nurses, who kept intermittent notes illustrating the degree to which patients were restrained from activity. "Advised absolute quiet," one record stated, "as she [the patient] appears greatly fatigued." Patients were required to stay in bed, and the quality and the quantity of their sleep was recorded. They took their meals, mostly just milk, in bed, and the amounts and the frequency of liquid nourishment were measured. Because bed rest might cause disorders of the muscular and digestive systems, massages and mild medications often accompanied the cure.[14]

Caught up in the broad reforms that called for psychiatry to become more aggressive in its therapies, many psychiatrists after 1900 began to criticize the rest cure. Herbert J. Hall, one of the participants in the Teachers College Educational Museum and later president of the American Occupational Therapy Association (1920–23), opposed the rest cure. Protesting "the almost universal application of rest in the treatment of neurasthenia and allied conditions," he based his critique on experimental work conducted at his workshop/asylum in Marblehead, Massachusetts, where patients daily made artistic crafts as part of his "work-cure medical treatment."[15]

Hall based his disapproval of the rest cure on Adolph Meyer's concept of mental illness and ill-directed habit formation. Meyer's ideas had influenced many American psychiatrists to view patients as mentally ill if they were unable to function well in their environment. Such patients, the theory went, had been debilitated by certain defective habits learned early in life that prevented them from adapting to adulthood. Meyer believed that patients with mental illness could be cured by "habit training" regimens that would restore them to a balanced, healthful life.[16]

Meyer and Hall promoted handcrafts as ideal activities for habit training. Hall claimed that patients could be "lift[ed] out of a tangle of nervous symptoms" when given work to do, and that giving them work was far better than "substituting another abnormality in the shape of unduly prolonged rest."[17] He reasoned that too much rest further endangered a patient's health instead of bringing it back into balance. He believed so strongly in work as a therapeutic measure, in fact, that he even said it was more important than medicine or "enforced rest" in helping patients regain their health.[18]

By the first decade of the twentieth century, the staff at the Adams Nervine Asylum had also renounced the rest cure, exchanging its near custodialism for more active therapies. A chapter authored by Daniel H. Fuller in Susan E. Tracy's book *Studies in Invalid Occupation* described a multitude of approaches used at the Adams Nervine Asylum, among them, drugs; massage; electricity; gymnastics; dietary regimens; hydrotherapy; light, heat, and fresh air; occupations; instruction in methods of self-help; and suggestion or psychotherapy.[19]

Fuller saw many advantages in engaging his "nervous invalid" patients in occupations. He agreed with Meyer's argument that patients were likely to focus too much on their own problems under enforced-rest regimens. Occupations diverted attention from illness and established new and healthier life habits. The occupations room created a "new environment," taking patients away from their "individual apartment" filled with the "suggestion of invalidism." Occupations also offered a "means of switching the attention from morbid introspection to ... normal interests, ... excluding abnormal habits of mind."[20]

Fuller hired Tracy in 1905, and for the next seven years she supervised the nursing school, developed the occupations program with Fuller, and conducted several postgraduate courses for nurses. Later Fuller wrote that he had "secured an excellent leader, [who was both] trained in teaching and conversant with the work to be taken up."[21]

In contrast to Fuller's reliance on theory, Tracy claimed that she based her approach to occupations on mere common sense and observation. She had spent seven years in private-duty nursing before going to the Adams Nervine Asylum. That experience had convinced her that patients were "happier when their hands and minds were occupied."[22] Even though she had studied at Teachers College, taking courses in crafts and hospital economics, she never acknowledged any formal training beyond traditional nursing school. She modestly said that she had learned many crafts in childhood and that when she became a nurse and "found herself responsible for removing the tedium of lagging hours," she reverted to occupations learned at her mother's side.[23]

Unlike psychiatrists such as Meyer and Fuller, Tracy never attempted theoretical explanations about when one ought to practice occupational therapy, nor did she feel the need to understand why one should. She simply designed a practical curriculum for her students at the Adams Nervine Asylum that would prepare them to work with patients with neurasthenia, as well as with the variety of cases that they would face when they graduated to become private-duty nurses. Her textbook was dominated by practical discussions of craft projects for convalescents of various age, sex, class, and medical categories. Each of her lessons required students to make a craft article, blending their arts and crafts skills with the medical knowledge that they had acquired in other courses. Her greatest concern was to develop judgment skills in students so that they could select appropriate activities for patients.[24]

Speaking from her own experience, Tracy declared that only nurses should practice occupations, for only they understood the limitations that different diseases imposed and the positive and negative consequences that various activities could produce. Nurses were able to notice "eye strain" and "fatigue" even before the patient became aware of them. Nurses were also able to recognize nervous disorders and temperamental differences among patients, and only nurses could produce individualized work plans to address these conditions, she claimed.[25] Tracy tried to make patient occupations a specialty within nursing, even offering a few courses at Teachers College in the early 1910s.[26] If nothing more, she hoped that the training in occupations would provide practitioners with skills that would ease the burdens of their daily practice. In offering the training, Tracy spoke to a problem that nursing leaders recognized: private-duty nursing was physically and psychologically exhausting.[27]

When speaking of Tracy in public, colleagues in psychiatry and nursing described her as a "caring" nurse devoted to serving society. They carefully commended her for contributing to nursing and occupational therapy while never projecting an image that in the least way might make her look self-interested, commercial, or "unladylike." Maryland psychiatrist William Rush Dunton, Jr., a strong supporter of occupational therapy and the editor of the *Maryland Psychiatric Quarterly*, devoted an entire issue to her work in occupations. In that issue he praised her for organizing the "first systematic training course for nurses in occupations" at the Adams Nervine Asylum, yet he deliberately wrote with restraint because he did not want to "embarrass the dear lady."[28] Another contributor to the special issue described interviewing Tracy in her home, depicted as an environment of domestic grace. Tracy reportedly greeted the writer at the door with "outstretched hands" and then "conducted [the writer] into her "quaint, old-fashioned home" with a "huge fire-place in the sitting room," for a meeting in which Tracy stated that she had decided to "devote the rest of her life to occupational therapy."[29]

Such mythologizing of Tracy can best be understood in the context of the history of nursing and the general predicament in which professional women found themselves in the early twentieth century. Tracy entered nursing during a period of reform in which leaders were struggling to gain recognition and power for the profession. Reverby has argued that professionalization presented several dilemmas to superintendent leaders in nursing and that Tracy was no exception. Nurses were expected to maintain a particularly feminine form of a service ethic; furthermore, they were commonly idealized as women with "natural" characteristics of self-sacrifice and patience. Thus they encountered difficulties in asserting concerns about professional autonomy or remuneration. Moreover, nurses were caught between traditional views of the "caring" nurse and the needs of hospital authorities moving toward efficient and scientific approaches to the care of patients. Nurses needed to "know" more; thus the profession pressed for higher educational criteria. Yet this greater knowledge did not guarantee nursing an authoritative position in the evolving medical hierarchy of the early twentieth century.[30]

Women aspiring to careers in Tracy's generation made it clear that their motives were based on altruism and service to society. If they held personal ambitions for or intellectual interests in work outside their traditional family duties, they rarely made public declarations of these motives. Such declarations would not have been socially acceptable. Rather, they commonly mythologized their calling to professional work by telling stirring stories of it: for example, Jane Addams's tale of being inspired to found the Hull House Settlement in 1889 after seeing the "wretchedness of East London" and the innovative work at Toynbee Hall;[31] and Lillian Wald's account of starting the Henry Street Settlement in New York City after witnessing the misery in the Lower East Side's immigrant neighborhoods.[32]

Women of the founding generation of occupational therapy told such stories as well. Eleanor Clarke Slagle claimed to have received her "inspiration and incentive" to work in occupational therapy during "a chance visit" to the Kankakee State Hospital in Illinois while taking courses in social economics, psychology, and recreation at the Chicago School of Civics and Philanthropy in the early 1900s. Slagle and others like Julia Lathrop were in fact conducting studies of such institutions to determine the state of patients' care. Slagle told how she noticed an "unkempt young" female patient unraveling her knitted underclothing from her waist in order to make a little shirt for a child. Slagle spoke to the woman, asking if she was making the garment for her daughter. The patient's "face lighted," so the story goes, and she exclaimed "that she actually had four children." Slagle left that day determined to help overcome the "appalling idleness of the mentally sick in the institutions [which was] a constant degenerating influence." With the help of some "Chicago women," she later established a community workshop under the auspices of the Illinois Society for Mental Hygiene, where persons with physical and mental disabilities were trained in occupations.[33]

Tracy too mythologized her calling to occupations. She described her days as a student nurse at the Massachusetts Homeopathic Hospital, where she had noticed that surgical patients who kept busy working managed to maintain their spirits. One courageous woman spent every last minute until surgery embroidering. Another woman recovered rapidly from abdominal surgery while lying on her back crocheting an elaborate piece of trimming. A young girl kept herself and others in the ward lively while she worked on projects, in spite of the fact that one of her legs had been amputated.[34] Tracy told and retold these anecdotes, thus explaining why she had become interested in occupations. More important, she accounted for her leadership in the field: it was all for the benefit of patients.

Occupational therapists and nurses were expected to demonstrate obedience and self-sacrifice. This cultural prescription of gender-specific personality attributes sometimes caused difficulties. For example, occupational therapists and nurses had to take orders from physicians, even though they possessed the executive skills to persuade patients to cooperate in the workshops and on the wards. Always taking orders obediently was no easy task, especially because many occupational therapists and nurses had accrued substantial practical knowledge and therefore were able to make intelligent observations about the care of patients. Yet cultural assumptions about the proper behavior of women prevented them from challenging the authority of physicians and certainly from being physicians' peers. Promoters of occupational therapy incessantly talked about the need for practitioners to be tactful, patient, mature, loyal, and observant of patients' behavior, as well as skilled in the crafts and knowledgeable about medicine. Herbert J. Hall made a point of saying that prospective occupational therapists needed to possess not only "good motherly instincts, an attractive personality, and some knowledge of the crafts," but also "careful preliminary training as complete as that required of the nurse or social service worker." He warned that "the medical subjects and handicrafts" could be learned by anyone, but "judgement and discretion" could "hardly ever be taught" and thus had to be innate characteristics, most likely found in women.[35]

Daniel H. Fuller expressed similar expectations for Tracy's performance at the Adams Nervine Asylum. He depended on Tracy to ensure that his orders were followed and that the patients would obtain the maximum benefit from his prescribed therapy. For example, Fuller had a rule never to allow any "talk of sickness, invalidism, treatment, past experiences, and symptoms" in the occupations room. Tracy had to enforce this exclusion of all gloomy subjects. She was to be a "tactful and watchful" teacher who set a good example of cheerful industriousness while encouraging healthy interactions among the patients at work. The success or the failure of an occupations room, he generalized, depended on the leadership and the example of the teacher or the nurse who ran it. "It is futile to put work into the hands of the sick and expect them to create an interest in it . . . The personality of the teacher and nurse therefore becomes an important factor."[36]

## FOUNDING OF THE EXPERIMENT STATION FOR THE STUDY OF INVALID OCCUPATIONS

The image of Tracy as a self-sacrificing lady and nurse suggests that she lived up to the cultural roles expected of turn-of-the-century American women. Yet Tracy was more than the demure lady that she chose to portray. In 1912 she broke her ties with the Adams Nervine Asylum to set up her own institution, which she called the Experiment Station for the Study of Invalid Occupations. There she instructed patients and public health and graduate nurses. She also created a resource center, claiming to keep complete records of all work done in the field.

One observer interpreted Tracy's leaving the Adams Nervine Asylum as its having been thrust on her because of lack of space.[37] In actuality Tracy planned the move years before. In a 1910 speech to the American Society of Superintendents of Training Schools for Nurses, she called for setting up "a bureau" for training "occupations nurses" in every large city so that nurses could gain control over practice. From their respective experiment stations, she argued, skilled occupations nurses could be sent to patients "of all sorts and conditions" to practice their specialization.[38]

Tracy's establishing the Experiment Station can only be interpreted as an autonomous act. She sought independence for herself and for other nurses who desired self-sufficiency in their workplaces and freedom from the confines of physician-dominated hospitals. Her true motive was to upgrade nurses' status by providing them with specialized skills. Although she may have claimed to be disinterested in theory, her establishment of the resource center, where she collected case studies for others to examine, proves her interest in gathering a body of knowledge. For Tracy, however, that knowledge was to be based in experience or practice, not theory. Did she leave the Adams Nervine Asylum in frustration because her ways of knowing went unappreciated? More likely she simply needed to free herself from the responsibilities of her nursing superintendency in order to create more opportunities for spreading the occupational therapy gospel.

As Tracy trained more and more practitioners, she in effect transported the practice of occupational therapy from its original, limited place in psychiatric institutions to many other arenas in which medicine was practiced. The nurses whom she trained at the Adams Nervine Asylum, who would later practice privately in the homes of patients, used occupational therapy to treat physical as well as mental illness. Many of her students went on to found their own institutions of practice or to head occupational therapy departments in hospitals as such departments slowly increased in number during the 1910s. Her visits to many other institutions, to give single lectures or complete courses to student and postgraduate nurses, ensured such a process. In

1911, for example, she gave lessons to the senior class at the nursing school at Massachusetts General Hospital. By 1916 she had given courses at the Newton and Children's hospitals in Boston and the Michael Reese and Rush-Presbyterian hospitals in Chicago, and she had lectured several times at Teachers College in New York, among other places. That year she taught a three-month course at Teachers College, dividing classes between ward patients and student nurses.[39]

Tracy did not attend the founding meeting of the National Society for the Promotion of Occupational Therapy, but her peers were aware of her important role in organizing occupational therapy professionally. To recognize her efforts in training practitioners, the founders declared her an honorary founding member and elected her chair of the Committee on Teaching Methods.[40] In those early years Tracy contributed several papers on teaching to the national association.[41]

During the 1910s, by introducing occupational therapy into general hospitals, where poor persons received health care, Tracy also exposed the work to a wider range of patients. Hitherto, mainly middle- and upper-class patients had received occupational therapy treatments, for only they could afford to hire private-duty nurses.

Tracy never saw occupational therapy become a specialty within nursing. Other occupational therapy leaders disagreed with Tracy's notion that practitioners had to be nurses. Eleanor Clarke Slagle and Susan Cox Johnson, both founding members of the National Society for the Promotion of Occupational Therapy, acknowledged that practitioners needed course work in medicine, as nurses did. They argued, however, that "occupations teachers," as Johnson called them, needed grounding in pedagogy and sociology too.[42] William Rush Dunton, Jr., agreed with Slagle and Johnson, saying that occupational therapy was a multidisciplinary profession that took a broad perspective from various fields such as "social science, mental hygiene, vocational education, and recreation"; he did not even mention nursing. Lamenting that occupational therapy was not considered "an exact science," he called for practitioners to devise "instruments or methods" by which outcomes could be measured so that the work could be brought into accordance with the contemporary scientific and systematic values of medicine.[43] Two efficiency experts, George Edward Barton, first president of the National Society for the Promotion of Occupational Therapy, and Thomas B. Kidner, vocational secretary of the Canadian Military Hospitals Commission, also attended the founding meeting. They pressed the neophyte profession to adopt efficiency routines that would help it gain the attention and the respect that Dunton felt it deserved, presumably from the world of medicine.

The will and the viewpoints of the other founders became the norm: occupational therapy found its own identity separate from nursing but including the perspectives of several other fields. Until her death in 1928, Tracy saw few new occupational therapy hospital departments or teaching institutions headed by nurses, although in many cases nurses worked alongside others representing the disciplines of medicine, teaching, psychiatry, social work, and arts and crafts. During World War I especially, several occupational therapy schools with representatives from multiple disciplines sprang up in major American cities, such as Boston, Chicago, Milwaukee, New York, Philadelphia, and St. Louis. A severe wartime shortage of nurses also accelerated the growth of nursing schools, but few, if any, included training in occupations. Such training was confined to schools for "reconstruction aides"—the wartime name for occupational and physical therapists who were involved in the movement to "reconstruct" wounded soldiers and sailors returning from the front.

The Philadelphia School of Occupational Therapy, for example, opened in spring 1918 with the purpose of furnishing an intensive course qualifying women to become reconstruction aides. The school's faculty represented the many disciplines from which occupational therapy was drawing its growing body of knowledge: Charles Watts Burr, a professor of mental diseases at the University of Pennsylvania, gave lectures on patients who were mentally subnormal (retarded) and abnormal. Lillian Clayton, a nurse graduate of Philadelphia's General and Children's Hospital and of Teachers College, and a former educational director of the Illinois Training School for Nurses, taught hospital economics. Several teachers from different studios and art schools offered instruction in a variety of crafts. An orthopedic surgeon, James K. Young, lectured on patients with disabilities. Beulah M. Johnson, a graduate of the Maryland State Normal School and the Sheppard-Pratt Hospital's Occupational Therapy School, where she later taught, stressed methods of teaching. Eleanor Clarke Slagle even participated during the school's first year, giving lectures on the history of occupational therapy that stressed its roots in mental hygiene and social work.[44]

## ALTRUISTIC LADY OR INDEPENDENT PROFESSIONAL?

Tracy's absence from the founding meeting in 1917 accurately pointed to the widening gap between her and many other leaders in occupational therapy. Were her focus on educating practitioners and her apparent rejection of theory based on a set of values particularly associated with women? The answer is yes and no.

In the context of American ambivalence toward women who stepped out of traditional domestic roles into public professional work, Tracy cautiously balanced the images of altruistic lady and independent professional. She exercised a form of altruism as she worked in nursing for the sake of her patients, and she played the expected role of dutiful woman as she practiced under the authority of others in private-duty nursing and at the Adams Nervine Asylum. In establishing her own institution, however, she gained a sense of autonomy that she had never before experienced. Tracy was ambivalent about independence, though. She located the Experiment Station in her own home in Jamaica Plain, shielding herself against possible criticism for leaving her traditional place as a woman in early-twentieth-century America.

Tracy was uncomfortable making public arguments on behalf of the profession of occupational therapy in the founding years. Her public writings leave no record of participation in the controversial theoretical discussions that male supporters of occupational therapy conducted, nor did she show enthusiasm for the turn toward efficiency that her male colleagues took. Whether she believed as they did or not, she was not willing to go public with her opinions.

She did believe, however, that occupational therapy deserved an independent place in the evolving medical hierarchy. Her attitude about occupational therapy is more comprehensible when compared with her opinion of the contemporary movement for women's suffrage. She believed in the struggle for suffrage, but thought it should be nonmilitant.[45] In other words, women deserved independence, but should not go into the streets to attain it.

Thus Tracy cast a deliberately female model for building the profession, one bound by contemporary gender-appropriate behaviors. Women did not need to focus energy on the national association, for which public arguments had to be fashioned.

Instead, they should build local institutions for teaching and practice, such as the one she founded in Jamaica Plain. Another example of Tracy's institution building was her helping to establish the occupational therapy department at Rush-Presbyterian Hospital of the City of Chicago in 1917. Financially supported by the women's auxiliary board of the hospital with members representing all of Chicago's Presbyterian churches, Tracy and the women with whom she worked drew on nineteenth-century traditions of women's volunteer and charity work. The department, a woman's space within the male medical hierarchy of the hospital, independently covered its own expenses and the salaries of the occupational therapists.[46] Hundreds of departments of occupational therapy backed by charity networks would be established during the next few years with the coming of World War I, resulting in the fledgling profession's having independent institutions in which to work.

Tracy was far from a passive woman. As she trained newcomers to the field, widened the settings in which occupational therapy was practiced, exposed a variety of patients to the new therapy, and encouraged the building of independent institutions, she significantly shaped the new profession's identity and place in early-twentieth-century America.

Not far from Tracy's Experiment Station in Jamaica Plain practiced another important figure in the early history of occupational therapy, Herbert J. Hall. Tracy had mixed feelings about Hall, privately complaining that he had made disparaging remarks about occupations and nursing in his book with Mertice M. C. Buck, *The Work of Our Hands* (1915).[47] Eleanor Clarke Slagle said that "Miss Tracy" saw Hall's words as a "direct slam at her work."[48] George E. Barton, first president of the National Society for the Promotion of Occupational Therapy, also criticized Hall. He feared that Hall projected too elitist an image for occupational therapy, claiming that the Devereux Mansion in exclusive Marblehead, Massachusetts, provided "little effort but amusement for neurasthenics—the richer the better."[49]

Much of the criticism of Hall was undeserved; he shared many ambitions for the new profession of occupational therapy. He may indeed have adopted "a very different standpoint from that of Miss Tracy" and William R. Dunton, as Dunton believed; but Hall, like Tracy, helped take occupational therapy from mental hospitals to other medical settings, and he shared with Dunton a multidisciplinary approach to the care of patients.[50] The next chapter discusses his contributions.

## NOTES

1. "Educational Museum: Special Exhibit of Occupations for Invalids" (May 16–June 10, 1910), pamphlet, History of Nursing Collection, microfiche 2374, Milbank Memorial Library, Teachers College, Columbia University, New York (hereafter History of Nursing Collection). Papers were presented by James E. Russell, dean of Teachers College; Susan E. Tracy, superintendent of nursing at the Adams Nervine Asylum; Mary Lawson Neff, of the Long Island State Hospital; Herbert J. Hall, director of the Devereux Workshops in Marblehead, Massachusetts; Livingston Farrand, of the National Tuberculosis Association; and Arthur Dow, professor at Teachers College. Later the papers were published in *Proceedings of the American Society of Superintendents of Training Schools for Nurses* (ASSTSN: 1910), 172–206.

2. Biographical material on Tracy can be found in Mary Barrows, "Susan E. Tracy, R.N.," *Maryland Psychiatric Quarterly* 6, no. 3 (Susan E. Tracy Number, 1917): 53–62; Sidney Licht, "The Founding and Founders of the American Occupational Therapy Association," *American Journal of Occupational Therapy* 21 (1967): 269–77; and Kathlyn L. Reed and Sharon R. Sanderson, *Concepts of Occupational Therapy* (Boston: Williams and Wilkins Company, 1983), 196–97.

3. Susan E. Tracy, *Studies in Invalid Occupation* (Boston: Whitcomb and Barrows, 1910).

4. See Licht, "The Founding," 275; and *Maryland Psychiatric Quarterly* 6, no. 3 (Susan E. Tracy Number, 1917), 51–67 passim.

5. Descriptions of the founding of the first national organization of occupational therapy can be found in Robert K. Bing, "William Rush Dunton, Junior—American Psychiatrist: A Study in Self" (Ed.D. diss., University of Maryland, 1961), 149–58; and Gerald N. Grob, *Mental Illness and American Society, 1875–1940* (Princeton, N.J.: Princeton University Press, 1983), 258–60.

6. In this book I define a profession as a vocation requiring specialized knowledge in some area of learning or science. To achieve status in the professional community, members must be trained in the science and the techniques needed for practice. Professional knowledge is exclusive, in order to eliminate the possibility of outsiders infringing on professional rights. Typically, training and membership in professional organizations instill a professional conscience and a group solidarity. This definition is based on that in Burton J. Bledstein, *The Culture of Professionalism: The Middle Class and the Development of Higher Education in America* (New York: W. W. Norton and Company, 1976), especially chapter 3 on the evolution of American professional mentality.

7. For an excellent discussion of women's entry into professional work and of conflicts between professional scientific ideology and women's purported subjectivity and irrationality, see Nancy F. Cott, *The Grounding of Modern Feminism* (New Haven, Conn.: Yale University Press, 1987), 215–39. An important study of women's professional work in the twentieth century is Penina Migdal Glazer and Miriam Slater, *Unequal Colleagues: The Entrance of Women into the Professions* (New Brunswick, N.J.: Rutgers University Press, 1987).

8. For information about the presidents of the National Society for the Promotion of Occupational Therapy, later called the American Occupational Therapy Association, see "Presidents of the American Occupational Therapy Association (1917–1967)," *American Journal of Occupational Therapy* 21 (1967): 290–98. For information about occupational therapy's professional journals, see Myra L. McDaniel, "Forerunners of the *American Journal of Occupational Therapy*," *American Journal of Occupational Therapy* 25 (1971): 41–52. George E. Barton served as the first president of the National Society for the Promotion of Occupational Therapy (1917), William R. Dunton as the second (1917–1919). Herbert J. Hall served as president of the National Society for the Promotion of Occupational Therapy, then the American Occupational Therapy Association, from 1920 to 1923. Subsequent male presidents of the American Occupational Therapy Assocation during this period were Thomas B. Kidner (1923–28), architect, efficiency engineer, rehabilitation expert, and president of the National Tuberculosis Association; and C. Floyd Haviland (1928–30), psychiatrist. Dunton edited the *Maryland Psychiatric Quarterly*, the association's first official organ. He then edited the *Archives of Occupational Therapy*, later called *Occupational Therapy and Rehabilitation*, from its founding in 1922 to 1946. According to Bing's biography, Dunton not only edited *Occupational Therapy and Rehabilitation* for all those years, but actually wrote many of its articles. Claiming that occupational therapists were "more concerned with doing than with thinking and writing," Dunton found himself begging speakers at state and national meetings to submit manuscripts. He would then "rewrite parts" that he considered "seriously deficient" (p. 187). Hall edited (and sometimes coedited with Elizabeth Greene Upham) a section called "Occupational Therapy and Rehabilitation" in *Modern Hospital*.

9. Daniel H. Fuller, "The Need of Instruction for Nurses in Occupations for the Sick," introduction to *Studies in Invalid Occupation*, by Susan E. Tracy (Boston: Whitcomb and Barrows, 1910), 3.

10. *Thirtieth Annual Report of the Managers of the Adams Nervine Asylum* (1907), 3, Faulkner Hospital Archives, Jamaica Plain, Massachusetts.

11. George M. Beard, *American Nervousness: Its Causes and Consequences* (1881; reprint, New York: Arno Press and the New York Times, 1972), 7–8.

12. George M. Beard, *A Practical Treatise on Nervous Exhaustion (Neurasthenia), Its Symptoms, Nature, Sequences, Treatment*, 2d ed. revised (New York: W. Wood and Company, 1880), 11–85.

13. Barbara Sicherman, "The Uses of a Diagnosis: Doctors, Patients, and Neurasthenia," in *Sickness and Health in America*, ed. Judith W. Leavitt and Ronald L. Numbers (Madison: University of Wisconsin Press, 1978), 25–39.

14. The records of the Adams Nervine Asylum are available to scholars on request at the Faulkner Hospital Archives, Jamaica Plain, Massachusetts. The quote is taken from a record dated in the 1890s.

15. Herbert J. Hall, "The Systematic Use of Work as a Remedy in Neurasthenia and Allied Conditions," *Boston Medical and Surgical Journal* 152 (1905): 29; Hall, "Work Cure—A Report of Five Years' Experience at an Institution Devoted to the Therapeutic Application of Manual Work," *Journal of the American Medical Association* 54 (1910): 12.

16. Adolph Meyer, "The Philosophy of Occupation Therapy," *Archives of Occupational Therapy* 1 (1922): 1–10. For a discussion of Meyer's career and his influence on American psychiatry, see Grob, *Mental Illness*, 112–18.

17. Hall, "The Systematic Use of Work," 29–30.

18. Ibid.

19. Fuller, introduction to *Studies*, by Tracy, 1.

20. *Thirtieth Annual Report of the Adams Nervine Asylum*, 11.

21. Fuller, introduction to *Studies*, by Tracy, 4–5.

22. Sarah E. Parsons, "Miss Tracy's Work in General Hospitals," *Maryland Psychiatric Quarterly* 6, no. 3 (Susan E. Tracy Number, 1917): 63.

23. Barrows, "Susan E. Tracy, R.N.," 53.

24. Fuller, introduction to *Studies*, by Tracy, 4–5.

25. Tracy, *Studies*, 16.

26. Course descriptions, mss., ca. 1911, History of Nursing Collection, microfiche 2374.

27. For an interesting discussion of private-duty nursing and its problems, see Susan M. Reverby, *Ordered to Care: The Dilemma of American Nursing, 1850–1945* (Cambridge: Cambridge University Press, 1987), 95–105.

28. William R. Dunton, "Editorial," *Maryland Psychiatric Quarterly* 6, no. 3 (Susan E. Tracy Number, 1917): 52.

29. Reba G. Cameron, "An Interview with Miss Susan Tracy," *Maryland Psychiatric Quarterly* 6, no. 3 (Susan E. Tracy Number, 1917): 65.

30. Reverby, *Ordered to Care*, 121–42.

31. Jane Addams, *Twenty Years at Hull House* (1910; reprint, New York: New American Library, 1960), 60–71.

32. Lillian Wald, *The House on Henry Street* (New York: Henry Holt and Company, 1915), 1–25.

33. "Founder of Occupational Therapy Work in Illinois," *Welfare Bulletin* (Official Publication of the Illinois State Department of Public Welfare) (June 1930), 2.

34. Barrows, "Susan E. Tracy, R.N.," 53–62.

35. Herbert J. Hall, *O.T.: A New Profession* (Concord, N.H.: Rumford Press, 1923), 11–13.

36. Fuller, introduction to *Studies*, by Tracy, 7.

37. Barrows, "Susan E. Tracy, R.N.," 59–61.

38. Susan E. Tracy, "The Training of the Nurse as Instructor in Invalid Occupations," in *Proceedings of the American Society of Superintendents of Training Schools for Nurses*, 181–82.

39. Susan E. Tracy, "Report of Classes in Invalid Occupation," n.d., History of Nursing Collection, microfiche 2374.

40. Licht, "The Founding," 275.

41. For example, "Report of Committee on Teaching Methods," in *Proceedings of the First Annual Meeting of the National Society for the Promotion of Occupational Therapy* (Towson, Md.: NSPOT, 1917), 34; Susan E. Tracy, "The Influence of Hospital Architecture on Methods of Occupational Teaching," *Proceedings of the First Annual Meeting of NSPOT*, 42–44; "Report of the Committee on Methods," *Proceedings of the Second Annual Meeting of the National Society for the Promotion of Occupational Therapy* (Towson, Md.: NSPOT, 1918), 20–25.

42. Susan C. Johnson, "The Teacher in Occupational Therapy," in *Proceedings of the First Annual Meeting of NSPOT*, 50.

43. William R. Dunton, "The Principles of Occupational Therapy," in *Proceedings of the Second Annual Meeting of NSPOT*, 27, 26–30.

44. "Prospectus of Second Course of the Philadelphia School of Occupational Therapy, 1918–1919," p. 12, Official Archives of the American Occupational Therapy Association, Wilma L. West Library, American Occupational Therapy Foundation, Bethesda, Maryland (hereafter AOTA Archives).

45. Cameron, "An Interview," 66.

46. *Thirty-fifth Annual Report of the Presbyterian Hospital of the City of Chicago with the 34th Annual Report of the Women's Auxiliary Board and the 15th Annual Report of the School for Nurses* (1917), 31, Medical Archives, Rush-Presbyterian–St. Luke's Medical Center, Chicago.

47. Herbert J. Hall and Mertice M. C. Buck, *The Work of Our Hands: A Study of Occupations for Invalids* (New York: Moffat, Yard and Company, 1915).

48. Letter, Eleanor Clarke Slagle to William R. Dunton, 12 November 1915, AOTA Archives.

49. Letter, George E. Barton to Dunton, 9 December 1915, AOTA Archives.

50. Letter, Dunton to Slagle, 17 November 1915, AOTA Archives. Dunton also wrote that Hall thought "parlor philanthropists" would appreciate occupational therapy more than those who were "actively engaged in helping others."

# Chapter 4

## A Patient *at* Work *is a* Patient Half Cured

Herbert James Hall, the Arts and Crafts Movement, and Early Occupational Therapy Theory

*A Patient
at Work
is a Patient
Half Cured*

In an article published in the *Boston Medical and Surgical Journal* in 1905, Herbert James Hall told his readers about the work-cure treatments for nervous patients that he directed in the nontraditional institution he called "the workshops" in Marblehead, Massachusetts. His patients, he said, were "clever and adaptable people, with a good deal of artistic taste, . . . critical ability, . . . and [an] inborn love of making things." He called his institution a "school of handcrafts," where patients became "artisans," tasting "the wholesomeness of a life of labor without the hardships and trials [of] the real industrial world." Hall hoped that the "treatment of work" at his institution would not only "side-track" patients from "vicious trains of thought, but rehabilitate them by introducing better "habits of living" that would lead to a "saner, more rational" way of life.[1]

Although he meant his message for a medical audience, Hall's holistic approach of engaging patients in arts and crafts activities would have been well received by a much broader segment of American society in the early twentieth century. Hall was using the rhetoric of the popular arts and crafts movement, which was made up of people who advocated returning to the idealized life of the craftsperson. Reacting to broad social and economic transformations in the early twentieth century, arts and crafts proponents rejected the growing dominance of machine production because they believed that such a process removed individuals from nature, alienated workers from products, and created poor-quality items. Simple hand production, they believed, was superior and, by extension, healthier because workers were physically more connected to their work and mentally more satisfied by it.[2]

Hall's work with so-called invalids was offering the American public a response to the widely held perception that chronic illness was on the rise. Middle-class persons with neurasthenia, workers made dependent by industrial accidents, and persons with tuberculosis were often cited as typical victims of industrial and urban life. Hall certainly expressed anxiety over the health-threatening effects of modern living. "A war goes on year after year between the machine and the man, between disease and the man," he and colleague Mertice M. C. Buck wrote, "keep[ing] our ambulances busy and tax[ing] our charities in no uncertain way." Being a physician with a social conscience, a strong work ethic, and a practical vision, Hall reacted to these social ills by adapting the arts and crafts movement to medical purposes. He advocated medically supervised training of invalids in crafts, to the point that they regained their health *and* their economic independence.[3]

Moreover, Hall's founding of the workshops in Marblehead fit historically with trends that had been growing in the psychiatric world since at least 1900. Psychiatrists and the public alike agreed that hospitalization was only one of several means by which persons could achieve and maintain mental health. Historian Gerald N. Grob has shown that during the first two decades of the twentieth century, proponents of the mental hygiene movement and members of several new professions such as occupational therapy, psychiatric social work, and clinical psychology worked together to safeguard mental health.[4] Hall simply harmonized with this coalition.

This chapter describes how the development of occupational therapy was connected to the expanding world of psychiatry and several social movements of the early twentieth century. It chronicles the work of Herbert J. Hall (see photograph 6) who, like Susan E. Tracy, helped popularize occupational therapy as well as promote its use in settings outside traditional mental hospitals. An analysis of his work and ideas, moreover, illustrates the multidisciplinary approach that has been a strong tradition in the profession of occupational therapy since the founding years. Hall's workshops in Marblehead, for example, were the result of a cross-pollination with other fields and disciplines. In the workshops he collaborated with craftswoman Jessie Luther, who had been at Hull House, and orthopedic surgeon Joel E. Goldthwait, his brother-in-law. In Marblehead, Hall tried to relieve patients of physical or psychological ailments and also to rehabilitate them to useful and meaningful lives, combining aims from medicine, psychiatry, the arts, and

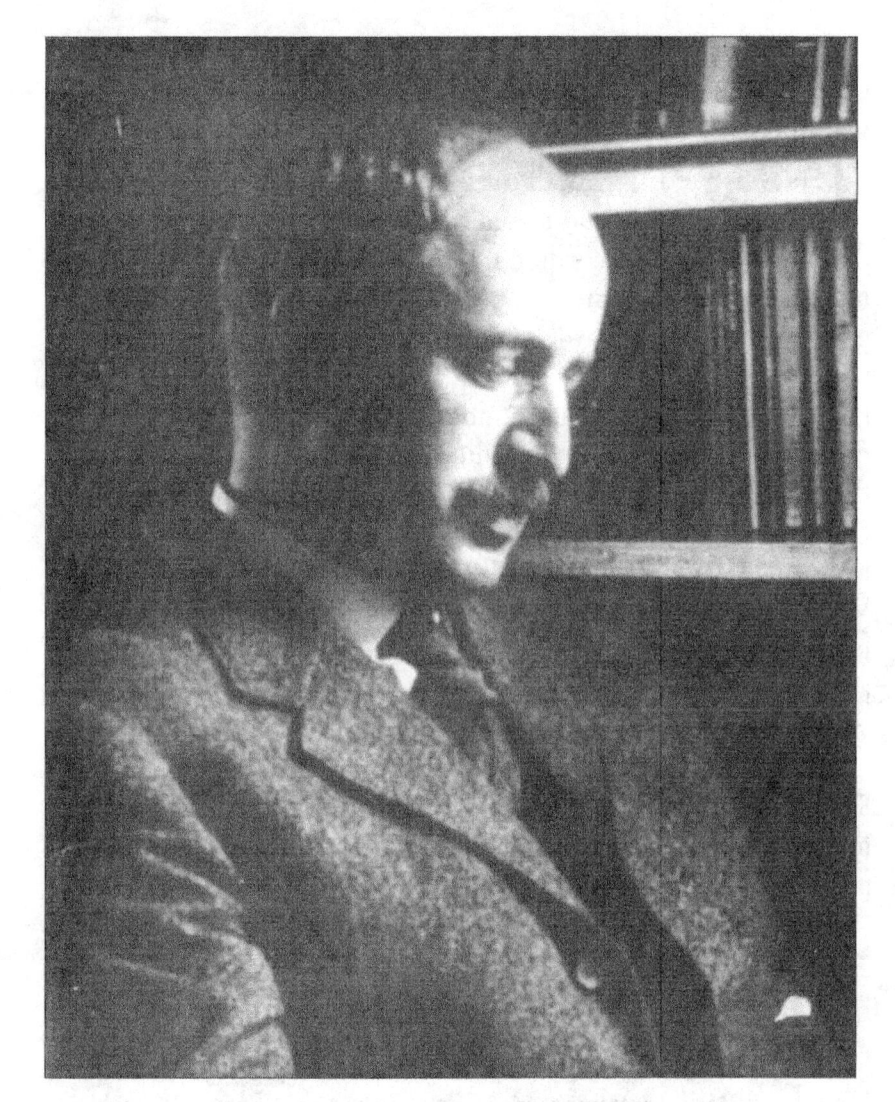

*A Patient at Work is a Patient Half Cured*

**Photograph 6:** Portrait of Herbert J. Hall. (AOTA Archives)

social work. Hall's work provided possible solutions to serious social problems; it did not reside within a medical vacuum.

Hall was of the same generation of American physicians as his colleague William Rush Dunton, Jr. He was born on March 12, 1870, in Manchester, New Hampshire, the son of Marshall Parker Hall and Susan Maria (James) Hall. He had one brother, Newton, who became a minister. Hall attended public schools and in 1895 graduated from Harvard University Medical School. He served internships at Children's Hospital and Massachusetts General Hospital, both in Boston. Although Hall worked largely with patients who had neurasthenia, he, like Dunton, had received no special training in psychiatry. From 1896 to 1912 he had a busy general practice in Marblehead. According to an obituary written after his death in

1923, during his years of private practice, Hall became interested in patients who were "handicapped in one way or another with the struggle of life."[5]

Hall married Elizabeth Pitman Goldthwait, who came from a wealthy and well-connected family that encouraged him to develop his career according to his interests. Hall especially had much in common with his brother-in-law Joel, who had also graduated from Harvard Medical School and was also affiliated with Boston's finest hospitals. As well as having similar academic and institutional backgrounds, Hall and Goldthwait agreed on a holistic approach to medicine, and this compatibility led them to collaborate often. They treated patients together at the Devereux Mansion, a sanatorium housed in a building that had been in the Goldthwait family for generations. During World War I, the physician brothers-in-law applied what they had learned at Devereux Mansion in the treatment of soldiers. They also advised United States government officials on wartime standards for occupational therapists. In 1918 they were instrumental in organizing the Boston School of Occupational Therapy, which had its modest beginnings in Goldthwait's home, where his wife Jessie called together volunteers to prepare for hospital war work.[6]

## THE DEVEREUX WORKSHOPS

Hall was not yet collaborating with his brother-in-law when he initiated his work-cure experiments with "invalids" in 1904. He joined with craftswoman Jessie Luther to open an "institution devoted to the therapeutic application of manual work," which they called the Devereux Workshops. Their ambition was to prove that "suitable occupation of hand and mind" would help maintain the "physical, mental, and moral health in the individual and in the community." Hall was certain that the only way to learn about the correct application of work therapy was to experiment in a setting explicitly devoted to it. He compared his experimental work with that of colleagues who investigated the "fullest usefulness" of drugs or other agents while working in the laboratory or the hospital.[7]

With the aid of a $1,000 grant from Harvard's Proctor Fund, Hall began his study of the use of work as a remedial measure in the manner that a good physician of his generation would. His institution was the laboratory; his patients were the subjects. Hall classified his cases so that he could later tabulate the results of treatment into the categories "improved," "much improved," and "no relief." Although he initially took a few "insanity" cases, his primary goal was to work with patients who had what he called "functional nervous diseases," or illnesses that could not be proven to have a gross pathological basis. Of the first 100 patients with whom Hall worked, 5 were diagnosed as "insane," 32 as mild or severe "neurasthenics," 18 as "hysterics," 17 as "neurotics," 8 as "psychotic or fixed idea," and 20 as "unclassified."[8]

Yet the institution was not a typical medical sanatorium; there was a great emphasis on exposing patients to training in the arts and crafts. Hall accurately called the sanatorium "primarily a practical industrial plant" where patients became "apprentices and pupils." The workshops consisted of a pottery, a blacksmith shop, a carpenter shop, and a weaving room. The products of the pottery were of high artistic value, largely because Arthur Eugene Baggs, a graduate of Alfred University, ran it. Baggs was a student of well-known British émigré and arts and crafts movement leader Charles Fergus Binns, the so-called father of American ceramics. So great was the emphasis on the arts and crafts that few other provisions were made for patients. Even food and lodging had to be obtained in a local hotel.[9]

Financially Hall's first institution was a shoestring operation. Beyond the original grant money, Hall depended on the gifts of charitable friends, small payments from patients, and the generosity of a staff that asked for little or no remuneration. By 1910, after five years of struggle, Hall claimed that the workshops were "nearly self-supporting" from the sale of the patients' products. Yet he was unsatisfied with the fact that the institution was run under what he called "somewhat unfavorable conditions." He believed that the lack of nursing care and living arrangements limited the institution's usefulness, making it suitable only for patients who could be categorized more accurately as "well people" than as "invalids." Hall aspired to create a more comprehensive institution, and he eventually did, with the generosity of the Goldthwaits.[10]

In spite of the original workshops' limitations, they may be credited with several accomplishments. First, Hall's strong position on the importance of work as a therapeutic tool helped eliminate the work cure's theoretical opposite, the faddish rest cure. Second, Hall set up efficient routines that divided each day into "changeable periods of work, rest and recreation, plenty of air, [and] wholesome food."[11] For work periods he chose not to use laundry, kitchen, or garden labor, typical options in old-fashioned moral therapy regimens.[12] Instead, Hall selected "artistic crafts" because they had "universal appeal" as well as "essential dignity." He probably also realized that such work would be more acceptable to his well-to-do patients and their families, who may have shared his interest in the arts and crafts movement.[13]

For Hall, crafts were the most suitable type of work in designing individualized therapy for patients. They made it possible to combine "mild mental effort with simple physical processes."[14] The "light manual occupations" that crafts provided helped "rouse interest" and "develop initiative" in patients who were permanently disabled or convalescing from illness or injury. Introduced early enough in individual cases, Hall wrote, crafts would prevent depression or discouragement, which so often interfered with patients' returning to the "work-a-day world." The simple skills that patients built while undergoing occupational therapy, such as concentrating, or sustaining activity, prepared them for the larger, more serious efforts that they would have to make to regain health and independence.[15]

Third, Hall's experiments in the original workshops provided a basis for several principles that were vital to early philosophy and theory in occupational therapy. At first, Hall built on the habit formation theories of contemporary psychiatrists Adolph Meyer and William R. Dunton. Patients with "functional nervous diseases," he wrote, were the victims of misguided habits, and the "right kind of work, properly carried on," would be a valuable remedy.[16] Patients with neurasthenia, in his opinion, no matter what the cause of their "original deviation from the norm," suffered because the "daily life of the individual ha[d] adjusted itself to the illness, . . . thereby forming a consistent but vicious cycle which [was] strengthened . . . by self-concern and fear." Hall noticed that many such patients suffered from fatigue and self-absorption. The work cure promised to "break into this ring [of symptoms] by instituting gradually . . . a new and absorbing interest" that would substitute for the old interests and habits, including the lack of productivity associated with the illness.[17] The work cure, Hall went on to say, "in a surprising number of cases" was the "*only* remedy needed to bring about satisfactory improvement [emphasis in original]."[18]

Hall further theorized that the occupations had to be "graded" to avoid exacerbating patients' fatigue and frustration. That is, patients should begin with tasks that were simple, physically and mentally undemanding, yet consistent, and graduate to more complex, strenuous ones. For example, a patient learned to cut a piece of wood repeatedly while gripping the saw in a moderate way instead of with great force. The idea was to have the patient "economize strength" while focusing on the simple task at hand. Hall argued that such a "mechanical education . . . cued . . . [the] mental processes" in such a manner that the patient "[found] himself thinking as well as acting in a simpler, more methodical way."[19]

From the time of his graduation from Harvard until the completion of these early experiments in the Marblehead workshops, Hall can easily be linked to a group of other psychiatrists such as William R. Dunton at the Sheppard-Pratt Hospital and Daniel H. Fuller at the Adams Nervine Asylum who were collectively attempting to bring psychiatry into step with the scientific changes occurring in medicine. Yet when Hall opened his new institution in 1912, he entered an awkward phase of his career during which he was temporarily estranged from his peers. Giving up his private practice, he devoted all his time to patients who entered the fashionably attractive Devereux Mansion, also in Marblehead, "in the midst of a beautiful park, with its face to the sea." The sanatorium consisted of a large white mansion and workshop buildings for weaving, pottery, and cement working. In Hall's words, it was "primarily a resort for people who need rest and medical treatment, combined with carefully prescribed manual work as a cure for nervous exhaustion and other disabilities." Hall openly admitted that the sanatorium was meant to serve "people of means who were broken down nervously or physically." Apparently he was not worried about how others might react to his claiming to own and run an elitist institution.[20]

In 1915, Hall published *The Work of Our Hands* with Mertice M. C. Buck, a teacher-craftswoman who had worked extensively with "handicapped" patients in charitable institutions in New York City. Hall wrote several chapters for the book; a very brief one titled "The Well-to-do Patient at Work" probably helped earn him the reputation of indulging the rich.[21] Devereux Mansion primarily catered to "nervously ill" female patients, whom Hall described as people whose lives lacked "dignity and purpose."[22] "The rush of social engagements, the stimulation of travel, and the search for amusement," Hall remarked, only satisfied his patients temporarily, leaving them to "go to pieces nervously . . . because there [was] no depth and substance to their lives." Although he agreed that "we would not always wish to make weavers or potters out of the daughters of society," he also believed that once "down to honest work with [their] hands," his patients would "make discoveries" and "find [their] way along new pathways."[23]

Hall also treated the "tired business man," who could find no true relaxation in trekking around Europe. "For real rest his mind must get down to primitive life," Hall advised. He described a patient who had tried the work cure using blacksmithing. The patient claimed to be totally "refreshed" because he had learned that whenever he allowed himself to think too much about his problems, he burned his fingers. Blacksmithing forced him to concentrate totally on hot iron and dismiss other thoughts.[24]

Hall described another male patient in *The Untroubled Mind*, also published in 1915. After carefully ruling out any organic causes for the patient's symptoms of sleeplessness, worry, indigestion, confusion, and headache, Hall concluded that the young man was suffering from "too much thinking." Hall took the patient to work with the blacksmith and prescribed that he be taught to make "hand-wrought nails," a relatively simple task. The patient was somewhat skeptical, but Hall convinced him that all he had to do was to "stop thinking" and go to work with his hands, which would "lead him to health." The patient acquiesced, and in time made many nails, and sets of pokers, shovels, and andirons for fireplaces. Hall reported that the patient had learned not only to handle the iron patiently and consistently without consciously thinking about it, but also to control himself. Eventually he returned to work in business in the city.[25]

Hall led a seemingly leisured life-style caring for the rich, but his visions for occupational therapy were not solely confined to that group. Increasingly he linked what he was learning about work and illness to people from other socioeconomic backgrounds. With a utilitarian outlook Hall devoted several chapters in *The Work of Our Hands* to the growing problem of caring for patients with chronic illness. He discussed and praised the innovative sheltered workshop at the Massachusetts General Hospital, finding that part-time work for persons with paralysis, rheumatoid arthritis, or injuries served both economic and social needs.[26] He spoke highly of the Burke Foundation's establishment of a special workshop for convalescing cardiac patients in Sharon, Connecticut, and in New York City, where men regained their health and earned livings as well.[27]

Aside from discussing several other such programs, Hall reviewed Massachusetts's workmen's compensation laws, which required manufacturers to pay workers through liability companies during periods of disability. Hall suggested that hospital workshops could reduce liability payments by providing injured workers with medically supervised work that would both treat the injuries and provide livelihoods. According to Hall, injured employees would benefit morally and financially because they would have the opportunity to learn a new trade in a "low pressure" industry, which would "save them from financial dependence."[28]

## "O.T. Equivalents, Immunities, and Substitutions"

After several years of practice in the workshops and at the Devereux Mansion, Hall elaborated on his earlier theoretical observations. He moved from focusing on habits, grading, and economizing strength to developing concepts called "O.T. equivalents, immunities, and substitutions." Hall explained these concepts in *O.T.: A New Profession*, written during the final years of his life.[29]

With the principle of equivalents, Hall tried to justify the use of occupational therapy, explaining that it was not merely "diversional" but integral to the full recovery of patients. If a patient was unable to be productive in his usual trade, Hall argued, occupational therapy encouraged the patient to make an "effort equal to that which would later be needed in his life outside the hospital." For example, the patient might learn concentration, which could later be applied in another setting. Hall went on to say that new forms of work, such as toy making or weaving, expedited the process because associations of failure and trouble were absent.[30]

According to Hall, patients typically began treatment with great difficulties in concentration: they were "often unable to read or to carry the thread of a simple story." After a period of medical treatment and rest, Hall would suggest a "simple problem in basketry" requiring patients to coordinate movements, think, and put thoughts into action. Patients succeeded because the work was "novel" and short-term. After careful "measured periods of work" and a gradual extension of time devoted to the craft work, patients would realize that they had regained their ability to concentrate, and would be able to transfer that skill to other tasks. Patients themselves, Hall argued, would then see the principle of equivalents "fully exemplified."[31]

The second principle, immunities, involved building patients' tolerance to irritations and disturbances, such as noise. Most nervous patients coming to the sanatorium, according to Hall, were intolerant of noise, which of course was a major characteristic of the workshop. Hall noticed that when patients were engaged in work, they were able to ignore not only the noise they made, but that created by other patients. "Gradually," Hall explained, "as O.T. progresses, the patient becomes immunized to noise, . . . and we may be sure that other tolerances . . . have been acquired . . . This," he said, "is the principle of immunity."[32]

Hall described a visit to a workshop during which he saw both the principle of equivalents and the principle of immunities clearly demonstrated. The patients were neuropsychiatric war veterans who were working in a highly noisy environment. Several jig saws, metal files, and a gasoline engine were running simultaneously while "a kind lady was singing with piano accompaniment." In the midst of this cacophony, ten "mental cases" were working "serenely" while paying "close attention" to their respective tasks.[33]

A third important principle that Hall identified was substitutions. "In O.T.," Hall wrote, "we substitute successful achievement in a small way for failure in a large way." He gave the example of a patient who had been unproductive for years and had internalized deep feelings of failure. Then, he said, the patient learned to make "a basket or a flower pot, a toy or a piece of homespun" with great skill, and felt "cheered and encouraged" by a sense of accomplishment. Finally, "a stranger, who [had] no personal interest in the patient" bought the product, reinforcing the patient's sense of accomplishment and success. Hall called the process of production, sense of accomplishment, and reinforcement "suggestion" and considered it the key to curing patients. In place of "hopelessness" patients experienced the "development of a will to do." No longer was there the "old sense of inadequacy"; "a new interest, a new belief in self" was substituted for it.[34]

Although Hall was able to identify and describe these principles of occupational therapy, he could not scientifically explain why they worked. When compared with the objective research that contemporary colleagues performed in other fields of medical science, Hall's observations probably appeared very subjective. Yet Hall made no apology for his approach. He even remarked that it did "little good to argue and explain the principles involved in these transactions [because] the demonstration is plain enough." The fact that his approach worked, in other words, was enough to make occupational therapy a worthwhile treatment to be offered alongside "the usual and necessary medical and surgical procedures."[35]

## The Influence of Emmanuelism

Hall never found an overarching theory that explained patients' improvement; probably this kind of work belonged in the domain of the new science of psychology, which had its roots in philosophy. Although Hall himself had not received any formal training in psychology, he seemed to have been influenced by persons who had. In *The Work of Our Hands*, Hall and Buck acknowledged Elwood Worcester, who promoted Emmanuelism, a popular self-help movement incorporating newly developed psychological methods.[36] Well-known in the first decades of the twentieth century, Emmanuelism posed a challenge to the medical model of disease and to physicians struggling to establish themselves as experts in medical science. It was founded in 1905 by Worcester, an Episcopal minister and the rector of Boston's Emmanuel Church.[37] The movement was closely followed by the lay population, judging by the vast coverage that it received in the newspapers and in women's magazines.[38]

Followers of Emmanuelism took both a scientific and a spiritual approach to somatic and psychological illnesses, among them, tuberculosis, nervous disorders, and alcoholism. Patients seeking help attended "classes" at the church, in which they learned about their disease from scientific and spiritual points of view. Ideally they learned how to take care of themselves. Emmanuelism, in other words, was based on an assumption that a partnership would develop between the minister, the physician, and the patient, which would result in a return to good health. It was, in short, a self-help movement.[39]

Worcester, the movement's leader, became interested in health issues while preparing for the ministry. Born in Massillon, Ohio, in 1863, he studied at Columbia University and the General Theological Seminary in New York. He then earned a doctorate in psychology at Leipzig. There he was the student of Wilhelm Wundt, the so-called father of experimental psychology. Wundt's most important work was on the "psychological laws of attention"; thus Worcester was exposed to the German work on habit training.[40]

Worcester also worked with Gustav Fechner, whose ideas so impressed the young student that he wrote a book, *The Living Word*, in which he explained his mentor's work.[41] Later he declared that he could barely separate Fechner's thinking from his own. Fechner's main interest was to develop a science that he called *Geistwissenschaft*, which considered both the material and the spiritual world. Worcester expanded on this idea, formulating a holistic conception of the individual. To Worcester, a person was a unified body, mind, and spirit that were interdependent and inseparable. Curing the diseased individual, then, required several approaches that addressed all aspects of the person.[42]

On his return from Germany, Worcester spent six years (1890–96) teaching psychology at Lehigh University. He was then ordained and became rector of St. Stephen's Church in Philadelphia, where he again became interested in developing a relationship between religion and medicine. One of his parishioners was S. Weir Mitchell, the neurologist who had popularized the rest cure.[43] According to historian Barbara Sicherman, Mitchell "appreciated the moral aspects of the rest cure." He ordered patients to be isolated from the stresses of work and family life and taught them to rely on their physicians. He saw such reliance as key to recovery.[44]

Mitchell and Worcester were friends; they took frequent walks together, sharing thoughts about establishing "a work on the basis of sound religion and sound science." They never accomplished this, for at least two reasons. First, by the turn of the twentieth century, habit training had gained more credence among physicians and psychiatrists treating mental illness, and the rest cure had lost its prominence as a useful therapy. Second, Worcester left Philadelphia in 1904 because he was offered the rectorship of Boston's Back Bay Emmanuel Church.[45]

Worcester thought that physicians were too "exclusive of the physical side of healing" and failed to appreciate its mental side.[46] In 1905 he had the opportunity to work with a physician to see how they might approach healing from both sides. Joseph H. Pratt, of Massachusetts General Hospital, came to Worcester with a plan to collaborate on an experimental program to treat indigent patients with tuberculosis from the Boston slums.

The program, which was implemented through a health class at the church, combined treatments such as nutritional and climatic therapies that promoted bodily cures, and treatments that addressed the "moral" or spiritual side. Patients were taught to monitor their own vital signs and record their observations on a "daily life chart." They were advised to eat properly and to sleep outdoors, even if that meant on a rooftop or a fire escape landing. Patients and staff met weekly to compare progress and to plan treatment together based on the patients' recorded observations. Patients and staff, in other words, established a reciprocal, cooperative relationship, and patients were expected to be responsible agents in the healing process. The patients in this church health class had a recovery rate equivalent to that of the best private sanatoriums.[47]

Worcester was soon joined by Samuel McComb, who was mainly interested in abnormal psychology. Born in Londonderry, Ireland, in 1864, McComb was a Presbyterian clergyman who had converted to Episcopalianism. After several years of serving as a pastor in England, Ireland, and New York City, and as a professor of ecclesiastical history at Queen's University in Canada, he began to think about working with patients who had psychiatric and nervous disorders.[48]

In 1906, after making an agreement with local Boston physicians, Worcester and McComb announced that they would be giving classes on Sunday nights at the church. Over 200 people showed up at the first meeting. Prominent physician and Harvard professor of neurology James J. Putnam spoke on "the power of control"; physician Richard C. Cabot talked about "the value and limitation of suggestion." The program consisted of several forms of therapy, including suggestion, explanation, education, rest cure, and work cure. In time it became notorious, for the sensationalist press began to criticize some of the procedures. Some thought that Emmanuelism was an imitation of the controversial Christian Science, an accusation that McComb denied emphatically.[49]

In 1909 an advisory medical board for the Emmanuel movement announced its support in the *Boston Medical and Surgical Journal*, underscoring the legitimacy of the movement's work in the community. Headed by several prominent Boston physicians, including Herbert J. Hall's brother-in-law, Joel E. Goldthwait, the board stated that there should be a relationship between clergy and physicians. It also approved of the class method developed by the Emmanuelists, which implicitly shared responsibility for health with patients themselves.

The board qualified its approval, however, making sure that medical authority was foremost in the patient-minister-physician relationship. For example, the board stated that patients had to be examined by their own family physicians before receiving any treatments from the Emmanuelists. It also stated that patients ought not to be referred to "specialists" without the consent of their family physicians and that patients who were not under a physician's care had "to put themselves in his care before they [could] receive instruction in the Emmanuel Church."[50]

Hall certainly shared many philosophical viewpoints with the Emmanuelists, which he expressed in *The Untroubled Mind*. In a chapter titled "Religio Medici," he described the all-too-common practice in medicine of physicians' being concerned "with the body only, and with its chemical and mechanical reactions." Although he agreed that such work was necessary, he expressed hope that physicians would not fail to address the "spiritual" side of care. "Both elements," he argued, "are necessary to our human welfare." Hall strongly believed that physicians should "see and treat the spiritual needs" of patients in order to "cure in the best sense." Physicians who saw medicine as completely separate from religion, he contended, were likely to see only "half the picture." Finally, Hall wrote, "There is much to be said for the religion of medicine, if it can be kept free from cant, if it can be simple and rational enough to be available for the whole world."[51]

Hall warned about the dangers of going too far into the religious side of healing, however. Discarding medicine for religion or philosophy, as the Christian Scientists did, courted "unnecessary suffering and even death." He scorned Christian Science faith healing because it was "unscientific" and because it made "untenable claims outside its own field."[52]

Hall called for curing and preventing disease through human agency, which he saw as part of a "divine plan." Research by "investigation and practice" was a "divine plan in action." Following the laws of nature, he reasoned, would lead to a "science of healing" that was not a "chance or irrational thing."[53]

Hall had ambivalent opinions about Freud, which distanced him from psychiatry even as they brought him closer to psychology. "Psychanalysis [*sic*]" was a new idea making "striking achievements," according to Hall. Studying the subconscious mind, helping patients recall mental experiences of the past, analyzing dreams, and clarifying "misconceptions and unfortunate impressions" that influenced patients' current lives were important aspects of practice among Freud's followers. Yet because all this took an "unbelievable amount of time and patience to accomplish," Hall said, he was not sure that the effort was worthwhile. Hall was more interested in behavior than in analysis, in helping patients deal with their current problems instead of analyzing causes. He even said, "The method does not appeal to me because I am so strongly inclined to take people as they are, to urge a forgetfulness that does not really forget, but which goes on bravely to the development of life."[54]

Like Dunton, Hall could not identify with the changes occurring in psychiatry with the onset of Freudianism. His multidisciplinary approach and his continued emphasis on arts and crafts and Emmanuelism dominated his thinking about care of patients. Continuing to assist in the development of occupational therapy, which addressed the social and economic problems created by chronic illness in a larger sense, seemed the most comfortable road for Hall to take.

As the next chapter shows, Hall and his Boston colleagues were not alone in their concern for patients with chronic illness. George Edward Barton in New York State, Philip King Brown in northern California, and Susan Cox Johnson in New York City were all experimenting with occupational therapy and chronic illness, indicating a growth of such concerns on a national level.

## Notes

1. Herbert J. Hall, "The Systematic Use of Work as a Remedy in Neurasthenia and Allied Conditions," *Boston Medical and Surgical Journal* 152 (1905): 30–32. See also Hall, "Neurasthenia: A Study of Etiology. Treatment by Occupation," *Boston Medical and Surgical Journal* 153 (1905): 47–49.

2. Eileen Boris, *Art and Labor: John Ruskin, William Morris, and the Craftsman Ideal in America, 1876–1915* (Philadelphia: Temple University Press, 1984), passim.

3. Herbert J. Hall and Mertice M. C. Buck, *The Work of Our Hands: A Study of Occupations for Invalids* (New York: Moffat, Yard and Company, 1915), vii–viii.

4. For a thorough discussion of the mental hygiene movement and the emergence of mental health professions, see Gerald N. Grob, *Mental Illness and American Society, 1875–1940* (Princeton, N.J.: Princeton University Press, 1983), 144–79, 234–66.

5. "Herbert James Hall, M.D.," obituary, *Boston Medical and Surgical Journal* 189 (1923): 326; Kathlyn L. Reed, "Herbert J. Hall, the Forgotten Founder" (Unpublished paper, Houston Academy of Medicine, Texas Medical Center Library, n.d.).

6. Joel E. Goldthwait was born in Marblehead, Massachusetts, in 1867. His family owned much of the property in the Devereux section of Marblehead. He graduated from the Massachusetts Agricultural College in 1886 and Harvard Medical School in 1890. He was a well-known authority on orthopedic surgery: in 1892 he began his work in the specialty as an assistant surgeon at Children's Hospital in Boston; in 1894 he established a clinic for the care of persons with disabilities at Carney Hospital; beginning in 1899, he headed the outpatient orthopedic service at Massachusetts General Hospital; he was a trustee of the Robert Breck Brigham Hospital for the care and the treatment of persons with disabilities; and during World War I, he was the chief of the orthopedic section of the American Expeditionary Forces. Goldthwait served on the board of directors of the Boston School of Occupational Therapy from its founding, and with Hall, he operated the Devereux Mansion from its opening in 1912 until his retirement in the late 1920s. Biographical information on him is taken from an obituary in *Marblehead Messenger*, 19 January 1961; and *Annual Report of the Boston School of Occupational Therapy*, 1920–29, Papers of the Boston School of Occupational Therapy, Wessell Library, Tufts University, Medford, Massachusetts (hereafter Papers of the Boston School of Occupational Therapy). For information on the founding of the Boston School of Occupational Therapy, see Terry Anne E. Litterst, "Boston School of Occupational Therapy, 1918–1930: The Formation of a Professional Educational Institution" (Paper presented at the Written History Seminar, Sixty-third Annual Meeting of the American Occupational Therapy Association, Portland, Ore., April 1983); Litterst, "Boston School of Occupational Therapy, 1930–1955: Transition to the University" (Paper presented at the Written History Seminar, Sixty-fourth Annual Meeting of the American Occupational Therapy Association, Kansas City, Mo., May 1984); and "Memorandum Regarding the Early History of Occupational Therapy in the United States," n.d., Papers of the Boston School of Occupational Therapy.

7. Herbert J. Hall, "Work Cure—A Report of Five Years' Experience at an Institution Devoted to the Therapeutic Application of Manual Work," *Journal of the American Medical Association* 54 (1910): 12.

8. Ibid., 13.

9. Ibid., 14; Gail Pike Hercher, "Marblehead Pottery," *Marblehead Magazine*, Fall 1980.

10. Hall, "Work Cure," 14.

11. Ibid., 13.

12. Hall cites several traditional moral therapy work programs that were then in existence in several state and county hospitals in "Manual Work for Patients in State and County Hospitals," in *The Work of Our Hands*, by Hall and Buck, 12–32. For a discussion of the history of moral therapy programs and the ways in which modern occupational therapy differed from them, see Hall, "What Is Occupation Therapy?" (Paper written for the General Federation of Women's Clubs, Biennial Meeting, Chautauqua, New York, 1922, Official Archives of the American Occupational Therapy Association, Wilma L. West Library, American Occupational Therapy Foundation, Bethesda, Maryland).

13. In "What Is Occupation Therapy?" Hall tried to convince wealthy club women that involvement in the occupational therapy movement was an appropriate "new form of service" (p. 1). In "Work Cure," Hall said that he recommended crafts to all patients, regardless of their social or economic background (p. 14).

14. Herbert J. Hall, *O.T.: A New Profession* (Concord, N.H.: Rumford Press, 1923), 3.

15. Herbert J. Hall, "Graded Effort in Convalescence," *Boston Medical and Surgical Journal* 185 (1921): 625–27.

16. Hall, "Work Cure," 12.

17. Herbert J. Hall, "Manual Work as a Remedy," in *Proceedings of the American Society of Superintendents of Training Schools for Nurses* (ASSTSN, 1910): 196–99.

18. Hall, "Work Cure," 12.

19. Ibid. Hall was also echoing the rhetoric and the ideology of the early-twentieth-century efficiency movement, which is discussed in more detail in chapter 6, on World War I's vocational training programs and their relationship to occupational therapy.

20. "The Work Cure at Devereux Mansion," *Nurse* (1917). Reprint.

21. Herbert J. Hall, "The Well-to-do Patient at Work," in *The Work of Our Hands*, by Hall and Buck, 57–60.

22. "The Work Cure at Devereux Mansion" states that most of the patients were female. To my knowledge, no records of the Devereux Mansion are extant. Hall made the remark regarding female patients lacking "dignity and purpose" in "The Well-to-do Patient," 57.

23. Hall, "The Well-to-do Patient," 57.

24. Ibid., 58–59.

25. Herbert J. Hall, *The Untroubled Mind* (Boston: Houghton Mifflin, 1915).

26. Herbert J. Hall, "Workshops in General Hospitals," in *The Work of Our Hands*, by Hall and Buck, 1–4.

27. Ibid., 4–7.

28. Herbert J. Hall, "Handicapped Labor and the Law," in *The Work of Our Hands*, by Hall and Buck, 66–69.

29. Hall, *O.T.: A New Profession.*

30. Ibid., 15–16.

31. Ibid., 16–17.

32. Ibid., 18.

33. Ibid., 19.

34. Ibid., 19–20.

35. Ibid., 20–21.

36. Hall and Buck, *The Work of Our Hands*, xxvii.

37. Ralph A. Adams, "The Emmanuel Movement: An Antecedent to Occupational Therapy" (Unpublished paper, n.d.); Katherine M. McCarthy, "Early Alcoholism Treatment: The Emmanuel Movement and Richard Peabody," *Journal of Studies on Alcohol* 45 (1984): 59–74; McCarthy, "Psychotherapy and Religion: The Emmanuel Movement," *Journal of Religion and Health* 23 (1984): 92–105. For more contemporary discussions of the movement, see John Gardner Greene, *Emmanuel Movement* (Boston: 1934); and Elwood Worcester and Samuel McComb, *Body, Mind and Spirit* (Boston: Marshall Jones Company, 1931).

38. McCarthy states in "Psychotherapy and Religion" (p. 96) that Worcester received more than "5000 unsolicited requests for help in response to one of his five articles [published] in the *Ladies Home Journal* in 1908."

39. Ibid., 93.

40. Greene, *Emmanuel Movement*, 495.

41. Elwood Worcester, *The Living Word* (New York: Moffat, Yard and Company, 1908).

42. Adams, "The Emmanuel Movement," 1–2; McCarthy, "Psychotherapy and Religion," 93.

43. Greene, *Emmanuel Movement*, 495.

44. Barbara Sicherman, "The Uses of Diagnosis: Doctors, Patients, and Neurasthenia," in *Sickness and Health in America*, ed. Judith W. Leavitt and Ronald L. Numbers (Madison: University of Wisconsin Press, 1978), 25–39.

45. Greene, *Emmanuel Movement*, 496.

46. Ibid., 498.

47. Ibid., 499–500; Adams, "The Emmanuel Movement," 2–4; Joseph H. Pratt, "The Home Sanatorium Treatment of Consumption," *Boston Medical and Surgical Journal* 154 (1906): 210–16. Pratt argued in this article that although sanatorium and climatic treatments of tuberculosis worked, he wanted to find a treatment for the poor in their own homes. He and Worcester took patients from Massachusetts General Hospital's outpatient department and tried a "large amount of care to a small number of patients." Every detail of daily life was supervised; nurses visited "class members" frequently; families were coun-

seled and "disciplined" tactfully. Disease was "arrested" in five of nine patients who began the program in July 1905 (pp. 211–12).

48. Greene, *Emmanuel Movement*, 500–01.

49. *Ibid*. For medical articles skeptical of Emmanuelism, see E. W. Taylor, "The Attitude of the Medical Profession toward the Psychotherapeutic Movement," *Boston Medical and Surgical Journal* 157 (1907): 843–50; and G. C. Smith, "The Psychic Factor in Disease," *Boston Medical and Surgical Journal* 157 (1907): 205–11.

50. "An Advisory Medical Board for the Emmanuel Movement," *Boston Medical and Surgical Journal* 160 (1909): 90–91. The authors of the letter were the four physicians who made up the board: Joel E. Goldthwait, James G. Mumford, Richard C. Cabot, and Joseph H. Pratt.

51. Hall, *The Untroubled Mind*, 18–19.

52. Ibid., 88–96.

53. Ibid., 93–94.

54. Ibid., 75–77.

# Chapter 5

## Education *of* "*the* Handicapped"

Occupational Therapy and Physical Rehabilitation Before World War I

*Education of "the Handicapped"*

As medical professionals began to turn their attention to chronic physical illness in the first decades of the twentieth century, occupational therapy became an important component of care. By World War I, promoters of occupational therapy had established clinics for patients with chronic physical illness. George Edward Barton had opened Consolation House, "a school, workshop, and vocational bureau for convalescents" in upstate New York.[1] San Francisco physician Philip King Brown had founded the Arequipa Sanatorium, where working women with tuberculosis "helped to cure themselves" while they produced museum-quality pottery.[2] At Teachers College, Columbia University, Susan Cox Johnson was sending students to the clinic at the Montefiore Home and Hospital for Chronic Diseases, for "practice-teaching" assignments.[3] On the Lower East Side, Evelyn Lawrence Collins made home visits to "shut-in" patients under the auspices of the Henry Street Settlement.[4]

All these practitioners agreed that craft work healed patients because its very authenticity provided physically and emotionally healthy activity. They also concurred that occupational therapy had a utilitarian purpose: it promised to return patients with disabilities to financial independence. Impatient with mere custodial care, promoters of occupational therapy adapted efficiency-engineering techniques to measure patients' productivity. The results in turn "proved" occupational therapy's efficacy. The step toward the vocational purpose of occupational therapy paved the way for participation in programs to "reconstruct" wounded soldiers and sailors returning from the World War I front.

Practitioners had to be careful not to tread too far into the field of vocational training, however. Placing occupational therapy squarely within medicine's domain was vital to its survival as a profession. George E. Barton, for example, called practitioners "occupational therapists," not "occupation workers," as they were sometimes titled, to be sure that they maintained a medical identity. Further, he insisted that promoters never "lose a single opportunity to rub in the word 'therapeutics.'"[5]

These leaders had adopted an ideology that historian T. J. Jackson Lears has called a "therapeutic world view."[6] In a world growing more modern and secular by the moment, this early-twentieth-century antimodernist ideology helped fill the vacuum previously inhabited by nineteenth-century religious values. The antimodernist movement was largely led by middle- and upper-class Americans such as Barton, Brown, Herbert James Hall, and other promoters of occupational therapy, who were trying to recapture "authentic living" through handcrafts.

This chapter illustrates how practitioners forged a vital link between occupational therapy and physical rehabilitation in the second decade of the twentieth century. Incorporating efficiency methods, observation, and empiricism, they broadened practice to encompass patients with physical disabilities. Further, practice expanded geographically during this period, from eastern urban centers to diverse settings.

## The Authentic Self: George Edward Barton at Consolation House

Studying George Edward Barton's career in occupational therapy is like trying to follow the course of a comet: after a moment of brilliance as it races across the night sky, it suddenly burns out. George Edward Barton was an occupational therapy zealot; he had personally been "cured" of "hysterical paralysis" by "occupation." Later, with a near-crusade mentality, he called and hosted the founding meeting of the National Society for the Promotion of Occupational Therapy, and in 1917 he served as the society's first president. Yet by the next year Barton had resigned from the presidency and was distancing himself from other members of the organization.[7]

What accounts for such a rapid rise and fall? Was Barton an enigma? Did his colleagues fear that his enthusiasm would damage occupational therapy's fragile public image? Barton was an architect; did his fellow founders disapprove of his lack of medical credentials? This section examines Barton's short-lived but significant relationship to occupational therapy during the age of efficiency and time-and-motion studies.

Born in 1871 in Brookline, Massachusetts, Barton became an architect in Boston at the height of the arts and crafts movement. He also studied in London under William Morris, a leader of Britain's arts and crafts movement. On his return, Barton helped incorporate the Boston Society of Arts and Crafts. He was its first secretary, and he was also active in professional architecture organizations. Barton, like William Rush Dunton, Jr., assumed that organizing a formal association was necessary to advance a profession.[8]

Barton's initial attraction to occupational therapy resulted from his being ill himself. In 1901 he discovered that he had tuberculosis. In 1912, needing to take periodic rests, he went to a Colorado sanatorium. On recovering, he undertook several architectural projects in Colorado, including redesigning the landscapes of the city of Pueblo and rebuilding a sanatorium in Colorado Springs. He also conducted a study of famine among farmers on the Kansas border, during which his left foot was frozen. Contracting gangrene, he had to undergo a partial amputation. Following the surgery, Barton suffered a "severe break in health," becoming paralyzed on the left side. In 1913 he went to the Clifton Springs Sanatorium in upstate New York, to rest.

Barton considered himself to be "well acquainted with the technicalities of many trades," but during his illness he was incapable of completing even the simplest tasks. He sought the advice of physicians regarding possibilities for rehabilitation, but was disappointed by their lack of encouragement. Nearly all of them cautioned that returning to work was "most dangerous and questionable."[9] Barton's experience with chronic illness and what he felt to be a lack of understanding on the part of physicians only induced him to try to overcome his disabilities.

Barton found new purpose in life after the Reverend Elwood Worcester visited the Clifton Springs Sanatorium and introduced him to occupational therapy in Emmanuelist classes for the patients.[10] On his release from the sanatorium, thinking that he could never return to a career in architecture, Barton set out to "devote the rest of his life to the reclamation of the sick and crippled."[11] He purchased a nearby two-story house built in the 1840s and in a state of disrepair. In 1914, after an extensive restoration, he opened Consolation House, where he hoped to realize a healthy and meaningful life for himself and others like him. He determined to "raise the cry that it is time for humanity to cease regarding the hospital as a door closing upon a life which is past, and to regard it henceforth as a door opening upon a life which is to come." He promised that the hospital would be not only a place "in which to get well," but one "filled with the joy of hope for a better job, or a job done better."[12]

Barton oversaw the initial stages of the restoration from his wheelchair, transforming the simple farmhouse into an arts and crafts showcase. His wife later said, "Barton's idea was not to 'modernize' the house, only to make it more comfortable and livable." He hired local craftsmen to tear down chimneys and reuse the bricks to give new fireplaces "an authentic air of age." He ordered a hob-grate from England for the dining room fireplace, where later "many an afternoon was cheered by toast and tea from the kettle boiling on the hob." Pottery, wrought-iron fixtures, and handmade clocks were abundant. In the living room window he had leaded stained glass installed that depicted a medieval lady with trailing draperies and headdress, riding a horse, a falcon on her arm. He had the front parlor converted into an office by installing bookshelves and glass cases and furnishing it with a mahogany rolltop desk, a typewriter, and file cabinets. He had new fixtures installed in the upstairs bathroom and had another bathroom built on the main floor for convenience. It too had a stained glass window, which showed a full-masted sailing vessel heading into the wind.[13]

In time Barton himself restored sections of farmland, bringing buildings and equipment to working order, even though the doctors warned that the project was "an absolute absurdity" that would result in "serious relapse or death." Ignoring their predictions, he dug gardens and built sheds and poultry houses, calling the work a "reclamation of waste land."[14] Whether Barton was referring to the restoration of the farm or to his own rehabilitation, for him, going back to the land and relearning basic skills for life were not just idealistic or symbolic goals; they were very real. His focus was beyond a return to the arts and crafts; he required a return to authentic rural life.

Barton converted the old red barn into a workshop and studio. Later his widow recalled that there he "used his own body as a clinic to work out the problem of rehabilitating himself."[15] He studied the body enthusiastically, taking courses with the nurses at the Clifton Springs Sanatorium Training School,[16] reading works, and corresponding with practitioners all over the country, including William R. Dunton and Susan E. Tracy.[17] He was determined to mimic other occupational therapy promoters' methods of systematic investigation in his own studies of occupations. In a narrative on his illness, for example, he described the importance of grading occupations and paying attention to fatigue, and he wrote of his failure to improve at first because he had not adopted these crucial principles. (He had even begun to believe the physicians' predictions of sure death.) Then he tried alternating work with rest periods: 10 minutes of light work, such as woodworking or weeding, followed by 15 minutes of rest; then 10 minutes of modeling or drawing, followed by another short rest period. With such a program he slowly began to gain strength without fatigue. In less than three years he was able to do "structural carpentry and heavy gardening for two or three hours at a time without deleterious results."[18]

Barton probably had no difficulty in adapting such efficiency methods to his own treatment in convalescence. Like medicine, architecture had been influenced by the turn-of-the-century efficiency movement. In fact, Barton thought that men like himself could teach the medical world more about efficiency than it already knew. Barton believed that American physicians had grown too "confined" within their own "specialty" and knew little of the "'inside' workings of life in the shop, the store, the office, the mill, factory, or foundry." As a result, he said, patients revolted against physicians' "advice concerning their welfare, especially as applied to their work." Moreover, Barton argued, the hospital system had a fatal flaw, discharging "not efficients, but inefficients." He read the literature of efficiency engineers Frank B. and Lillian M. Gilbreth to cull information about motion studies so that the patients at his institution could avoid waste.[19]

It might be said that Barton was to the care of persons with physical disabilities as Clifford W. Beers was to the care of persons with mental illness. Both men started their quest to reform the medical system as lay patients victimized by its limitations. In several publications written between 1914 and his death in 1923, Barton pressed in particular to reform hospital care for persons with physical disabilities. Speaking from his own experience, he argued, "Few patients are sick one day and well the next."[20] Sick men, he reasoned, needed and wanted a restoration of their ability to work so that they could live independently. Hospitals should be used "not as an educational but as a reeducational institution through which to put" what he con-

*Education of "the Handicapped"*

sidered to be "the waste products of society back and into the right place."[21] With proper supervision, Barton contended, patients would be guided through their illness, and once cured, steered away from work with potential for causing a relapse. Occupational therapy, provided in hospitals or convalescent facilities, could resolve such difficult issues.[22]

Yet Barton's writing accomplishments cannot be compared with those of Beers, whose remarkable autobiography, *A Mind That Found Itself*,[23] helped galvanize activists from medicine and the general public to form the mental hygiene movement. Indeed, some of Barton's writings may have created more foes than allies to the cause. In a paper that he wrote for the professional journal *Modern Hospital* to describe the work at Consolation House, he patronizingly adapted medical language to convince readers of occupational therapy's legitimate place in medicine. He described cases in which he had made an "occupational diagnosis" after receiving the "physician's diagnosis of physical or mental condition." His first step, he wrote, was to "isolate" a "latent" patient "interest" by using "psycho-analysis." Once he had isolated it, he would "handle it in much the same way that the physician prepares a bacillus for an autogeneous vaccine." That is, he would "try to surround that interest with a mental condition which acts as a culture in which the germ can grow." He would then "inoculate . . . the patient with . . . the 'bacillus of work.'" Depending on the difficulty of the patient's condition, Barton said, one had to rely on either "superficial stimulation" or the more intense alternative of getting into "the blood or the muscle." Barton may have gone too far when he declared that sometimes "hypodermics" or "lumbar punctures" had to be used in certain difficult cases. One wonders how the readers of *Modern Hospital*, most of whom were physicians, nurses, social workers, administrators, laboratory technicians, and other medical professionals, reacted to these analogies.[24]

Barton was undoubtedly an unusual if not eccentric character, who occasionally had difficulty knowing his own identity. This peculiarity he revealed in letters exchanged with William R. Dunton between 1914 and 1917.[25] Barton initiated the correspondence in an effort to contact others interested in occupational therapy.[26] Dunton responded immediately, telling Barton about his use of occupational therapy at Sheppard-Pratt Hospital.[27] Barton then replied that he was not a physician, but could make "a slight claim to being a socialist" whose "great aim [was] to use the hospital as a re-educational institution."[28]

In a much later letter, however, he claimed to be a "sociologist" who had a "horrid vision" of what might "occur if [the term] therapeutics" was not included in the name of the new national professional organization that the two men would later found.[29]

Barton's lack of medical credentials never affected his aggressive pursuit of leadership within the movement. He zealously and unrelentingly demanded to be in the forefront. For example, he proposed the first occupational therapy conference and urged that it be held at Consolation House. When Dunton suggested holding it concurrently with the meeting of the American Medico-Psychological Association scheduled for 1914 in Baltimore, Barton rejected the idea. He wanted the organization to be founded on his terms and in his territory. "Thank you for your offer of assistance in regard to my proposed conference," he answered; "however, I have received such attractive offers from citizens of New York, that I should hardly be justified in calling it elsewhere."[30]

A similar exchange occurred about a year later when an enthusiastic Dunton tried gently but firmly to advance the scheduling of the conference. He offered to set up a meeting in Maryland between Christmas and New Year's "in order to bring the matter definitely to a head."[31] Barton took offense, saying he was surprised at Dunton's calling a conference. Dunton had given him the responsibility to "take the lead in [the] matter" of calling the group together, he claimed. In a manipulative manner he said further, "I shall send word to those individuals whose co-operation I asked to collaborate with me, at your request, to transfer their allegiance to you provided you have asked them to do so."[32] Dunton responded immediately in a conciliatory tone. "I think you must have read my letter rather hurriedly or I expressed myself badly," he wrote. "My intention was to invite you as head of this movement to extend to others the invitation provided it met with your approval," he explained. "It was with the idea of helping that it was offered."[33] Barton replied that he was "very glad indeed" to find that his impression of the November 17 letter was "not correct." He also claimed to be pleased that they did not have to begin the "conference with a division."[34]

Barton and Dunton did not correspond about organizing nationally until nearly a year after this incident, although both attended conferences and continued working in the field. In December 1916, Dunton wrote Barton about "considerable local [Baltimore-area] activity going on to organize practitioners of occupation therapy." Dunton felt strongly that a national association should be organized first so that local and state groups could follow its example.[35] During the next few months Barton and Dunton corresponded frequently. With little disagreement they settled on a March 1917 organizational meeting at Consolation House, chose the members of the founding group (see photograph 7), proposed and revised a constitution, and made several other decisions regarding the internal organization of what would soon be called the National Society for the Promotion of Occupational Therapy.[36]

During the March meeting, the papers of incorporation were signed by George Edward Barton, Eleanor Clarke Slagle, William Rush Dunton, Jr., T. B. Kidner, Susan C. Johnson, and Isabel G. Newton, Barton's secretary. The constitution was accepted, and Susan E. Tracy, not in attendance, was declared an active member. The founders elected officers and chairs of five standing committees. Barton was elected president and chair of the Committee on Research and Efficiency because he had developed connections with domestic and foreign efficiency

**Photograph 7:** NSPOT Founders. Seated, left to right: Susan Cox Johnson, George Edward Barton, Eleanor Clarke Slagle; standing, left to right: William Rush Dunton, Jr., Isabel Newton, Thomas B. Kidner. (AOTA Archives)

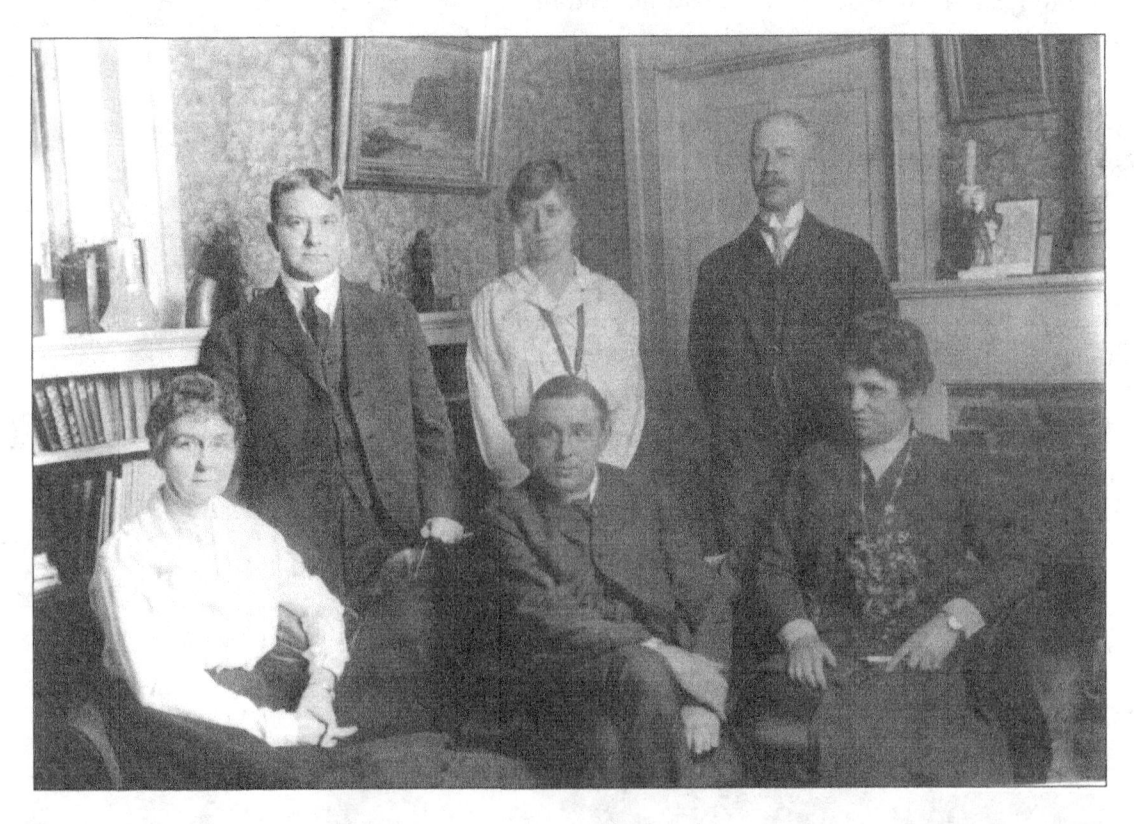

engineers who were working on the physical rehabilitation of soldiers wounded in the war. Slagle was chosen vice-president and chair of the Committee on Installations and Advice, given her experience in promoting mental hygiene, conducting research, and setting up clinics. Dunton was voted treasurer and chair of the Committee on Finance, Publicity and Publication. Johnson, then at Teachers College and very involved in establishing educational standards for practitioners and an employment placement center, was chosen to lead the Committee on Admissions and Positions. Tracy was elected to oversee the Committee on Teaching Methods. (Her election was a gesture of tribute more than anything else. Eventually Tracy realized that her primary identification as a nurse did not fit the goals of the evolving profession of occupational therapy, and she distanced herself from the association.)[37]

Barton's connections with various efficiency experts help explain Dunton's willingness to overlook Barton's sometimes irrational behavior. In Dunton's mind, Barton represented a link between occupational therapy and physical rehabilitation that was to be crucial in the advancement of the profession in the immediate years ahead. Barton had several accomplishments in the field. More than having cured his own physical disability through occupation, he had established an institution for patients, and students were even taking courses at Consolation House to prepare themselves to work with persons with physical disabilities.[38] Most important, because of Barton's personal experience with physical disability and his background in the building trades, he had had the interest and the foresight to look into the work of efficiency engineers such as Frank B. Gilbreth of the United States and Jules Amar of France, who were already dealing with thousands of war-wounded men needing rehabilitation.[39] Barton had even invited Gilbreth to attend the first meeting of the National Society for the Promotion of Occupational Therapy, but Gilbreth had declined because of war-related duties. Moreover, Barton had been asked to direct a school in Antwerp, Belgium, for persons with disabilities, and thus was presumed to be an expert in the field. Barton did not take the position, but he formulated an education plan for Belgian workers with disabilities.[40] Barton had also established connections with Thomas B. Kidner, who was educated in architecture and building construction like himself. In 1917, when Barton asked Kidner to serve as a founder of the National Society for the Promotion of Occupational Therapy,

Kidner held the important position of vocational secretary of the Canadian Military Hospitals Commission.[41]

In spite of the important contribution that Barton made to the establishment of the new profession's first national organization, by the following year he had resigned from the presidency and declined to attend the annual meeting. A recurrence of idiosyncratic behavior partly accounts for this change in commitment. Barton never directly explained his withdrawal from activity, but in correspondence with Dunton following the first meeting, he expressed annoyance that members of the group planned to have the next meeting of the National Society for the Promotion of Occupational Therapy in New York City instead of at Consolation House. Susan Cox Johnson had written to Dunton in June 1917 saying that she did not want to go back to Clifton Springs and proposing the more convenient location of the city for most members of the group. Barton disagreed with the idea of meeting in New York, arguing that the society had no money to spend for accommodations. Johnson suggested using her own apartment at Nine Livingston Place as the meeting site, promising to reduce expenses to a minimum.[42]

This did not satisfy Barton. He then protested that he did not "have the price" to come to New York City and that "the Society [had] already cost [him] a good deal of money, to be perfectly frank." Overlooking the fact that he was the one who had insisted on locating the headquarters of the National Society for the Promotion of Occupational Therapy at Consolation House, he complained about the cost of paying his secretary and of housing the founders when they came for the first meeting.[43] Facing this litany of complaints, Dunton again acquiesced to Barton, offering to pay him for any of the expenses incurred during the first meeting.[44] Whether Barton accepted or refused Dunton's offer is not recorded in the dwindling number of letters that passed between them after this point.

Such pettiness makes Barton appear to have been an egocentrist who would associate with the National Society for the Promotion of Occupational Therapy only on his own terms. This assessment may be unfair. He was a sick man, with limited strength and energy; perhaps he was actually unable to travel to New York City for meetings. He had also made some personal commitments that might have caused him to distance himself from the organization. In 1918 he had married his secretary, Isabel Newton, and shortly thereafter they had had a son, George Gladwin.[45]

Yet as he promised Dunton when he resigned from the organization, he continued to promote occupational therapy.[46] For the next two years he sent reports of the Committee on Research and Efficiency to the annual meetings. They outlined the training of occupational therapists at Consolation House and listed important new publications and contributions to the field.[47] When the war emergency ended, Barton spent his final days at Consolation House. He died in 1923 because of a "return of his old laryngeal tuberculosis," according to his wife.[48]

Barton was undoubtedly a difficult person with whom to work in the organizational phase of the national association. Nonetheless, his short-lived career with occupational therapy was significant. By drawing on his own life experience, he helped to set self-help and craft work as basic values for occupational therapy. Barton actually embodied such values as he transformed himself from a person who was sickly and disabled into a productive and independent citizen. His most important contribution was his role in promoting the use of occupational therapy with persons who were physically disabled, many of whom, like him, had tuberculosis.

Yet Barton did not possess the interpersonal skills that he needed to maintain successful professional relationships with his would-be colleagues in occupational therapy. Nor did he seem to have the ability to conduct scientific research. His work was not original, and thus he was more a student of occupational therapy than an innovator in the field. Because occupational therapy was on the defensive in having to convince the medical world of its efficacy in healing patients, Barton's emphasis on experience rather than scientific credentials proved to be a problem. He simply did not fit the profile of what his contemporaries considered to be a professional leader.

As the next section shows, Philip King Brown, like Barton, saw the value of occupational therapy in the care of patients with physical disabilities, and he too was influenced by the arts and crafts, efficiency, and Emmanuelist movements. Unlike Barton, however, Brown had outstanding medical credentials.

## Philip King Brown and the Care of Patients With Tuberculosis

In 1912, Boston physician Richard C. Cabot traveled to San Francisco to study methods of combating the dreaded disabling disease tuberculosis. While he was there, he visited the newly founded Arequipa Sanatorium, located an hour from the city, near a small town called Fairfax. In Cabot's view Philip King Brown, the director of the sanatorium, had managed to overcome a serious "character problem" that often afflicted persons with tuberculosis. The length of the illness, Cabot wrote, often caused an idleness that "pulled down" many patients. Some victims became "despondent," and others got involved in "every sort of vice and folly." At the Arequipa Sanatorium, Cabot noted, patients "conquered these evils" by working to earn money for their own support.[49]

Brown would certainly have agreed with Cabot's assessment of the Arequipa Sanatorium. Echoing the arguments made by reformers who disagreed with the rest cure therapy for patients with mental illness, he criticized tuberculosis sanatoriums that promoted "absolute rest." In such places, Brown wrote, lack of work "brings about a habit of idleness which the patients never overcome." He found a "moral advantage . . . in requiring work of the patients." For Brown, work was as important to patients as providing medical care.[50]

Born in 1869 in Napa, California, Brown had family and professional connections to the Bay area's medical elite. His mother, Charlotte Blake Brown, was one of California's first female physicians, a well-known surgeon, and a founder of San Francisco's Children's Hospital. Brown completed his A.B. at Harvard University in 1890 and graduated from Harvard Medical School in 1893. After studying for a short time in Germany, he returned to California, where he completed postgraduate work in nervous disorders at the University of California in 1894. He was an associate professor of clinical medicine at the university from 1896 to 1898, he studied veterinary medicine at the university's Institute of Animal Pathology from 1896 to 1899, and he was a consulting pathologist to several San Francisco institutions, such as Mt. Zion Hospital, California Eye and Ear Hospital, and the French Hospital. He read several papers at state and local medical society meetings, and he published articles in local, state, and national journals, on topics ranging from hemorrhagic meningo-myelitis in dogs to blood findings in bone tuberculosis cases in children.[51]

In the first decade of the twentieth century, Brown became particularly interested in reforming San Francisco's system of caring for persons with tuberculosis. He was convinced that recent conditions in San Francisco, especially those prevailing since the 1906 earthquake and fire, were causing an alarming rise in tuberculosis. He pointed to poorly built homes, irritating dust in the air, and crowded working quarters as all contributing to the problem. For Brown, such an unhygienic environment and continued employment in trades dangerous to the lungs exacerbated individual cases. Looking at the wider causes of tuberculosis, Brown declared that he could not "treat TB by medicine or by a cough mixture." Other solutions had to be found.[52]

Brown and reformer Jesse W. Lilienthal, president of the San Francisco Association for the Study and Prevention of Tuberculosis, were appalled by the inadequate care offered by the municipal authorities. They agreed that tuberculosis was a preventable disease causing a "needless loss of life." Sharing an optimistic view prevalent among Progressive reformers, they thought that with proper study and effort, the problem of tuberculosis could be eradicated. The first step, Lilienthal argued, was to inform the city's citizens about the extent of the problem so that they would know more "about existing conditions," "what may be done to improve them," and "how they [might] help." Next, with the help of the citizens and the Department of Health, an energetic campaign would be waged against tuberculosis by instituting both preventive and curative measures.[53]

In 1908, by this time affiliated with the San Francisco Polyclinic Hospital, Brown began experimental "tuberculosis class work" in a special clinic. Modeling his program after those of his colleagues Joseph H. Pratt in Boston and Charles Minor in Asheville, North Carolina, Brown sought to "educate" his patients to "treat themselves." Such an approach, he argued, gave patients the "greatest chance of recovery" and eliminated the possibility of their continuing to be "a source of danger to others."[54]

In the tuberculosis classes at the San Francisco Polyclinic Hospital, patients learned to observe and record their daily condition and anything that might influence it, such as "unusual symptoms, weather conditions, hours of work, blocks walked, or appetite." Once a week, they met to compare notes. According to Brown, such comparison assisted them in seeing what helped them improve. More important, peer review kept potential backsliders from returning to bad habits. Nothing was more impressive, said Brown, than the testimony of a fellow patient about the positive "effects of sleeping outdoors or the greater gains under absolute rest." Using a team approach, the patients, the physicians, and the visiting nurses exerted a "rigid discipline and optimistic influence" bringing "decided success."[55]

Brown's classes served a population of patients who were deemed to be "early or hopeful" cases of tuberculosis; the staff declared most of them to be "independent" or self-supporting. To keep them on the road to recovery, the staff scrutinized their physical, social, and economic lives. At times the staff even helped wives of ill husbands find jobs. Further, the staff encouraged patients to find work in less dangerous trades. In spite of this supervision and support, many patients could not adhere to the program's rules. At least half of the patients dropped out in the first three years.[56]

During the time that Brown worked with the tuberculosis class patients at the San Francisco Polyclinic Hospital, he realized the importance of founding a country sanatorium particularly devoted to working women. Brown often prescribed a six- to eight-month stint of light outdoor work for his patients. For single men, finding such work seemed simple. For women, he claimed, it was difficult if not impossible. Brown listed "young mothers, clerks, stenographers, shop-girls, seamstresses, and school teachers," mainly experienced in indoor work, as particularly having problems. He found a solution by setting up the Arequipa Sanatorium immediately adjacent to Hill Farm, an outdoor charity home for "sickly and feeble children," thus providing mothers and children with an opportunity to escape the city's unhealthy conditions together.[57]

Brown wanted the Arequipa Sanatorium to be a healthy, morally wholesome, and financially sound operation. Different from Herbert J. Hall, who catered to the well-to-do at the Devereux Mansion, Brown tried to make it possible for working-class patients to "earn the cost of their maintenance" while living "out of doors" and making pottery "so finished and so exquisite that the demand for it exceed[ed] the supply."[58] He admitted only "first stage cases" to the sanatorium, and this policy helped hold daily costs per patient at one dollar. Moreover, he planned healthful work for the patients, keeping them self-supporting. He also persuaded employers and social and labor organizations to help cover the patients' expenses.[59]

To build the sanatorium in the first place, Brown relied on charitable contributions. Wealthy Marin County philanthropist Henry Bothin gave a tract of land adjacent to Hill Farm and the nearby Bothin Convalescent Home. Noted San Francisco architect John Bakewell donated plans designed to provide maximum fresh air and sunshine.[60] To obtain funds for a laundry, Brown approached his wealthy aunt, Phoebe A. Hearst, who had supported some of his other undertakings. In a letter written to her shortly before the opening, Brown exclaimed, If we are truly "teaching that 'cleanliness is next to godliness,'" then the sanatorium has to have its own laundry.[61] Hearst was probably one of the three anonymous donors who together gave $10,000 for the project.[62]

In setting up the Arequipa Sanatorium, Brown offered a solution to the problem of dealing with the "physically handicapped," a problem perceived by many Americans in the 1910s. "Science," Brown stated, had made "wonderful progress" in increasing the average life span by twenty years, but what, he asked, had "science done to make th[o]se extra years of life worth living?"[63]

In harmony with a cohort of occupational therapy promoters, Brown adopted craft work as the ideal activity for realizing a healthy life. From 1911 to 1918 the sanatorium ran a pottery under the directorship of nationally renowned ceramicists Frederick H. Rhead and Albert Solon and the lesser-known Fred Wilde. The pottery attained a national reputation, especially after its exhibition at the Panama-Pacific Exposition in 1915. Its art pieces were sold in such places as Marshall Field in Chicago; John Wanamaker in New York; Bigelow, Kenard, and Company in Boston; and several San Francisco stores. One observer was convinced that the vases provided Arequipa patients with "a way out" of "poverty, ill health, and despair" because the pottery-making skills that the women learned gave them "independence and health." Rising costs during the war forced the pottery to close in 1918, but many patients continued working as potters in other places after their discharge from the hospital.[64]

Brown was not the only person in the San Francisco Bay area to combine arts and crafts with the care of persons with chronic physical illness, nor was he the only occupational therapy promoter to associate craft work by patients with self-support. Susan Cox Johnson lived and taught in Berkeley, California, during this time of arts and crafts enthusiasm. An aspiring professional and design specialist, she published *Textile Studies* in 1912.[65] By 1916, under the auspices of the Department of Public Charities, she was directing a program of occupations for patients in New York City's municipal hospitals. There she too attempted to demonstrate the positive relationship between craft work, rehabilitation, and financial independence.

## Susan Cox Johnson and Evelyn Lawrence Collins in New York City

Susan Cox Johnson arrived in New York City on the eve of World War I, a crucial period in the history of occupational therapy. During a short stint in the city hospitals, Johnson tried to show that occupation was worthwhile as both a "therapeutic agent" and an "economic factor" in the lives of "heavily handicapped" patients.[66] Later she took a faculty position at Teachers College in the Department of Nursing and Health and gave courses in "occupations for invalids" with Evelyn Lawrence Collins, a self-identified teacher associated with the Henry Street Settlement. They taught their subject from the "psychological, medical, and economic viewpoint," they said, in order to prepare nurses and social workers to work with patients at home, in hospitals, or in workshops. They hoped that basketry, chair caning, leather work, pamphlet binding, and other such "practical work suitable for many classes of patients" would be of "commercial value" so that previously dependent citizens could regain self-sufficiency.[67]

Johnson's appointment as director of occupations at Blackwell's Island Hospital attests to a growing interest in more aggressive treatments for patients with chronic illness. In 1916 a "committee of private citizens" experimented with introducing occupations to "aged and infirm" inmates of the almshouses and to the "chronic sick in the public hospitals." Johnson produced a study of these efforts and then initiated several programs: one for patients with mental illness, at the Neurological Hospital; a second for patients with physical disabilities, at the Manhattan Home for Women; a third for patients with tuberculosis, at the Metropolitan and Sea View hospitals; and a fourth for patients with cardiac and orthopedic problems, at the Metropolitan Hospital.[68]

During 1916–17, Johnson could not demonstrate profitable "financial returns" from any of these programs, but she could give evidence of patients' improvement. Patients who typically quarreled with one another, turned their backs on the director, refused to work, or daily threw fits of hysteria changed for the better. After treatment, she said, "laughter, smiles, and a spirit of helpfulness and friendliness prevail[ed]" in the same wards. Physicians "who knew the old conditions sp[oke] of the change as 'wonderful.'"[69]

Giving case histories, Johnson described the particulars of patients' recoveries, ranging from change in attitude to improvement of bodily function. A melancholic young woman partly paralyzed on one side constantly cried. Johnson warned her that the tears would "spoil the work," so the patient promised not to cry. Soon, Johnson said, the patient "smile[d] and laugh[ed] habitually" and took evening walks with her to the docks. The patient ran messages for Johnson within the hospital and even spoke of getting a job outside. A patient with paraplegia learned to make tennis nets. The exercise of his abdominal muscles improved a chronic intestinal inactivity, making it possible for him to stop taking daily tonics. Another patient with paralysis, after mastering the making of tennis nets, gained so much "confidence" that he took a job as a night telephone operator at the City Home.[70]

Johnson believed that no one had to "prove" the therapeutic value of occupation; mere observation made the point. Lay persons and medical professionals alike saw the humanitarianism inherent in the work. Even "hard-headed businessmen," she said, recognized occupational therapy as a "rational treatment" that appealed "to their philanthropy and to their business sense."[71] Patients' productivity was the measure by which Johnson won converts to the cause.

Collins, like Johnson and Susan E. Tracy as well, claimed that she came to understand the value of occupational therapy by both observation and experience. She solicited potential allies for the cause by reminding them of their own sense of illness. "If you have ever been shut up for any length of time," she stated, "you know a little bit about the value of having something to do." Collins modestly claimed that "close personal experience" had best trained her for the work. Describing her own career, she denied any ability to present a "formal paper" or a "scientific treatise." She could only try to take her audience through some "mental pictures" in which they might see what she had seen, feel what she had felt, and be moved to do "much more" to develop the field of occupational therapy.[72]

Collins sentimentalized the plight of the "shut-in" patients whom she visited under the auspices of the Henry Street Settlement. One patient with heart disease, previously a "lady's maid" who had "travelled extensively" and therefore had superior "mental resources," was fighting her "battle" with illness "bravely" from a "spotlessly clean little room on the East Side." Bringing handiwork to this patient was "her salvation." Hearing about Collins's work, persons experiencing illness corresponded with her, seeking relief from their "pathetic" lives. Some were "courageous"; others sought "freedom from dependence." Some asked for "instruction by mail"; one pleaded for escape from her struggle in "shadowland."[73]

Such sentimentalizing of work in the tenements of the Lower East Side helped Collins and other aspiring professional women of her generation justify their involvement. Collins built on the tradition of women's charity work, even likening her efforts to the work of the city's Shut-In Society, an organization of volunteer visitors.[74]

At the same time Collins distanced herself from that tradition by mildly criticizing the Shut-In Society. She described its work as "beautiful, noble, and social," but "not scientific." By contrast, she and her "trained occupation teachers" entered patients' homes by official medical authority. They followed Henry Street Settlement nurses, whose services addressed acute needs of patients. District and Board of Education physicians referred cases to the occupation teachers after making diagnoses and prescriptions. The teachers, she argued, had a "broad educational background" and expertise in crafts. Referring briefly to theory, she mentioned the teachers' knowledge of "habit forming," which she related to "character building" in patients. For Collins, teachers had to be able to transmit to patients a "spirit of independence and courage to overcome difficulties" so that they could regain the goal of freedom—"freedom from disease first if possible, if not then freedom won by surmounting the obstacle or handicap."[75]

Like other occupational therapists, Collins represented a transitional generation of American women, one that drew on the traditions of volunteer charity work but looked forward to professional status. Furthermore, Collins embodied the tension within the profession born of trying to establish a medical identity and a body of aims somewhere between utilitarianism and humanitarianism.

This tension was particularly evident on one occasion when Collins discussed the remuneration of occupation teachers. Seemingly trapped in an ideology of service and altruism, Collins claimed to be "dismayed" by discussing money. She felt "inappropriate and mercenary" addressing the issue during the war, she said, when "half the world [was] giving it all in sacrifice." Ideal teachers of occupation, just like ideal physicians and nurses, gave freely of "that which money [could] not buy"— "vitality, faith, hope, courage, broad human sympathy and understanding." However, she continued, she and hospital authorities did not live in an ideal world; it was therefore important to grapple with the topics of how workers could "provide for their own living" and how occupational therapy could establish a "sound financial basis."[76]

Collins's comfort level rose when she talked about patients earning money. Declaring that the "commercial value" of products enhanced the therapeutic effect of occupations, Collins agreed with physician Richard C. Cabot's view that there was "a spiritual value in being paid in hard cash." She had formed a philosophy, she reported, which held that patients' courage and self-respect rose in proportion to their productivity. She had then transferred that philosophy to practitioners: "As with the patient so with the teacher," she said, "courage and self-confidence must be protected by freedom from financial strain."[77]

In the mid-1910s, with the field of occupational therapy well established in the area of mental health and growing more important in the care of persons with physical disabilities, Collins and Johnson tied many social, educational, craft work, medical, and economic threads together in their courses at Teachers College. Growing numbers of reformers in health care accepted occupational therapy's validity. By 1917 many would-be practitioners were ripe for training in occupational therapy to prepare for work with returning "crippled and disabled men" who would need to be "restored to physical and mental health before they [could] be made self-supporting."[78]

Attempting to attract "eager" and well-prepared women wanting to give "some form of personal service to the sick and wounded," Johnson called for teachers, supervising nurses, and social workers to apply to Teachers College. Indeed, Johnson planned to create an elite corps of practitioners capable of supervising occupations departments in private, state, and military hospitals.[79] The students coming from the various professions would spend a majority of their training time learning crafts. Women with backgrounds in craft work had to be willing to concentrate on developing their education and social work skills. The program was flexible, but there was a common curriculum. All the students were required to enroll in Education 175, a course taught by Johnson that dealt with methods of teaching in occupational therapy and included lectures to prepare students for supervisory positions in occupations departments.[80] In addition, all the students had to conduct observations and practice-teach in a variety of city hospitals.

Johnson sympathized with the wounded soldiers whom her students would help, but she did not view the work sentimentally. She realized that the war emergency provided opportunities for occupational therapy firmly to establish itself as a profession. Therefore she took her role in preparing women for war emergency work very seriously and on more than one level. In a letter to Major Henry R. Hayes of the Office of the Surgeon General, she made it very clear that she, her colleagues, and her twenty-eight enrolled students took "a professional standpoint" and were not just "a group of well-intentioned but unprepared women actuated wholly by sentiment and romantic ideas of helping the wounded soldier." Her students, she assured Major Hayes, gave "promise of becoming successful" professionals. Her greater concern was whether she could supply enough capable practitioners to meet the growing demands of the government hospitals. She complained of a "dearth of competent teachers," saying that she could not even answer recent "calls from four [New York City] civil hospitals."[81]

Occupational therapy expanded greatly during the war emergency, and Johnson's concerns about quality versus numbers came to be shared by a number of her colleagues. During and immediately following World War I, many women entered the field as schools, hospital departments, and independent therapeutic workshops were established across the nation. The coming together of several medical and nonmedical fields, the influence of social movements, and the unprecedented entrance of women into professional work all helped to form the new profession of occupational therapy. Medicine's continued and growing attention to chronic illness, which required a workforce of health care practitioners, also fueled the expansion of occupational therapy as a profession. Men in the movement tended to concentrate on theory as a way of legitimizing the field, while women concentrated on developing practice and training. Such a division of labor by gender endured through the next phase of occupational therapy's development as a profession.

# NOTES

1. "Consolation House Announces a Series of Classes in Occupational Therapy to Begin October, 1917," pamphlet, Official Archives of the American Occupational Therapy Association, Wilma L. West Library, American Occupational Therapy Foundation, Bethesda, Maryland (hereafter AOTA Archives).

2. Philip K. Brown, "Tuberculosis Class Work in the San Francisco Polyclinic," pamphlet, Philip K. Brown Papers, Bancroft Library, University of California, Berkeley (hereafter Philip K. Brown Papers).

3. *Thirty-Fourth Annual Report of the Montefiore Home and Hospital for Chronic Diseases and Country Sanatorium for the Tuberculous* (1918), 35, Archives of the Montefiore Hospital and Medical Center, New York City.

4. Evelyn L. Collins, "Occupational Therapy for the Homebound," *Archives of Occupational Therapy* 1 (1922): 36–38.

5. Letter, George E. Barton to William R. Dunton, 20 December 1916, AOTA Archives.

6. T. J. Jackson Lears, *No Place of Grace: Antimodernism and the Transformation of American Culture, 1880–1920* (New York: Pantheon Books, 1981), 47–59.

7. Biographical information about George Edward Barton is drawn from "George E. Barton," obituary, *Geneva Times*, 30 April 1923; "George E. Barton," obituary, *Rochester Democrat*, 30 April 1923; "George Edward Barton," editorial, *Archives of Occupational Therapy* 2 (1923): 409–10; Isabel G. Barton, "Consolation House Fifty Years Ago," *American Journal of Occupational Therapy* 22 (1968): 340–45; and Sidney Licht, "The Founding and Founders of the American Occupational Therapy Association," *American Journal of Occupational Therapy* 21 (1967): 269–71.

8. George E. Barton, *Teaching the Sick* (Philadelphia: W. B. Saunders Company, 1919), 51.

9. Ibid., 52.

10. I. Barton, "Consolation House," 340–45; George E. Barton, "A View of Invalid Occupation," *Trained Nurse and Hospital Review* 59 (1914): 329.

11. I. Barton, "Consolation House," 340.

12. G. Barton, "A View," 336–37.

13. I. Barton, "Consolation House," 340–42.

14. G. Barton, *Teaching the Sick*, 50.

15. I. Barton, "Consolation House," 342.

16. G. Barton, "A View," 329.

17. The correspondence is on file in the AOTA Archives.

18. G. Barton, *Teaching the Sick*, 52–53.

19. George E. Barton, "The Movies and the Microscope," *Trained Nurse and Hospital Review* 62 (1917): 193–97.

20. George E. Barton, "The Existing Hospital System and Reconstruction," *Trained Nurse and Hospital Review* 69 (1922): 320.

21. George E. Barton, "Occupational Therapy," *Trained Nurse and Hospital Review* 60 (1915): 139–40.

22. Publications by George E. Barton referring to hospital reform include "The Existing Hospital System," 317–20; "The Movies," 193–97; "Occupational Therapy and the War," *Trained Nurse and Hospital Review* 61 (1916); *Teaching the Sick*; and "A View," 327–30.

23. Clifford W. Beers, *A Mind That Found Itself: An Autobiography* (New York: Longmans, Green, and Company, 1908).

24. George E. Barton, "Inoculation of the Bacillus of Work," *Modern Hospital* 8 (1917): 399–403.

25. The correspondence is on file in the AOTA Archives. Parts of this exchange of letters were published by William R. Dunton in "An Historical Note," *Occupational Therapy and Rehabilitation* 5 (1926): 427–39.

26. Letter, George E. Barton to William R. Dunton, 15 November 1914, AOTA Archives.

27. Letter, Dunton to Barton, 18 November 1914, AOTA Archives.

28. Letter, Barton to Dunton, 30 November 1914, AOTA Archives.

29. Letter, Barton to Dunton, 20 December 1916, AOTA Archives.

30. Letter, Barton to Dunton, 15 November 1914, AOTA Archives; also in Dunton, "An Historical Note," 428.

31. Letter, Dunton to Barton, 17 November 1915, AOTA Archives.

32. Letter, Barton to Dunton, 1 December 1915, AOTA Archives; also in Dunton, "An Historical Note," 430.

33. Letter, Dunton to Barton, 2 December 1915, AOTA Archives.

34. Letter, Barton to Dunton, 7 December 1915, AOTA Archives; also in Dunton, "An Historical Note," 431.

35. Letter, Dunton to Barton, 7 December 1916, AOTA Archives; also in Dunton, "An Historical Note," 432–33.

36. See other letters in Dunton, "An Historical Note," 433–39.

37. "Report of the Secretary: Minutes of the First Consolation House Conference," in *Proceedings of the First Annual Meeting of the National Society for the Promotion of Occupational Therapy* (Towson, Md.: NSPOT, 1917), 19.

38. "Special Courses in Invalid Occupations, Bedside Occupations, Occupational Therapy, Reeducation," pamphlet, 1918, AOTA Archives; "Consolation House Announces."

39. Barton held Gilbreth in very high esteem. In a letter to Dunton dated February 19, 1917, Barton suggested naming Gilbreth the

First Honorary Member because he saw Gilbreth as "probably the most foremost efficiency engineer in the U.S., and who by his discovery of autostereochronocyclegraphology and the motion cycle charts, [had] made possible the Re-education of wounded soldiers on a large scale in Europe." Barton continued, "He certainly knows more than anyone else in the U.S., possibly in the world, about the needs of the maimed, and has since the beginning of the war crossed the frontier some eighteen times, is personally acquainted with Dr. Amar and all leaders of the work in Europe, both for the Allies and for Germany." Barton cites Gilbreth's work in "The Movies," 193. Amar's work is cited in Part II of this book.

40. Editorial, *Archives of Occupational Therapy* 2 (1923): 409–10.

41. According to "Presidents of the American Occupational Therapy Association (1917–1967)," *American Journal of Occupational Therapy* 21 (1967): 292–93, Thomas B. Kidner was born in England, then went to Canada in 1900 to develop "practical forms of education" and to improve school buildings. He began his work as vocational secretary for the Canadian Military Hospitals Commission in 1915, and he worked as a special advisor to the United States Federal Board for Vocational Education in 1918. He later worked with the National Tuberculosis Association, and he served as president of the American Occupational Therapy Association from 1923 to 1928.

42. Letter, George E. Barton to William R. Dunton, 8 August 1917, AOTA Archives; letters, Dunton to Susan C. Johnson, 14 July 1917, 4 August 1917, AOTA Archives.

43. Letter, Barton to Dunton, 7 August 1917, AOTA Archives.

44. Letter, Dunton to Barton, 10 August 1917, AOTA Archives.

45. Editorial, 410.

46. Letter, Barton to Dunton, 7 August 1917, AOTA Archives.

47. "Report of the Committee on Research and Efficiency," in *Proceedings of the First Annual Meeting of NSPOT*, 24–27; "Report of the Committee on Research and Efficiency," in *Proceedings of the Second Annual Meeting of the National Society for the Promotion of Occupational Therapy* (Towson, Md.: NSPOT, 1918), 35.

48. Letter, Mrs. Barton to Dunton, 12 July 1923, AOTA Archives.

49. Richard C. Cabot, "Arequipa Sanatorium Where a Tuberculous Patient Can Be Cured without Expense to Himself or Anyone Else," *Survey* 21 (1912): 311–14.

50. Brown, "Tuberculosis Class Work."

51. Biographical information on Philip King Brown is taken from Lynn Alison Downey, "Philip King Brown and the Arequipa Sanatorium," *The Pacific Historian* 39 (1986): 47–55; and Thomas Francis Harrington, *The Harvard Medical School: A History, Narrative, and Documentary* (New York: Lewis Publishing Company, 1905), 1602–3.

52. Brown, "Tuberculosis Class Work."

53. San Francisco Association for the Study and Prevention of Tuberculosis, "A Report of the Tuberculosis Situation in San Francisco," July 1915, pp. 4–23.

54. Brown, "Tuberculosis Class Work."

55. Philip K. Brown, "The Opening of a Sanatorium for Early Cases of Tuberculosis in Wage-Earning Women. San Francisco Polyclinic Tuberculosis Class," pamphlet, n.d., Philip K. Brown Papers.

56. Brown, "Tuberculosis Class Work."

57. Brown, "The Opening."

58. Brown, "Tuberculosis Class Work."

59. Downey, "Philip King Brown," 49–50. As well as having these goals for the sanatorium, Brown planned to continue his educational efforts among San Francisco's 40,000 working women in order to lower the death rate among them, which was twice as high as the death rate in the population of working men (ibid.).

60. Ibid., 48.

61. Letter, Philip K. Brown to Phoebe A. Hearst, 27 July 1911, Phoebe A. Hearst Papers, Bancroft Library, University of California, Berkeley.

62. Downey, "Philip King Brown," 48.

63. Philip K. Brown, "The Problem of Our Physically Handicapped," *Archives of Occupational Therapy* 2 (1923): 178.

64. Robert Blasberg, "Arequipa Pottery," *Western Collector* 6 (1968): 8.

65. Susan C. Johnson, *Textile Studies* (Berkeley, Calif.: W. R. Morris, 1912).

66. Susan C. Johnson, "The Teacher in Occupation Therapy," in *Proceedings of the First Annual Meeting of NSPOT*, 46.

67. Columbia University, Teachers College, School of Practical Arts, Department of Nursing and Health, "A Course in Occupations for Invalids Consisting of Lectures and Laboratory Work by Evelyn Collins," pamphlet, n.d., AOTA Archives.

68. Johnson, "The Teacher," 45.

69. Ibid., 46.

70. Ibid., 46–47.

71. Ibid., 47.

72. Collins, "Occupational Therapy for the Homebound," 33–34.

73. Ibid., 34.

74. Ibid., 35.

75. Ibid., 40.

76. Evelyn L. Collins, "Remuneration of the Teacher," in *Proceedings of the Second Annual Meeting of NSPOT*, 31.

77. Ibid.

78. Columbia University, Teachers College, School of Practical Arts, Department of Nursing and Health, "Course for Teachers of Occupational Therapy Beginning October 9, 1917," pamphlet, AOTA Archives.

79. Columbia University, Teachers College, School of Practical Arts, Department of Nursing and Health, "Courses for Reconstruction Aides in Physical Therapy and Occupational Therapy Beginning by April 10, 1918," pamphlet, AOTA Archives.

80. Susan C. Johnson, "Outline of Education 175 B," History of Nursing Collection, microfiche 0152, Milbank Memorial Library, Teachers College, Columbia University.

81. Letter, Susan C. Johnson to Major Henry R. Hayes, 4 March 1918, Surgeon General's Office Correspondence, 1917–27, National Archives, Washington, D.C.

# PART II

## WORLD WAR I *and* OCCUPATIONAL THERAPY

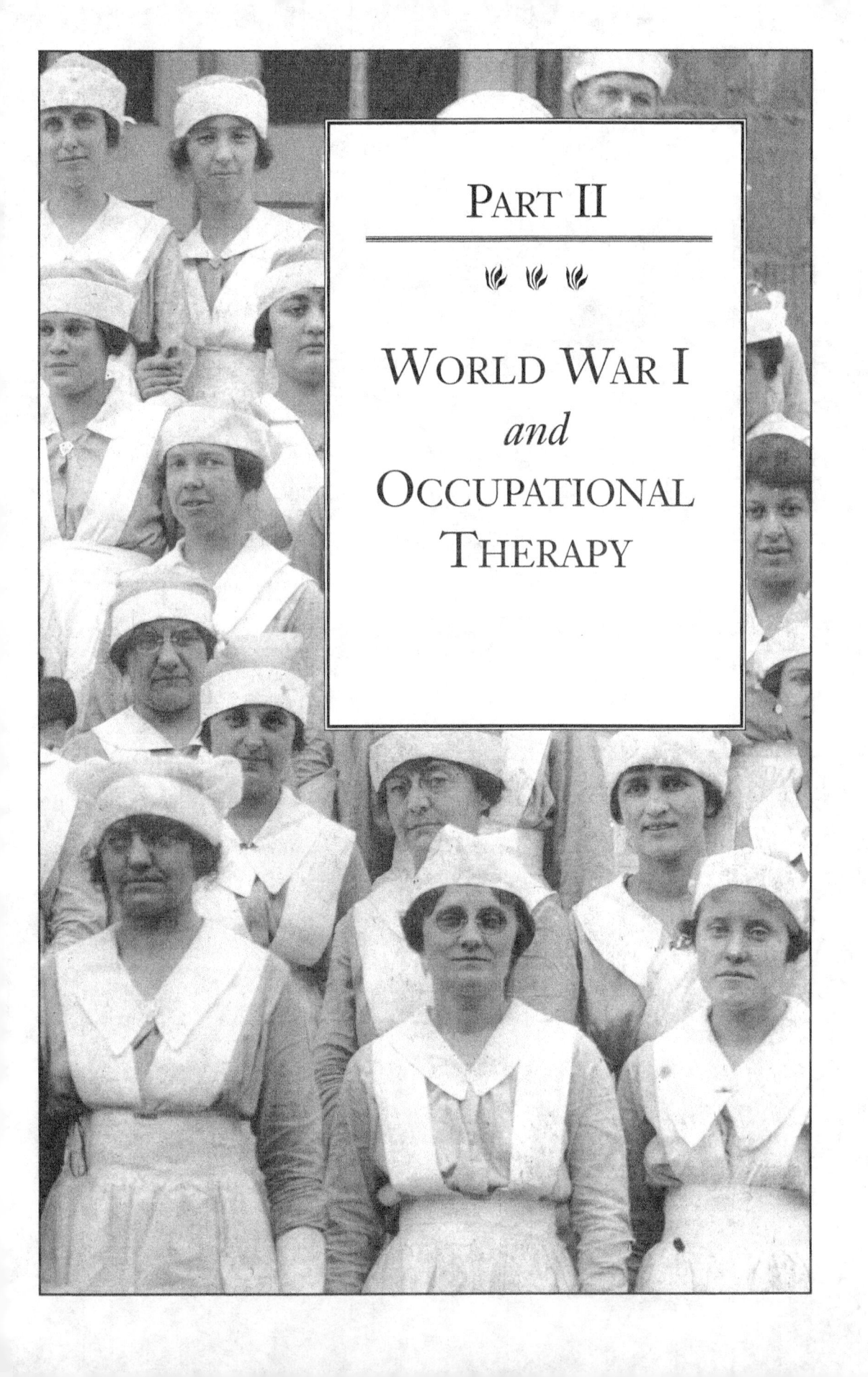

> The millions of wounded and crippled soldiers in the belligerent countries of Europe present to the world the greatest problem it [has] ever had to face in the care of human beings. It is a medical problem, a social problem, and perhaps most of all an economical problem.
>
> *G. Canby Robinson, physician, in a paper read at the Sixty-first Annual Meeting of the Missouri State Medical Association, 1918*

> These war experiences showed us what was obvious before, that idleness is a dangerous thing. Every maimed soldier was likely to become a centre of social unrest and no nation can stand that. There were numerous cases of wounds in the hand. Three or four months were lost by these during ordinary medical treatment; with occupational therapy available, the time was brought down to as many weeks, and the men returned to the front. This is entirely possible in civil life.
>
> *Joel E. Goldthwait, orthopedic surgeon, in a lecture given at the meeting of the Massachusetts Association for Occupational Therapy, 1921*

## Introduction

Meeting the medical, social, and economic needs of returning World War I soldiers propelled the American armed forces and public into a surge of organizational activity. Government and private citizens mobilized personnel to work with an expected 123,000 soldiers and sailors with disabilities returning to the United States by May 1919.[1] Most agreed that many soldiers needed surgical, medical, nursing, and educational or vocational services to return successfully to a productive civilian life. Thus the postwar period prompted many "experts" representing these several aspects of recovery to establish themselves professionally. In the climate of fear created by the war emergency, numerous competing professions found fertile ground in which to take root and thrive.

Occupational therapy vied for an authoritative position in the postwar movement known as the "reconstruction of the disabled soldier." Most Americans felt as President Woodrow Wilson did: "No subject . . . deserves more immediate or earnest consideration than the subject of the physical reconstruction of disabled soldiers."[2] Occupational therapy leaders capitalized on this general concern by stressing the utilitarian value of the work.

Yet from the outset of the war, occupational therapy had to explain its potential usefulness in the reconstruction of soldiers. Few Americans, except those working with patients who were mentally ill, understood what occupational therapists actually did. The formation of the National Society for the Promotion of Occupational Therapy in 1917 indicates the extent to which occupational therapists had to define the field to the public and

*Part II: World War I and Occupational Therapy*

the medical world. (It was no coincidence that the word "promotion" appeared in the name of the group.)

Part II describes the World War I watershed era in the history of occupational therapy, when the emergency forced the field to clarify its role and standardize training and practice. While developing a clearer self-identity and public image for the profession during the war, leaders in the occupational therapy movement established many clinics, workshops, and training schools all over the nation. An ethic to serve the nation drew many women into the field. As the so-called reconstruction aides "did their bit for the boys," they also consciously strove to establish the profession.

During the war, occupational therapy defined a practice field between acute illness, the domain of physicians and nurses, and return to economic self-sufficiency, the responsibility of vocational educators. Occupational therapy claimed that its expertise lay in the critical period of convalescence.[3] Although it was closely aligned with physical therapy during these years, the two fields defined distinct boundaries.

As the war progressed, occupational therapy's supporters united in a near-crusade mentality to further the cause. Feeling defensive, practitioners formed a group consciousness, bonding themselves to their work, to their individual institutions, and to one another. The two chapters in Part II describe this critical period. Chapter 6 analyzes occupational therapy's relationship to the domestic and international efficiency and rehabilitation movements of World War I. It also discusses the actual experience of reconstruction aides and their attitudes about their work. By the end of the war, the novice profession had laid a permanent institutional foundation for itself. Chapter 7 discusses how leaders used the strategies of selection and networking to sustain the momentum gained during the war. Leaders placed only the most highly qualified practitioners in positions where their work would be noticed, praised, and broadcast. Leaders also formed a unique community-based organization of women that supported institutions for training and practice. Drawing on a nineteenth-century tradition of women's charity networks to expand the field, they built independent institutions while seeking coalitions with male physicians and mainstream medicine's institutional base, the hospital. Unlike nursing, which by the 1920s was finding itself more and more sealed within hospital walls and therefore under the direct authority of male physicians, occupational therapy enjoyed a highly unusual autonomy. Occupational therapists depended on physicians to refer patients and prescribe treatments, but in many cases the training of practitioners and the actual treatment of patients took place in independently run institutions funded by women's community networks. ❦

## Notes

1. Glenn Gritzer and Arnold Arluke, *The Making of Rehabilitation* (Berkeley: University of California Press, 1985), 39.

2. *Carry On* 1, no. 2 (August 1918): 3.

3. Office of the Surgeon General, War Department, *Abstracts, Translations and Reviews of Recent Literature on the Subject of the Reconstruction and Re-Education of Disabled Soldier and Sailor*, Bulletin No. 2, 15 March 1918.

# Chapter 6

## "No More Cripples"

### The Reconstruction Movement

*"No More Cripples"*

The rehabilitation of World War I soldiers and sailors was not an exclusively American concern; it was an international movement that built on prewar concerns for persons who were chronically ill or physically disabled. In Belgium, France, and Russia several trade schools for the reeducation of "crippled victims of industrial accidents" had been established between 1890 and 1910. To avoid paying compensation to injured workers for extended periods, authorities in these nations established programs in which men were "fitted by special training" in an appropriate trade to become "self-supporting in spite of . . . disability."[1] The programs emphasized both the economic and the medical problems associated with disability. In these European institutions, orthopedic surgeons worked side by side with male technicians, "experts" in their respective trades. In 1917, after two inter-Allied conferences on "disabled combatants" were held in Europe, several countries, including Belgium, France, Great Britain, Portugal, Russia, and the United States, set up a permanent institute to study the problem, variously called "reeducation" and "reconstruction."[2]

## THE WARTIME RECONSTRUCTION MOVEMENT

A loose coalition of American and European engineers, physiologists, and orthopedic surgeons struggled for a central role in the wartime reconstruction movement. Defining the term "reconstruction" literally to mean rebuilding of bodies, they furthered prewar knowledge gleaned from their work with "industrial cripples." They expanded on American engineer Frederick W. Taylor's scientific management methods in analyzing the health problems of workers in industrial settings.

Taylor, likening the human body to a machine, called for exact measurement of labor processes and human fatigue and activity as a means of improving workers' output and industrial efficiency.[3] French physiologist Jules Amar, an expert in prosthetic devices, reflected Taylorism in his study *The Human Motor*, in which he brought together "all the physical and physiological elements of industrial work."[4] Amar took precise motion and strength measurements of limbs; he also tested for fatigue by recording respiration and other bodily functions.[5] Influenced as well by the arts and crafts movement, Amar wrote of combining the "art of labour" with engineering principles and scientific physiology to ensure the "re-education of war cripples."[6]

Many Americans interested in the reeducation of persons with disabilities looked to Canada's system, which had gotten under way early in 1915 when wounded soldiers began to return from the front.[7] George Edward Barton studied the work of Amar and also of Vocational Secretary of the Canadian Military Hospitals Commission Thomas B. Kidner, inviting the latter to the founding meeting of the National Society for the Promotion of Occupational Therapy in March 1917.[8] Frank B. Gilbreth, America's foremost efficiency engineer, studied Canada's injured workers and soldiers while doing research on reeducation.[9] He then suggested a number of innovations in machines that allowed workers with disabilities to produce efficiently. In other words, he tried to adapt machines to men rather than make men fitted with prosthetic devices adapt to machines, as Amar was doing.[10]

In May 1917, one month after President Woodrow Wilson declared war, the Medical Department of the United States Army initiated its reconstruction program by sending newly commissioned Colonel Joel E. Goldthwait to study and report on the British Army's orthopedic work.[11] Goldthwait, a Harvard Medical School graduate and the chief of orthopedics at Massachusetts General Hospital, was a leader of this recently defined medical specialty, which combined surgery with mechanical devices. He also chaired an American Orthopedic Association committee formed in 1916 that was charged with estimating the orthopedic needs of the United States if it entered the war. He and his colleague Elliot G. Brackett, another Harvard Medical School graduate and Massachusetts General Hospital orthopedist, sought to use the crisis to promote their specialty. Having treated patients with disabilities for decades in special hospitals that they had founded in the Boston area, the two men conceived of their work as handling acute surgical emergencies and restoring patients functionally and economically. In other words, in civilian life, orthopedic surgeons had followed patients from incapacity to restored independence, and Goldthwait and Brackett hoped that they might now do so in the military.

On receiving Goldthwait's recommendations, the surgeon general created a Division of Orthopedic Surgery in the Medical Department of the Army and appointed Brackett, commissioned as a major, to recruit orthopedic surgeons for service and to set up proper equipment and hospitals at home and abroad. It seemed as though orthopedic surgeons would dominate the reconstruction service.[12]

However, after some conflict among medical specialties within the Surgeon General's Office over professional authority, a Division of Special Hospitals and Physical Reconstruction was created. This development indicated that medical officers representing general surgery, head surgery, and neuropsychiatry would share control with orthopedic surgeons over the reconstruction of soldiers.[13]

Civilians also competed for authority in the reconstruction movement. In 1917 the newly organized American Federal Board for Vocational Education assigned to Douglas C. McMurtrie, the director of the Red Cross Institute for Crippled and Disabled Men, the job of studying worldwide national systems of vocational reeducation for disabled soldiers and sailors. In his recommendations to leaders of the American reconstruction movement, vocational educator McMurtrie emphasized remaking the men into civilians. He outlined several principles of rehabilitation specifically designed for wounded soldiers.[14] The soldier's state of mind had to be considered if the soldier was to be brought back into civilian life as a complete man. Typical soldiers, McMurtrie claimed, were mentally dependent because they were distant from home influences and because the military had provided them with "every necessity of life." Moreover, each soldier had been "given every care which the medical corps" could offer, and "every effort ha[d] been made to minimize worry or exertion on his part." Such experience, McMurtrie reasoned, "deadened initiative and [a] sense of social responsibility," which reconstruction meant to restore.[15]

McMurtrie recommended that the men be restored to trades appropriate to their abilities, interest, and background. Whenever possible, he thought, they should be returned to their former type of employment. Further, unskilled workers should receive training in a viable trade. Men from the city should be trained as "mechanics," whereas rural dwellers should be instructed in "agriculture." Most important, the men had to be persuaded to take courses voluntarily because reluctant students "learned little." Accurate success stories of other men in similar situations, McMurtrie maintained, would help encourage the most distressed individuals.[16]

When he was asked if the "support and direction of the after-care of war cripples" ought to be in public or private hands, McMurtrie emphatically stated they were a "national responsibility."[17] Representing the Federal Board for Vocational Education, he argued for civilian authority in all phases of rehabilitation. This view ran counter to the surgeon general's plan to create a primarily medical system of orthopedic reconstruction hospitals that included vocational training.[18] In June 1918, with the passing of the Soldiers (Veterans) Rehabilitation Act, popularly known as the Smith-Sears Act (Public Law 65-178), Americans finally adopted a system that placed the rehabilitation of returning soldiers under the dual stewardship of the army's Division of Physical Reconstruction and the civilian Federal Board for Vocational Education.[19]

Responding to a warning by McMurtrie that the "attitude of the public toward the returned soldier w[ould] make or mar" the success of the reconstruction movement, the Surgeon General's Office mounted a public relations campaign.[20] It used the popular World War I colloquial phrase "Carry on," which referred to heroic efforts made by all Americans during the adverse conditions of wartime. Surgeon General William C. Gorgas vowed that the Medical Department of the Army would "carry on" its treatment of soldiers with disabilities until they were cured or at least until they were in the best-possible condition that modern medicine could provide.[21]

Reconstruction leaders developed an ideology that called for transformation of soldiers from military personnel to civilians and from dependents with disabilities to citizens. Many Americans agreed that it was one problem to make a soldier out of a citizen, but a "greater problem [to make a] citizen out of a soldier," especially a wounded one.[22] Former president Theodore Roosevelt, for example, reminded all Americans of their "plain duty" to stand behind the returning soldiers and sailors and give intelligent and generous help. The same efficiency that had made a strong armed service and built ships to "hurry men and supplies overseas," he contended, had to be applied to the restoration of the men. "What the men need," Roosevelt declared, "is an opportunity to make good as straight citizens."[23] Labor leader Samuel Gompers stated that failure to rehabilitate the men would have "detrimental economic consequences."[24] The "Creed of the Disabled" best exemplified America's expectations of returning soldiers and sailors:

> Once more to be useful—to see pity in the eyes of my friends replaced with commendation—to work, produce, provide, and to feel that I have a place in the world—seeking no favors and given none—a MAN among MEN in spite of this physical handicap.[25]

This ideology also stressed American women's crucial supportive role in bringing the men to full recovery. Mothers, sisters, and wives were urged to see the soldier through all stages of reconstruction, preventing him from "losing hope," while stressing responsibility. The Surgeon General's Office reminded women that recovery depended on the soldier's "state of mind" and that because his state of mind reflected his wife's or his mother's, it was up to her to convince the soldier that he had a future.[26] The "best reason for reconstruction," according to one issue of the surgeon general's magazine *Carry On*, was the soldier's sweetheart, illustrated as a beautiful, young woman (see figure 1).[27]

Such romantic images of American women's role in reconstruction were vastly outnumbered by less sentimentalized ones, such as the photograph (photograph 8) accompanying an article by a soldier who was "re-weaving the web" of his life. In the photograph, female occupational therapists concentrated on weaving, and the caption read: "In every hospital here and overseas women are doing a wonderful work. These reconstruction aides at Lakewood are teaching handicrafts that hasten the cure by giving the soldier something to divert his mind from himself. It is called occupational therapy."[28]

By publishing such a photograph, the Surgeon General's Office asserted two fundamental elements of reconstruction policy: first, that reconstruction must include psychological as well as orthopedic aspects; and second, that women could play an important role in reconstruction work. Psychiatrist Thomas W. Salmon, formerly medical director of the National Committee for Mental Hygiene, helped move the Surgeon General's Office along these lines. He studied the care and the treatment of "mental diseases and war neuroses" in England and then set up neuropsychiatric units in France and the United States, recommending that professional occupational therapists work with patients in these units. In Salmon's opinion, "shell shock cases suffered from a disorder of will as well as function," and "rest in bed and simple encouragement" would not suffice to help them regain "manhood and self-respect." Salmon believed that women had a knack for raising the men's morale and persuading them to start on the road to recovery.[29] However, he was not looking for mere "cheer-up" workers, as certain female volunteers were called in England. He expected his patients to be treated by trained practitioners, like those with whom he had worked in the mental hygiene movement. As part of his effort to secure such women, he tried to recruit

Figure 1: The best reason for reconstruction. (Cover of *Carry On* 1, no. 10)

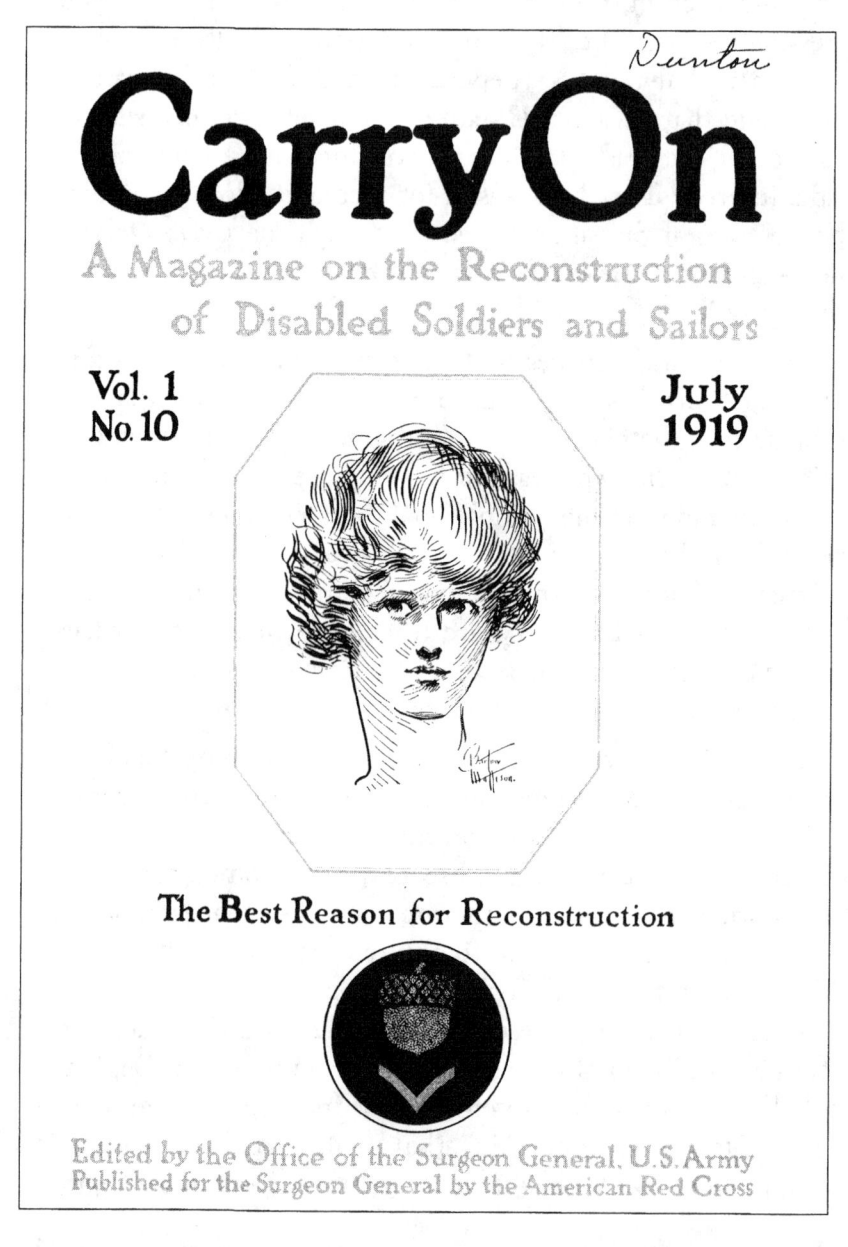

# Carry On

A Magazine on the Reconstruction of Disabled Soldiers and Sailors

Vol. 1
No. 10

July
1919

The Best Reason for Reconstruction

Edited by the Office of the Surgeon General, U.S. Army
Published for the Surgeon General by the American Red Cross

Eleanor Clarke Slagle for the position of Director of Re-educational Work in the overseas reconstruction aide service.[30]

## The Reconstruction Aides

The reconstruction movement in America adopted a clearly gender-defined division of labor. Male physicians performed the medical and surgical services, assisted by 21,480 mainly female army nurses serving in hospitals all over the United States by November 1918.[31] Growing numbers of male orthopedic surgeons and psychiatrists called on female reconstruction aides (occupational and physical therapists) to take patients beyond acute care to a stage called "curative occupations," which ensured the "maintenance of good morale and . . . discipline."[32] Occupational therapy, according to the rhetoric, offered "a new way for women to aid the wounded." Women would "win the wounded back to health" by providing "interest for the mind," considered more important than "ministering to [the] body."[33]

Initially the United States military planned to duplicate the European model of reconstruction by using military men as teachers in newly established "reconstruction hospitals," but the idea failed dismally. Few men had the teaching expertise, and even fewer wished to remain in the army once the war ended. The army then tried to recruit male civilians for the job. A few recruits held pending commissions for service, which the military canceled when the armistice agreement was signed in

**Photograph 8:** Some of the Weavers. (*Carry On* 1, no. 4, 1918, p. 23)

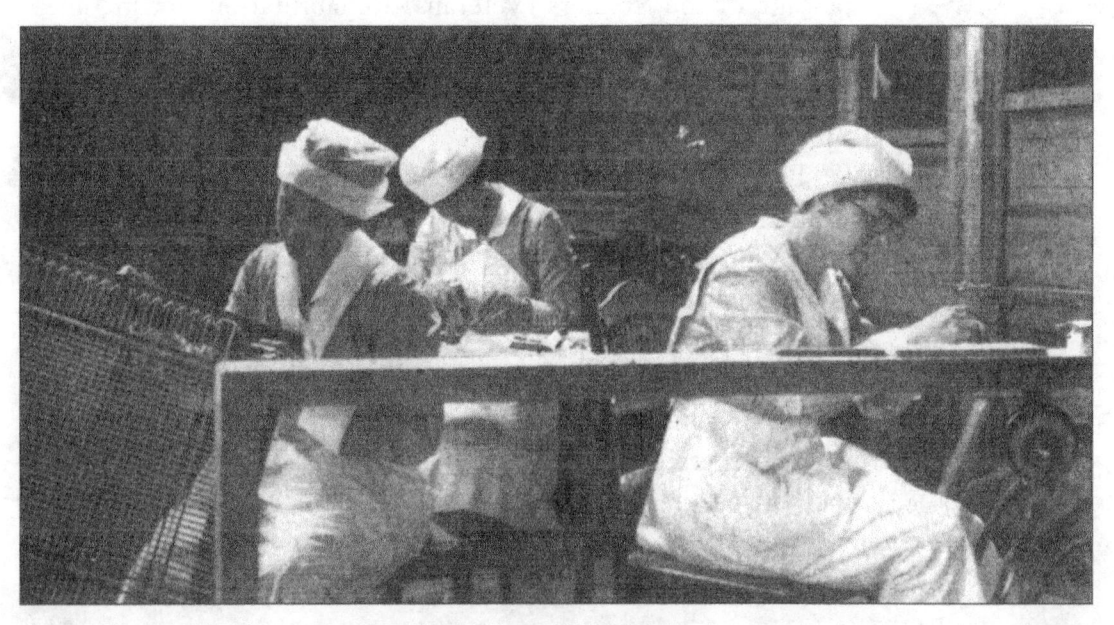

November 1918. In the end, women turned out to be the superior recruits: they surpassed their male counterparts in educational background, teaching experience, and special training. Moreover, the women were willing to take "modest salaries," some even accepting "war service at financial loss and great personal inconvenience."[34]

Early in 1918 the Surgeon General's Office began recruiting reconstruction aides from a ready and willing pool of American women wanting to "do their bit" for the war emergency. Research conducted by Elizabeth Greene Upham at the Federal Board for Vocational Education in Washington helped secure a superior group of practitioners. Upham, well-known in vocational education circles in Canada and the United States, had initiated courses in "invalid occupations" at Milwaukee-Downer College in Wisconsin and was vocally promoting *trained* women's potential contribution to reconstruction. The task that women "occupational therapeutists" had to undertake, according to Upham, was "the conservation of life," which could be fulfilled only by "the fit, the trained, and the ready."[35]

In October 1917, when Upham was called to Washington by Charles Winslow, the director of research at the Federal Board for Vocational Education, she undertook to ensure that occupational therapists would have an important role in reconstruction. She spent two years forming official reconstruction policy and writing official bulletins pertaining to the recruitment, the training, and the service of reconstruction aides. She also gathered data for congressional inquiries that led to the passage of the Soldiers (Veterans) Rehabilitation Act in June 1918. The law guaranteed retraining and/or compensation under the War Risk Insurance Act to soldiers and sailors with disabilities.[36]

Elliot G. Brackett and Joel E. Goldthwait also helped bring women into official reconstruction work.[37] Like psychiatrists and other physicians treating patients with chronic illness, the newly identified specialists in orthopedic surgery had grown to depend on the assistance of occupational and physical therapists. Brackett's sister Minnie, an occupational therapist, helped him in his clinic at Massachusetts General Hospital, and occupational therapists worked with Goldthwait in the Marblehead institution that he ran with his brother-in-law, physician Herbert James Hall. In January 1918, Goldthwait placed his long-time Massachusetts General Hospital assistant Marguerite

Sanderson, a physical therapist, in the position of Supervisor of Reconstruction Aides in the Surgeon General's Office.[38]

In early January 1918 the Surgeon General's Office released a decidedly medical set of official specifications for occupational therapy reconstruction, intending to set it apart from work with a strictly vocational purpose. Occupational therapy had a "purely medical function," the specifications read, to be prescribed in "early stages of convalescence" in order to "occupy" patients and prevent their hospitalization. Occupational therapy "prepare[d] the mind for subsequent vocational treatment" and was not to be "in any sense vocational." Patients' activities were to be simple, quickly done, and commercially valuable, but only to motivate patients, for no one planned to sell patient-made products.[39]

The army began its first trial of occupational therapy at Walter Reed Hospital in February 1918 (see photograph 9). Bedridden patients knitted squares for blankets and reportedly "welcomed the opportunity to do something." Ambulatory patients participated in chair caning, woodworking, printing, rug making, and several other crafts. The Walter Reed authori-

**Photograph 9:** Walter Reed Hospital, February 1918. [Reprint from the *New York Times* (Milwaukee–Downer College Records, 1852–1964, Milwaukee Manuscript Collection L, Milwaukee Urban Archives, Golda Meir Library. University of Wisconsin–Milwaukee)]

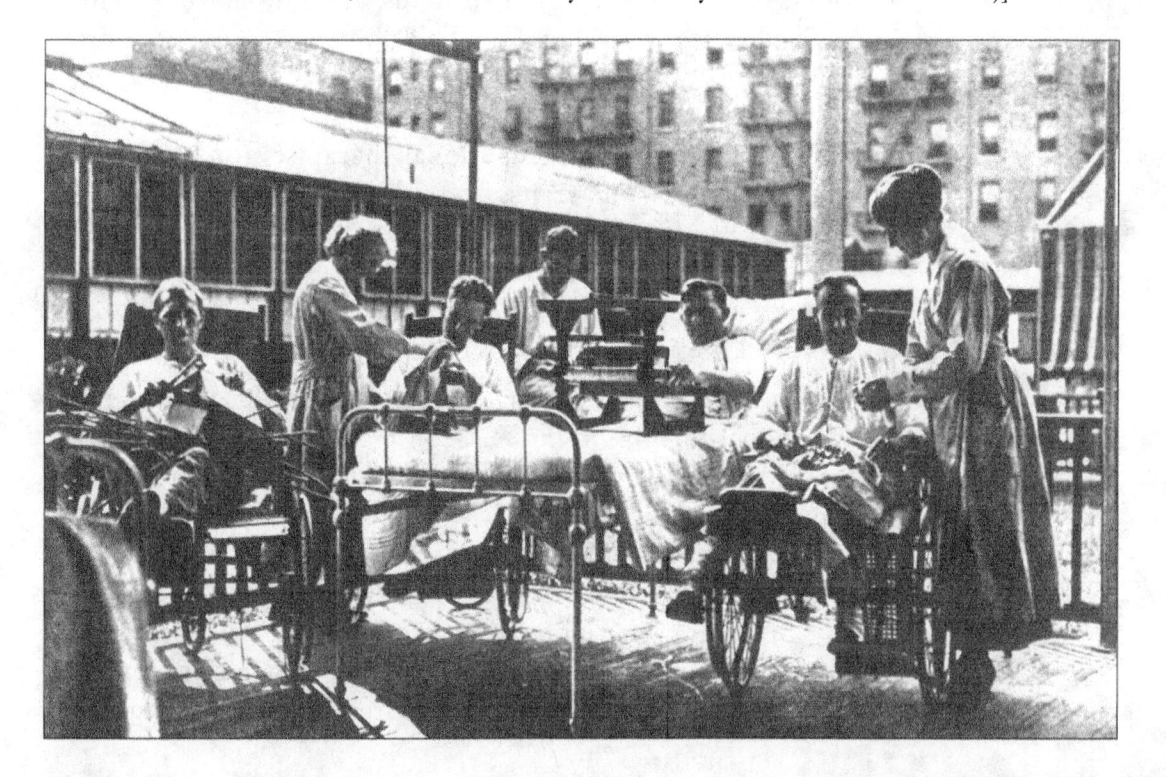

ties characterized the work as "palliative," keeping the men "cheerful and in good spirits." As well as discouraging "idleness" and developing a "desire for useful forms of work," the therapy had a "remedial" purpose. It physically improved finger, wrist, and shoulder dexterity, and psychologically tranquilized the men, prevented depression, and controlled attention. In a typical case, Private S. R. F., age twenty-six, with shrapnel wounds to his right arm and lower chest, took "curative" as well as "vocational" activities. In the morning he worked in the jewelry shop for "flexion-extension of the thumb, fingers, and wrist." In the afternoon he worked at a nearby farm, where "the vocational was united with the curative." Closely monitoring the jewelry shop work, Private S. R. F.'s physician prescribed "pulling of copper wire" to strengthen the flexion of the patient's fingers. The releasing of the tool helped his extension. The "hammering out of rings from French coins" improved his elbow extension and flexion. The patient's work was changed every 15 minutes so that he would "avoid fatigue." As he gained strength, the work assignment in the shop became heavier, and the afternoon farm work was canceled for full days in metal work.[40]

Reconstruction aides in January 1918 were of two types, physical therapists and occupational therapists, and they worked side by side in clinical settings. A lack of clear boundaries caused each type to define its respective area of expertise. Leaders explained that the two fields' training and focus for practice differed widely but both fields were vitally important to reconstruction. Physical therapists studied physical education, corrective exercise, and massage. Their practice largely emphasized body motion.[41] Occupational therapists, on the other hand, in using arts and crafts, stressed combining the mind and the body. Physical therapists had developed their greatest strength in working with orthopedic patients. Occupational therapists also worked with orthopedic patients, but had the additional experience of working with psychiatric patients.

In anticipation of a rising demand for both physical and occupational therapists, the Surgeon General's Office immediately tried to establish recruitment methods and centers for training. In her first days on the job, Supervisor of Reconstruction Aides Marguerite Sanderson took charge of the nearly 100 applications pending for service as a physical therapist.[42] She sent each candidate a Circular of Information, which declared "an immediate need" for "trained women to give massage and exercises and other remedial treatment to the returned soldiers." In the circular she recommended five schools for short emergency courses, three of which were in her own city of Boston.[43]

A later circular strongly emphasized "the type of woman necessary to do this work." Character and personality seemed more important than academic background or even health fitness. Different from nurses, reconstruction aides were categorized as civilian employees. Even without military status, the women had to have "powers of personal subordination," be "amenable to military discipline," and be cooperative and capable of "team play." Such a "spirit" was the "one thing" on which the "physical re-education of the returned soldiers depend[ed]." Expected to be mature women, candidates had to be between twenty-five and forty years of age. Single women could serve overseas, married women only in the United States.[44]

Competition reigned in the organizational phase of the reconstruction aide service. In January 1918, ignoring Elizabeth Greene Upham's work at the Federal Board for Vocational Education, Major M. E. Haggerty, a member of the surgeon general's reconstruction staff, recommended Martha Wadsworth for the position of Supervisor of Occupational Aides, as a counterpart to physical therapist Sanderson. Perhaps Haggerty wanted to capitalize on Wadsworth's impressive political and philanthropic connections. Wadsworth had grown up in a prominent family in Western upstate New York and was actively involved in the Red Cross and the Junior League. She had previously placed Junior League volunteers in overseas work. Her husband Herbert was a senator in Maine and a relative of United States Senator James Wadsworth, a conservative antisuffragist. (Mrs. James Wadsworth led the antisuffrage movement in New York State.) Martha wanted to do her part in reconstruction, and she claimed to have a thorough knowledge of handcrafts. In a memo to Major Elliot G. Brackett (who was from Boston and had worked with Sanderson), Haggerty also recommended Wadsworth to head a planned training program for occupational therapists at the Walter Reed Hospital in Washington, D.C. Further, he urged that she be given the responsibility of selecting practitioners for service. He even hinted that she could raise the funds for the Washington school if they were not "appropriated by the Medical Department" of the Army.[45]

Haggerty may have been the only one to endorse Wadsworth for the position of Supervisor of Occupational

Aides. Interested in establishing their own specialty of orthopedic surgery, Brackett and Goldthwait may have judged Wadsworth to be more a liability than an asset. Elizabeth Greene Upham certainly disagreed with Haggerty's choice: she tried to bring Eleanor Clarke Slagle to Washington to head the proposed Walter Reed Hospital training school. Slagle held more than adequate credentials for such a conspicuous and prestigious position, but she turned it down because of her commitment to start a war emergency course at the Henry B. Favill School of Occupations in Chicago. She and other active members of the National Society for the Promotion of Occupational Therapy consulted with Upham frequently about the proposed project, however.[46]

During spring 1918, Wadsworth did serve in a limited capacity as an advisor to the Surgeon General's Office, but she found this low-profile status irritating. In several communications she demanded an official supervisory position. Further, she complained about the procrastination of the Surgeon General's Office in setting up a training center in Washington. Also she objected to the Surgeon General's Office asking women such as Susan Cox Johnson of Columbia University's Teachers College for advice on standards for training and qualifications for practice, and she squabbled with others at Teachers College over who should rightfully recommend candidates for service.[47]

Although there is almost no direct evidence of occupational therapy leaders criticizing Wadsworth publicly or privately, it might be surmised that they too perceived her as more a threat than an ally. Wadsworth embodied a tradition of American womanhood rooted in charity and volunteer work. Although Americans valued volunteer service, especially during wartime, occupational therapy promoters with ambition for the profession were discreetly distancing them from that tradition in order to establish their authority. If occupational therapy was to claim autonomous professional ground, it needed to find space between traditional charity networks and the government. Another matter for speculation is that Wadsworth's antisuffrage family exacerbated her stormy relationship with the surgeon general's staff and leaders of the occupational therapy movement.

The Surgeon General's Office, on the whole, often worked cooperatively with "professional types," and occasionally did so with "charity types" if they seemed to support the development of women's professional work. Surgeon General's Office authorities frequently corresponded with Adelaide Nutting and Susan Cox Johnson, Teachers College leaders in nursing and occupational therapy, respectively, about plans for training courses in New York City. Marguerite Sanderson wrote to Johnson often for advice on a "model school" so that she could respond to groups all over the country planning to open emergency schools. Authorities called on William Rush Dunton, Jr., Herbert James Hall, George Edward Barton, and other members of the National Society for the Promotion of Occupational Therapy for names of candidates for service. Surgeon General's Office staff corresponded as well with Jessie Goldthwait, married to the orthopedic surgeon, and Helen Mansfield, active in settlement work, suffrage, and art circles, regarding the emergency schools that these charity workers founded in Boston and New York City, respectively.[48]

In late 1917 and early 1918, scores of practitioners prepared for service. Placing them proved to be a difficult task, however. Joel E. Goldthwait found that many of his colleagues viewed occupational therapy as a fad. Few understood its therapeutic value. Their attitudes began to change, though, when Goldthwait brought several occupational therapy reconstruction aides to Base Hospital 114 in Bordeaux, France. At first there was sneering at the aides, but after only two weeks the commanding officer and the hospital staff showed appreciation for the occupational therapists' work. They noted "that the discipline of the hospital [had] been changed completely by the presence of these aides" because the men were doing work to keep themselves occupied and not brooding "over things that had happened to them."[49]

Another important medical figure to situate occupational therapists in the reconstruction effort was psychiatrist Frankwood E. Williams, associate medical director of the National Committee for Mental Hygiene. Williams participated in a planning committee for the establishment of neuropsychiatric Base Hospital 117 in France. As early as February 1918, he tried to persuade authorities in the Surgeon General's Office to send six highly qualified occupational therapy reconstruction aides overseas: Mrs. Clyde M. Myres, a teacher of crafts at the Bloomingdale Hospital in New York who had graduated from the Boston School of Fine Arts and had taken postgraduate courses at Teachers College; Laura B. LaForce, a teacher of occupations at the New York Neurological Institute; Reba G. Cameron, a graduate nurse who had been supervising occupations for years at the Taunton State Mental Hospital in

Massachusetts; Amy Drevenstedt, a craftswoman who instructed students at Hunter College in New York City; Mabel C. DeZeller, a New York City teacher who had a strong academic background in psychology; and Eleanor H. Johnson, his prize candidate, who had graduated from Smith College and Teachers College, had taught New York City "defective school children," and had just completed a special course at the Phipps Clinic in Baltimore in preparation for war service. Unable to overcome the biased opinions of his colleagues, Williams offered his candidates the opportunity to go to France in the category of "civilian aide," which gave them no official rank or authority. The women, for their part, viewed the experience as a chance to prove themselves.[50]

In June 1918 these first women to serve in the American Expeditionary Forces arrived in France to a cold reception. Determined to succeed, they set up shop with tools and materials carted from home and a few "saw horses, planks and mess tables" that they borrowed locally.[51] The army considered it impractical to set up vocational or therapeutic workshops in France; therefore the majority of the reconstruction work that the women conducted focused on physiotherapy and bedside occupations. The overseas reconstruction aides worked with two types of soldiers: those temporarily unfit for combat duty, but expected to become fit within six months; and those permanently unfit for combat, but fit for other overseas duty.[52] By sheer tenacity the women won over patients and military personnel. Within weeks Colonel Thomas W. Salmon, by this time chief of the Psychiatric Division of the Surgeon General's Office in France, declared that reconstruction aides were "worth their weight in gold." Later General John J. Pershing sent a cable saying, "Send over a thousand of these aides as soon as you can get them ready." By December 1918, at least 200 reconstruction aides were serving in twenty base hospitals in France.[53]

They found their experience exhausting yet exhilarating. Gertrude Reilly, serving with four other women in Base Hospital 85 in Angers, had charge of two wards of bed patients and the shop. She supervised the other women, ran the shop, prepared designs for crafts, kept accounts and reports, and made rounds of the wards to "get to know the men." The women worked from 8:30 in the morning until late at night, and generally spent their only afternoon off buying materials for the shop or catching up. The work was interesting, Reilly wrote, but too much. Hoping for more help, she sent an

"S.O.S." to Marguerite Sanderson. Lillian Link felt that the months of training and service were the happiest she had ever spent. Helen Therese Damrisch wrote of her work with the soldiers, "It's been one of those wonderful experiences that no matter how much you give, you *get* a great deal more [emphasis in original]." Elizabeth Preston Cocke reported, "I really love the work, and have enjoyed it every day since I got here." Dorothea Macomber was "heartbroken to leave" Red Cross Base Hospital 109 at Evreux, despite the fact that materials were in such short supply that the reconstruction aides had resorted to using cigar boxes for projects for the men. Expressing a worry of many reconstruction aides, she wrote, "If it isn't too much trouble, I would love to know if there is still occupational work to be done [back in the United States]."[54]

The overseas reconstruction aides had nothing to fear: Between 1917 and January 1, 1920, nearly 148,000 sick and wounded men were placed in hospitals on their return to the United States. Thousands more from domestic cantonments were hospitalized. At the time of the armistice, seventeen reconstruction hospitals were functioning; by mid-1919, the height of the reconstruction period, fifty-two such hospitals had received nearly 111,000 men taking some form of "educational service" as they recovered from a range of disabilities, such as tuberculosis, orthopedic problems, heart disease, and mental disorders.

In setting up the reconstruction service, Surgeon General's Office authorities overcame many problems. They quickly found instructors, equipment, and space to serve the vast numbers of men in need. They learned to reach men whose educational backgrounds ran the gamut from functional illiteracy to college graduation. (The median education of the men was the sixth grade.) With limited time and money they served a population that ranged widely in intelligence and vocational background.[55]

The occupational therapy reconstruction aides helped accomplish all of this with little status or pay and few allowances. Unable to achieve parity with army nurses during the war, they at least convinced the military, medical, and public worlds of the effectiveness of occupational therapy.[56] By April 1919, physician Eleanor Rowland Wembridge had become the Supervisor of Occupational Therapy Reconstruction Aides in the Surgeon General's Office. She spoke matter-of-factly about the accomplishments of the nearly 1,200 occupational therapy reconstruction aides who had served actively in the reconstruction effort: the war had given occupational therapists the opportunity to "prove what they were for."[57] Now leaders would try to ride the momentum of growth.

## NOTES

1. Douglas C. McMurtrie, *The Evolution of National Systems of Vocational Reeducation for Disabled Soldiers and Sailors* (Washington, D.C.: Federal Board for Vocational Education, May 1918), 11–12.

2. Office of the Surgeon General, War Department, *Abstracts, Translations and Reviews of Recent Literature on the Subject of the Reconstruction and Re-Education of Disabled Soldier and Sailor*, Bulletin No. 2, 15 March 1918, passim.

3. Frederick W. Taylor, *The Principles of Scientific Management* (New York: Harper and Brothers, 1919).

4. Jules Amar, *The Human Motor, or the Scientific Foundations of Labour and Industry* (London: George Routledge, 1920), v.

5. William R. Dunton, *Reconstruction Therapy* (Philadelphia: W. B. Saunders Company, 1919), 107.

6. Jules Amar, *The Physiology of Industrial Organization and the Re-employment of the Disabled* (London: London and Norwich Press, 1918). See especially chapter 6, "The Art of Labour," pp. 125–67.

7. Military Hospitals Commission—Canada, Bulletin, November 1917, Official Archives of the American Occupational Therapy Association, Wilma L. West Library, American Occupational Therapy Foundation, Bethesda, Maryland (hereafter AOTA Archives).

8. Barton cites Amar in George E. Barton, *Re-education* (Boston: Houghton Mifflin, 1917), 66–69, 103, 117; and *Teaching the Sick* (Philadelphia: W. B. Saunders Company, 1919), 31–42.

9. Frank B. Gilbreth, "The Engineer, the Cripple and the New Education," *Journal of the American Society of Mechanical Engineers* 1 (1918): 51, as cited in Dunton, *Reconstruction Therapy*, 106.

10. Dunton, *Reconstruction Therapy*, 107.

11. A. G. Crane, *The Medical Department of the United States Army in the World War*, vol. 13, pt. 1, *Physical Reconstruction and Vocational Education* (Washington, D.C.: U.S. Government Printing Office, n.d.), 3; Glenn Gritzer and Arnold Arluke, *The Making of Rehabilitation* (Berkeley: University of California Press, 1985), 53.

12. Gritzer and Arluke, *The Making*, 40–41.

13. Ibid., 43–45. In May 1918 the name was shortened to Division of Physical Reconstruction, and the division's functions were more clearly defined [Robert S. Anderson, ed., *Army Medical Specialist Corps* (Washington, D.C.: Office of the Surgeon General, Department of the Army, 1968), 70].

14. Douglas C. McMurtrie, *The Evolution*; McMurtrie, *The Disabled Soldier* (New York: Macmillan, 1919); McMurtrie, "The High Road to Self-Support," *Carry On* 1, no. 9 (June 1919): 4–9.

15. McMurtrie, *The Evolution*, 13–14.

16. Ibid., 15.

17. Ibid., 20.

18. Office of the Surgeon General, War Department, *Civilian vs. Medico-Military Control of the Disabled Soldier during His Rehabilitation and Placement*, Bulletin No. 2, n.d.

19. Ibid. For a detailed discussion of debates surrounding authority in the rehabilitation movement in the United States during and following World War I, see Gritzer and Arluke, *The Making*, 28–60.

20. McMurtrie, *The Evolution*, 17–18.

21. *Carry On* 1, no. 1 (June 1918): 3.

22. Student notebook, unidentified emergency school in Michigan, AOTA Archives, unprocessed materials.

23. Theodore Roosevelt, "For Their Soul's Desire," *Carry On* 1, no. 2 (August 1918): 5.

24. Samuel Gompers, "Labor Stands Ready," *Carry On* 1, no. 3 (September 1918): 3.

25. Cover, *Carry On* 1, no. 8 (May 1919).

26. Alice Duer Miller, "How Can a Woman Best Help?" *Carry On* 1, no. 1 (June 1918): 17.

27. Cover, *Carry On* 1, no. 10 (July 1919).

28. Photograph, *Carry On* 1, no. 4 (January 1919): 10.

29. Dunton, *Reconstruction Therapy*, 109–12.

30. "Experience of Eleanor Clarke Slagle," resumé, 1922, Papers of the American Occupational Therapy Association, AOTA Archives.

31. Crane, *The Medical Department*, 290.

32. A. G. Crane, *Education for the Disabled in War and Industry* (New York: Teachers College, Columbia University Press, 1921), 1.

33. "A New Way for Women to Aid the Wounded," *Literary Digest* 58 (September 1918): 32–33.

34. Gritzer and Arluke, *The Making*, 45; Crane, *The Medical Department*, 80.

35. *Milwaukee-Downer College Bulletin*, series 1, no. 2, *Occupational Therapy* (Milwaukee, Wisc.: November 1918), 3, Papers of Milwaukee-Downer College, University of Wisconsin–Milwaukee (hereafter Papers of Milwaukee-Downer College).

36. "Elizabeth Upham Davis," resumé, ca. 1948, State Historical Society of Wisconsin, Madison. For more information on the War Risk Insurance Act, see Gritzer and Arluke, *The Making*, 47.

37. Gritzer and Arluke, *The Making*, 53.

38. Myra L. McDaniel, "Occupational Therapists before World War II (1917–40)," in Anderson, ed., *Army Medical Specialist Corps*, 70. Sanderson and the reconstruction aide program were initially assigned to the Division of Orthopedic Surgery. They were transferred to the Division of Physical Reconstruction in May 1918.

39. As quoted in Crane, *The Medical Department*, 58.

40. Bird T. Baldwin, *Report of the Department of Occupational Therapy, Walter Reed General Hospital* (Takoma Park, Washington, D.C.: Walter Reed Hospital, 30 January 1919), 11–15. For more information, see Baldwin, *Occupational Therapy Applied to Restoration of Function of Disabled Joints* (Takoma Park, Washington, D.C.: Walter Reed Hospital, 1919). Major Baldwin was director of occupational therapy and chief psychologist at Walter Reed Hospital beginning on April 25, 1918.

41. Gritzer and Arluke, *The Making*, 52–56.

42. Weekly Report, Week Ending 26 January 1918, Marguerite Sanderson to Major E. G. Brackett, Surgeon General's Office Correspondence, 1917–27, National Archives.

43. Medical Department of the United States Army, Circular of Information, 22 January 1918, Papers of the Surgeon General's Office, National Archives, Washington, D.C.

44. Medical Department of the United States Army, Circular of Information, 27 March 1918, Papers of the Surgeon General's Office, National Archives.

45. "Bedside Occupational Aides," memo, Major M. E. Haggerty to Major E. G. Brackett, 11 January 1918, covering resumé of Mrs. Herbert (Martha) Wadsworth and memos "A"–"D," Surgeon General's Office Correspondence, 1917–27, National Archives; Anderson, *Army Medical Specialist Corps*, 72.

46. Letter, Elizabeth Upham to President Ellen Sabin, 22 June 1918, Papers of Milwaukee-Downer College.

47. Letters, Martha Wadsworth to Major E. G. Brackett, 13 February 1918, 18 February 1918; letters, Wadsworth to Major Henry R. Hayes, 9 April 1918, 13 April 1918, Surgeon General's Office Correspondence, 1917–27, National Archives.

48. Correspondence between officials of the Surgeon General's Office and Adelaide Nutting, Susan Cox Johnson, William Rush Dunton, Jr., Herbert James Hall, George Edward Barton, Eleanor Clarke Slagle, Jessie Goldthwait, Helen Mansfield, and others is on file in the Surgeon General's Office Correspondence, 1917–27, National Archives.

49. "Extract of a Letter of Colonel Joel Goldthwaite [sic], N.C., Base Hospital 114, Bordeaux, France," 1918, History of Nursing Collection, microfiche 1052, Milbank Memorial Library, Teachers College, Columbia University.

50. Letter, Frankwood E. Williams to Major Pearce Bailey, 27 February 1918, Surgeon General's Office Correspondence, 1917–27, National Archives; C. M. Meyers, "Pioneer O.T.s in World War I," *American Journal of Occupational Therapy* 2 (1948): 208.

51. Meyers, "Pioneer O.T.s," 209. At times the American Red Cross furnished equipment. Very often the aides themselves financed the work ("Report of the Work of Reconstruction Aides, Hospital Center, Savenay," 29 December 1918, Surgeon General's Office Correspondence, 1917–27, National Archives). Another report stating that reconstruction aides or the Red Cross provided materials is the Padre [pseudonym], *Base Hospital No. 9, A.E.F.: A History of the Work of the New York Hospital Unit During Two Years of Active Service* (New York: n.p., 1920), 75–88.

52. Crane, *The Medical Department*, 63; Anderson, *Army Medical Specialist Corps*, 84.

53. Meyers, "Pioneer O.T.s," 209.

54. These narratives are taken from correspondence from reconstruction aides to Mrs. Howard (Helen) Mansfield, the director of the New York War Service Classes for Training Reconstruction Aides in Occupational Therapy. The letters are among unprocessed materials in the AOTA Archives.

55. Crane, *Education for the Disabled*, 1–5.

56. Crane, *The Medical Department*, 60.

57. Eleanor Rowland Wembridge, "How the Reconstruction Aides Have Proved What They Are For," *Carry On* 1, no. 7 (April 1919): 10.

# Chapter 7

## "Do Your Bit *for* *the* Boys"

Occupational Therapy's
Response
to the
Call for Service

*"Do Your Bit for the Boys"*

Small numbers of occupational therapy reconstruction aides served in seventeen domestic reconstruction hospitals that the United States Army established before the armistice agreement was signed in November 1918. Yet they managed to convince the reconstruction authorities that their work had the potential to shorten the hospital stays of the men, thus making the whole effort less expensive. By June 1919, nearly 700 reconstruction aides, approximately half of whom were occupational therapists, served in forty hospitals across the United States, giving "ward occupations" to men confined to beds or wheelchairs, and "shop occupations" to ambulatory patients.[1]

Leaders in the occupational therapy movement adopted the strategies of selection and networking to establish the work as a legitimate health profession during the war. Realizing that the emergency offered unprecedented opportunities to educate the public and showcase occupational therapy's benefits, but fearing negative judgments about the new profession, leaders selected only their finest candidates to serve. Building on momentum gained during the war, promoters and practitioners initiated a drive to expand the field by networking with sympathetic physicians, army personnel, and citizens. They pulled political strings and supported institutions on both the local and the national level to guarantee the profession of occupational therapy continued growth beyond the war years. They tried to attract upper-class well-educated women to the field in order to support its still-fragile public image.

When General John J. Pershing sent the telegram in summer 1918 asking that 1,000 reconstruction aides be sent overseas as soon as possible, occupational therapy promoters responded with both exhilaration and anxiety. All over the nation they scrambled to provide a supply of workers to meet the expected demand while they also agonized over the quality of practitioners. Emergency schools, organized in several major cities such as Boston, Chicago, Milwaukee, New York, and St. Louis, struggled to balance quantity and quality in this period of institutional establishment.

## THE NATIONAL SOCIETY FOR THE PROMOTION OF OCCUPATIONAL THERAPY

Central to occupational therapy's growth and success during the war was the role played by the National Society for the Promotion of Occupational Therapy. The organization served as a clearinghouse of information on domestic and overseas reconstruction efforts, domestic training programs, and federal government policy shifts. Members of the organization exchanged information, shared ideas, developed strategies to promote the field, and debated issues critical to occupational therapy's further development. Conference attendance soared: whereas fewer than 10 persons participated in the founding meeting, in Clifton Springs, New York, in March 1917, nearly 300 attended the third annual meeting, in Chicago in fall 1919.[2]

By the time the membership met in Chicago in 1919, many felt that the profession had achieved acceptance by the general public and medicine. William Rush Dunton, Jr., declared that occupational therapy was "coming into its own."[3] At the next annual meeting, President Eleanor Clarke Slagle discussed removing the word "promotion" from the name of the group.[4] In 1921, with new self-assurance, the membership voted to change the organization's name from the National Society for the Promotion of Occupational Therapy to the American Occupational Therapy Association. During 1920 the journal *Modern Hospital* launched a regular column on occupational therapy, which Elizabeth Greene Upham and Herbert James Hall would edit, sometimes individually, sometimes cooperatively. In 1921 the association started its own professional journal, the *Archives of Occupational Therapy*, under the editorship of Dunton.[5]

On the other hand, the overwhelmingly female membership was not completely convinced that occupational therapy had acquired legitimacy. During these early years a pattern of electing men to the office of president emerged. Further, with the exceptions of George Edward Barton (1917) and Thomas B.

Kidner (1923–28), both of whom held close connections to reconstruction circles, all the men elected were physicians.[6] Only one woman served as president before World War II—Eleanor Clarke Slagle (1919–20), after a very close election.[7]

Susan Cox Johnson, chair of the 1919 elections committee, articulated the problem in simple language. She told the membership that the committee recommended Herbert J. Hall for the office of president because he was "one of the leading physicians interested in occupational therapy" and active in the field. Furthermore, she said, "placing a physician as president will have the tendency to stimulate interest and confidence on the part of physicians in general, and emphasize the therapeutic purpose of our work." The committee slated Slagle for the vice-presidency, but members of the association nominated her for the presidency as well. When the votes were counted, Slagle had fifteen to Hall's thirteen.[8]

Slagle certainly possessed the organizational skills and the self-confidence to preside over the neophyte association. For nearly a decade before her nomination for the presidency, she had worked indefatigably in the field. After completing her course at the Chicago School of Civics and Philanthropy in 1911, she conducted a six-month survey of the care of patients with mental illness and then organized a school of occupational therapy for nurses, attendants, and patients at the Upper Peninsula State Hospital in Newberry, Michigan. From there she accepted employment at the state hospital in Central Islip, Long Island, to organize reeducation classes under the auspices of the Russell Sage Foundation. Next she went to the prestigious Phipps Clinic at Johns Hopkins Hospital to work with Adolph Meyer. She stayed for two years, returning to Chicago in 1914 to start a community workshop under the auspices of the Illinois Society for Mental Hygiene and to lecture at the Chicago School of Civics and Philanthropy. In 1916 she took a summer leave to attend courses at Columbia University's Teachers College in New York City. By 1917 she had taken the position of general superintendent of occupational therapy for all the state hospitals in Illinois. Then, after turning down at least two offers to serve in reconstruction work in Washington, she directed a war emergency school at the Chicago School of Civics and Philanthropy, called the Henry B. Favill School of Occupations.[9]

Unlike many of her occupational therapy peers, Slagle had adopted a professional persona modeled after her Hull House colleagues Jane Addams and Julia Lathrop. She saw many Chicago women take on positions of authority in their fields, so it is no surprise that she internalized self-assurance in pursuing professional work. Perhaps not coincidentally, Slagle was elected to the presidency of the National Society for the Promotion of Occupational Therapy during the third annual meeting, held at Hull House in Chicago. On the very day that Slagle won the election, Jane Addams addressed the membership on the topic of mental hygiene and its relationship to occupational therapy.[10] Women's rightful authority in professional work permeated the national meeting in 1919.

That authority was fleeting, however, at least as far as its being expressed through the presidency of the organization. At the next annual meeting, in 1920, Herbert J. Hall won the office after another close race with Slagle. The nominating committee had recommended Hall for the presidency. From the floor a member of the association pleaded with Slagle to consider serving another term, and Slagle agreed to run. Thomas B. Kidner took the chair and called for a discussion on whether the election should be run by open or closed ballot. The delegation decided on a closed vote. The final tally was Hall, thirty-three; Slagle, thirty-two. After the official voting ended, a late vote came in for Slagle, which could not be counted.[11]

As president-elect, Hall explained to the delegates that he and Slagle had decided one year before to "fight for the presidency" of the association. "The best compliment that a man can show a woman," he said, was to "play the game with her and offer no odds at all."[12] Apparently Slagle felt strongly enough about taking authority in her chosen vocation to compete for the highest leadership position. Strangely, though, she never ran for the presidency again.

For the next fifteen years Slagle served as secretary-treasurer, a position that she made sure wielded great power. In addition, she traveled extensively all over the country to speak and to launch dozens of new occupational therapy schools and occupational therapy departments in hospitals and private institutions. Occupational therapy lore has it that although Slagle was no longer the official head of the association, she was nonetheless its heart and soul. In 1922 she moved to New York, the state in which she was born and in which her family still resided. In New York City she established the headquarters of the American Occupational Therapy Association, where it remained for years because Slagle was there to run the majority of its business.[13]

Also crucial to the advancement of occupational therapy as a profession in the World War I era were the schools that trained practitioners to serve during the emergency. In some places, existing schools and hospitals added special courses to train women quickly for service; for example, Teachers College did so, under the supervision of Susan Cox Johnson, as did Massachusetts General Hospital, under the supervision of Susan E. Tracy. In other places, completely new schools sprang up, such as the War Service Classes for Training Reconstruction Aides in Occupational Therapy, in New York City under the leadership of Helen Mansfield. In all these schools, promoters of occupational therapy worried about quality versus quantity.

## The New York War Service Classes for Training Reconstruction Aides in Occupational Therapy

In spring 1918, Helen Mansfield of New York City, a consummate diplomat in her interactions with the Surgeon General's Office, founded one of the only emergency schools to be endorsed by the government.[14] Wanting to produce at least "100 well-trained aides in six months," Mansfield drew on her political skills and social contacts to accomplish this ambitious task.[15] She corresponded with Major Henry R. Hayes and Marguerite Sanderson, making sure that her planned school met the soon-to-be-articulated standards of the Surgeon General's Office.[16]

Mansfield understood that lines of authority in the Surgeon General's Office during the first months of 1918 were fluid. She knew of recent friction between the office's controversial representative Martha Wadsworth and Teachers College administrators. Wadsworth had complained to the Surgeon General's Office that Teachers College was accepting students into its emergency courses without waiting for her approval. Worried that emergency schools might produce inferior practitioners, Wadsworth wrote letters to Hayes in March and April 1918. Claiming to be "confused" about her role in the government reconstruction service, she questioned how she could "assure the service the very best material in the country" unless she and some "reliable and interested friends" had clear authorization to "gather together a really 'selected' reserve" of students.[17]

Mansfield took a neutral stand, promising Hayes the "friendliest of relations with Teachers College, because," she explained, "we should all be working towards the same end."[18] She demonstrated similar tact in handling relations when Wadsworth demanded the right to interview applicants whom Mansfield and her cofounder Helen Sanborn Sargent Hitchcock planned to accept into their proposed school. Mansfield graciously (but probably untruthfully) told Wadsworth that she had no list of prospective students because she had not told anyone of her plans to open a school in New York. She was waiting, she said, for approval from the Surgeon General's Office before publicizing the opportunity to interested students.[19] Wadsworth left Mansfield to her own decisions, going on to Boston and Philadelphia to meet with committees planning for emergency schools in those cities.[20]

Mansfield moved in social circles that helped her bring together a group of women who could build a school surpassing all necessary expectations. As a feminist and an activist in settlement work, she had the personal, familial, and political commitment to promote women's professional work. She was the president of both the New York Music School Settlement and the National Association of Music School Societies. She held memberships in the Women's Political Union, the Women's Suffrage Party, and the New York State Suffrage Association, and she was the president of the Equal Women's Suffrage Association. Her husband was an attorney and a well-known patron of the arts. During the war he had served as the chair of the Advisory Board on Compulsory Service, and later he was a trustee of the Metropolitan Museum of Art.[21]

The women whom Mansfield gathered to start the school were no less socially prominent. Culturally sophisticated, wealthy, and active in women's charity activities, they also promoted women's professional work. Mrs. Cornelius J. Sullivan, who became supervisor of textile work at the school, was, like Mansfield, married to a well-to-do New York attorney. One of the three originators of the movement that led to the founding of the Museum of Modern Art in New York City, she had studied in London, had taught classes in secondary schools and at Pratt Institute, and had been instrumental in establishing occupational therapy at Blackwell's Island Hospital, where Susan Cox Johnson worked.[22] Mrs. Charles Sprague Smith directed art work at the Veltin School for girls and taught many New York City artists in her private studio.[23] Mansfield's cofounder Hitchcock, an artist, had studied at the Art Student's League, was the founder and the president of the Art Worker's Club and the Art Alliance of America, and had organized Art War Relief. Her husband was Ripley Hitchcock, author and editor of many works on art and history.[24] Mrs. Willard Straight, whose husband worked for J. P. Morgan, helped finance the school. She was president of the Junior League and chair of the Mayor's Commission on National Defense.[25] Mrs. John D. Rockefeller, who served on the board, donated space in one of her Fifth Avenue buildings for classes.[26]

By May, Mansfield had obtained the approval that she sought from the Surgeon General's Office. After she persuaded *New York Times* publisher Adolph Ochs to publish for free an article calling for students to come to the "War Service Classes for Training Reconstruction Aides for Military Hospitals," hundreds of applications poured in. Forty-two women entered the first course of study, completing it by September 1918.[27]

Mansfield's committee closely screened students before accepting them into the war service classes.[28] Most of the students had been educated in the arts; many called themselves teachers of art, teachers of arts and crafts, or artists. Applicants claimed to be adept at several crafts; regardless, they learned new ones during their time at the school. According to the standards of the Surgeon General's Office, reconstruction aides had to be skilled in at least six crafts: weaving, wood carving, basketry, block printing, knitting needlework, and cordwork knotting.[29] They also had to receive medical instruction and do practical work in hospitals. Mansfield persuaded several prominent New York physicians to volunteer their time to give lectures to the students.[30] The students heard twelve medical lectures on nervous and mental states and on the application of occupational therapy in other medical situations. They also heard lectures on hospital etiquette and personal hygiene. They did practice training in the Presbyterian Hospital, the New York Orthopedic Hospital, the Rockefeller War Reconstruction Hospital, and the Bloomingdale Hospital, all in New York City.[31]

The school's selectivity continued in placement of the graduates. When the first group of students had completed the course, Mansfield proudly sent twenty-five applications to the Surgeon General's Office and promised to send another twelve as soon as another group finished its hospital training. Mansfield's assistant director, Mrs. Cornelius J. Sullivan, wrote personal recommendations for each student, stressing personal and technical skills.[32]

Mansfield and Sullivan tried to persuade the Washington authorities to visit the school and to participate in a proposed conference on the training of reconstruction aides. They and Eleanor Clarke Slagle had discussed the need for such a conference in a recent meeting in New York. The three women planned to analyze the existing training programs and work together in improving them.[33] Mansfield requested continuous feedback from the government regarding the needs of the reconstruction hospital authorities so that students would receive adequate preparation for service. She maintained regular communication with other emergency school leaders as well.[34]

Even though she had no definite information from the Surgeon General's Office that demand for occupational therapists would continue, Mansfield prepared for a second group of students to begin classes in September 1918. "Doing this work is very much like shooting an arrow into the air and not knowing just where it is going to fall," she complained in a letter to Marguerite Sanderson.[35] As the armistice drew near, she expressed even more concern about whether or not there would be continued opportunity for her students. Should she not continue to train reconstruction aides, she wrote General Ireland, given the reports in the newspapers on the return of wounded men and the large number of base hospitals being set up? She reminded him that only months before, the surgeon general had accorded status to occupational therapy by supporting General Pershing's cable for 1,000 aides for overseas duty, and then she implored him to "establish [occupational therapy] in this country in the same way." Carefully choosing her words to show patriotism, she promised him "the well trained women such as we can supply, and if you say we are needed, we shall go on." In the meantime Mansfield put the nearly 1,000 applicants for the January 1919 class on hold by sending each of them a letter explaining that additional aides might not be needed.[36] She also collected testimonials from prominent medical figures such as Everett S. Elwood, of the State of New York Hospitals Commission; Charles H. Johnson, of the State of New York Board of Charities; Pearce Bailey, of the State of New York Commission for Mental Defectives; and Thomas W. Salmon, then of the National Committee for Mental Hygiene. All spoke positively about the value of occupational therapy.[37]

Concern about continued demand for practitioners pervaded the occupational therapy movement, especially after the Surgeon General's Office, in June 1918, began requesting emergency schools to stop using the office "as an authority for the continuation of the schools."[38] This development did not stop school leaders all over the United States from launching a massive recruitment drive. Wanting to maintain momentum, they placed advertisements in local newspapers quoting Surgeon General William C. Gorgas's call for 1,000 aides. In Milwaukee, flyers and newspaper articles announcing "a new field of military and civilian service" claimed that "1000 reconstruction aides [were] wanted immediately."[39] An advertisement said that the "demand" was "far in excess of the supply."[40]

Hundreds of women applied to emergency schools to prepare for service in returning the country to "normal conditions after the great world catastrophe."[41] In schools all over the country, students learned how to work with men suffering from "complete nervous exhaustion." Lecturers convinced future reconstruction aides that the soldiers returning from the front had "used up" all their "reserve force of nervous energy" and that the "building up of this reserve" was a "slow process, but it [could] be done." Students internalized the responsibility to encourage patients and instill confidence in them so that they would get well. "The importance of optimism," one student wrote, "is supreme."[42]

Caught up in the enthusiasm of reconstruction, occupational therapy promoters used organizational strategies similar to Mansfield's in New York to establish, virtually overnight, schools attracting women to the new profession. Founders carefully attempted to ensure quality. Jessie Goldthwait, wife of Colonel Joel E. Goldthwait, regularly communicated with the Surgeon General's Office in the founding period of the Boston School of Occupational Therapy, to be sure that course offerings met standards.[43] She and her cofounders Minnie Brackett (sister of Elliot G. Brackett) and Mrs. Horace Morrison (an arts and crafts enthusiast well studied in European reconstruction) used their social and family ties to the elite of Boston to open by April 1918.[44] In Philadelphia and St. Louis, founders of new schools organized similarly.[45]

Further, school leaders experimented with the number and the length of courses needed and with the entering qualifications of students in order to standardize training for the profession at large. By the time the National Society for the

Promotion of Occupational Therapy met in fall 1918, Eleanor Clarke Slagle could announce that "two months craft training and three months practice teaching in hospitals made an ideal arrangement for a short course."[46]

As much as leaders wanted to meet the expected demand for practitioners, two vocal occupational therapists, Susan Cox Johnson and Elizabeth Greene Upham, worried about the quality of practitioners entering the field. Johnson felt that before the war, "occupation for convalescents" had "fallen short of its possibilities," and she hoped that the war work in military hospitals would "set a higher standard" to be followed later in civilian hospitals. She also feared that reconstruction aides trained in emergency schools might not have an adequate background to meet the challenge.[47] Upham surveyed hospitals and institutions offering training for occupational therapists early in 1918 while she was still working at the Federal Board for Vocational Education. She concluded that "though there [were] numerous schools of mushroom growth for this subject," none "adequately" met "the situation." Privately she opposed Johnson's Teachers College emergency course, even when Adelaide Nutting added courses to the originally planned program, and she only tacitly approved of Eleanor Clarke Slagle's course at the Henry B. Favill School of Occupations, although she felt that it was the best in the country at the time.[48] Upham wanted occupational therapists to be college graduates. Few women in the founding generation of occupational therapists held college degrees, even among the leadership. Slagle, Johnson, and Upham had completed some college work, but they attributed most of their preparation for occupational therapy to experience and practice. Seeing this lack of college credentials as a weakness, Upham planned to establish a degree program at her alma mater, Milwaukee-Downer College, after finishing her duties at the Federal Board for Vocational Education.

## Elizabeth Greene Upham and Milwaukee-Downer College

Born in 1890 to a wealthy Milwaukee family, Elizabeth Greene Upham had influence at Milwaukee-Downer College, which she planned to use for promoting the profession of occupational therapy. The women in Upham's family had strong ties to this women's college. Her grandmother had served on its board of trustees in 1874, and her mother had been serving on the board of trustees since 1902. Further, her mother was a graduate of the class of 1880, and over the years the family had donated a considerable amount of money to the institution.⁴⁹

Upham began her career at Milwaukee-Downer College as an art student. Because of a serious eye condition, she temporarily dropped out of school, risking her opportunity to obtain a degree. After a year of struggling with her sight, Upham went to Chicago to take classes in jewelry making at Hull House, where she personally became interested in occupations and applied arts. She then went back to Milwaukee and persuaded Emily Parker Groom, the chair of the Art Department, to allow her to teach a course in jewelry and metal work, even though the college's president, Ellen Sabin, did not approve. President Sabin was trying to upgrade the college's reputation, and she discouraged Upham by saying that her proposed invalid occupations/applied arts course was a luxury having little place in an academic institution.⁵⁰ Upham persisted, and the course succeeded. Groom took a leave of absence, putting Upham in charge of the department, even though she had not yet earned a bachelor's degree.

In the early 1910s two students who were disabled came to Milwaukee-Downer for "manual training" in Upham's classes, and this marked the beginning of occupational therapy training in Milwaukee. Other students "in need of special understanding and training" soon entered the classes. According to Upham, their presence inspired many of the regular college students to study invalid occupations. Rachel Horner and Irene Grant, two particularly devoted students having a "keen social sense together with a desire for service," grew interested in the responses of the "disabled members in the class," studied material that Upham had gathered, and decided to make "service to the handicapped their profession."⁵¹

After graduation, Upham placed Horner in several local sanatoriums to study care of patients with tuberculosis. With the help of Hoyt Dearholt of the Anti-Tuberculosis Society, Upham managed to get Horner hired at the Muirdale Hospital in December 1915 as Director of Industrial Recreation. Horner later admitted that she was self-conscious about such a "high sounding title," especially because she felt that she did not know "beans when the bag was open" about her new career. In autumn 1916, at a Milwaukee-Downer teachers' convention banquet, she gave a talk about her work at the Muirdale Hospital. On that occasion President Sabin demeaned Horner's work, saying that "there was TEACHING,—and teaching."

*"Do Your Bit for the Boys"*

According to Horner, the only thing to "convert" Sabin to the "cause" was $25,000 that the Upham family donated to the college in 1918 to establish a department of occupational therapy.[52] Upham's memory was that the relationship with Sabin was far more amiable; her autobiography documents a long-term friendship, including at least one shared vacation.[53] More important, in 1917, while Upham was working in Washington, Sabin granted her a bachelor's degree after examining her complete college records. For this Upham was eternally grateful; "the desire to be a college graduate [was] always in the back of my mind," she related.[54]

During the two years (1917–19) that Upham served in Washington at the Federal Board for Vocational Education, her devotion to Milwaukee-Downer College only deepened. In regular correspondence she kept President Sabin abreast of the debate about the status of occupational therapy in Washington and in the reconstruction movement in general, and the possible effect of the outcomes on their beloved institution. As Upham wrote government bulletins pertaining to the training of occupational therapists, she and Sabin secretly planned to open a high-quality degree-granting course of study at Milwaukee-Downer that would rival the course at any other school.[55]

From her vantage point in Washington, Upham perceived that war emergency training courses might compete with one another: the government was refraining from funding such courses because many universities, colleges, and organizations were eagerly funding courses themselves. In a letter to Sabin, Upham cited Eleanor Clarke Slagle's school in Chicago, Dean James E. Russell's program at Columbia University's Teachers College, Helen Mansfield's school in New York City, and a proposed school in Dayton, Ohio, funded by "some wealthy person," as just a few examples of the competition in the marketplace of training institutions.[56]

Upham and Sabin aspired to make Milwaukee-Downer's program the best in the United States, both during the war emergency and afterward. They obtained financial backing and a high-quality faculty. Following a study tour of Canada's reconstruction program, Upham recommended her recent acquaintance Hilda B. Goodman, formerly of the Strathcoma Military Hospital in Edmonton, to organize and supervise practice teaching for Milwaukee-Downer's program. She and Sabin recruited their former student Esther Mabel Frame when

Frame completed her postgraduate studies at Teachers College. Upham invited Eleanor Clarke Slagle to lecture, as well as Milwaukee's finest physicians, social workers, and nurses. Upham's mother, still a Milwaukee-Downer College trustee, persuaded the board to establish not only a war emergency course but a permanent department of occupational therapy. Upham's family provided the money for it. Upham herself then filed for a leave of absence from the Federal Board for Vocational Education and anxiously awaited her return to Milwaukee to launch her own school.[57]

After a barrage of publicity in the Milwaukee papers, the war emergency course opened at Milwaukee-Downer College in fall 1918, just one month before the armistice agreement was signed. In an attempt to turn out only high-quality practitioners, the short course was open to college graduates only. It included six months of "intensive work in crafts" and then a series of lectures covering the "medical, psychological, sociological, economic and theoretical aspects of the work," followed by three months of hospital practice training.[58]

## PHILANTHROPIC SUPPORT AND THE SERVICE ETHIC

Many local chapters of charity and philanthropic organizations supported the opening of the Milwaukee-Downer College war emergency course. The Red Cross, the Junior League, the Russell Sage Foundation, the Milwaukee Community War Chest, and the National League for Women's Service sponsored scholarships for students and encouraged young women to take the course. The Junior League even provided for the establishment of a department of occupational therapy at Milwaukee's civilian Columbia Hospital. In a later newspaper article, the Junior League made it very clear that the department was under the league's authority, not the hospital's. "Though located at the hospital," the article stated, "the department is in no way connected with that institution, and is to be fostered and maintained solely through the work and efforts of the Junior League."[59]

Occupational therapy activities were supported by women's and charity organizations in other cities as well. From 1918 to 1919, Eleanor Clarke Slagle oversaw emergency courses in occupational therapy for the Chicago Chapter of the Red Cross.[60] In 1919 the School of Nursing at the Hospital of the University of Pennsylvania established an occupational therapy department in which several Philadelphia School of Occupational Therapy students volunteered their time.[61] In a few short years, charity money ensured the growth and the permanence of that department. Wealthy Philadelphian Mrs. Sabin W. Colton, Jr., funded a separate building to provide a "laboratory" for the department, which was "developing rapidly and . . . proving its value."[62] The newly founded Missouri Association for Occupational Therapy provided a workplace for its members, funding an occupational therapy department at the St. Louis City Hospital itself.[63]

The war emergency schools of occupational therapy conducted continuous publicity campaigns, acting while opportunity lasted. Milwaukee-Downer's occupational therapy department published several press releases stressing three important themes that were meant to ensure the department's future. The first theme centered on the importance of occupational therapy's role in adjusting soldiers to their "industrial responsibilities" in civilian life. The second theme underscored the scientific basis of occupational therapy, explaining how it alleviated "mental suffering" and relieved the "depression of slow convalescence."[64] The third theme stressed the appropriateness of such work for women, particularly women from the upper classes. In Wisconsin, society women with a history of civic volunteerism—or perhaps more accurately the daughters of such women, many of whom held an additional interest in the possibility of a professional career—found the opportunities offered by the reconstruction movement extremely compelling. "Society," one press release stated, is taking up a "new study to aid the wounded." In 1918 one wealthy Milwaukee woman said that "winning the wounded back to health" fast became the "task of the hour" among the women of "our social set."[65]

In Jamaica Plain, Massachusetts, Anna Wheelright Codman, the daughter of a wealthy mill owner, felt that she simply "must do something for these boys" when she volunteered to serve during the war. She was following the influential example of her "sympathetic" mother, who had frequently "visited" patients at the nearby Adams Nervine Asylum during Codman's early life. Codman was one of fourteen students enrolled in the Boston School of Occupational Therapy's second class; her mother was a friend of Marjorie Greene, the "leading light" of the school. Codman later said that many of her society peers thought that she and her friends who had decided to "do something" were "crazy," but her mother's "tremendous personality" and determination to allow Codman to go her own way sustained her commitment to the cause.[66]

Many reconstruction aides based their commitment to reconstruction work on examples given by their politically active families. Both of Elizabeth Greene Upham's parents, for example, were active in the women's suffrage movement in Wisconsin. They frequently attended and spoke at suffrage meetings, drawing their daughter into political life at an early age. Upham interpreted her parents' political activity to be part of their "sense of responsibility for the community." Their political activity also undergirded her basic belief in women having an equal place with men in public life.[67]

Other reconstruction aides saw no consistency between women's suffrage and public service. Lois Clifford of Pennsylvania came from a family of "rabid anti-suffragists." Her mother was the secretary of the Western Pennsylvania Anti-Suffrage Association. Young Clifford traveled all over the state with her mother on antisuffrage campaigns; she even helped chair a booth at the Exposition Hall in Pittsburgh. Yet Clifford's mother was also very active in settlement and club work during Clifford's formative years. By the time Clifford turned eighteen in 1910, she regularly taught crafts at a club for young working-class women in Pittsburgh and had joined her mother in membership in the Twentieth Century Club, the largest women's organization in the city.[68]

The Boston School of Occupational Therapy, founded during the war emergency as well, actively sought to attract wealthy "girls" to its doors. The society pages of many Boston newspapers reported that "society girls" had volunteered to "go overseas to teach wounded soldiers bedside occupations" after completing their training at the newly organized Boston School of Occupational Therapy. One group of four women who had been notified to be ready for immediate service felt that it was a "great honor" to do their part in the reconstruction effort.[69]

Service and patriotism attracted women to the field of occupational therapy, but so did its implicit elitism. Most of the schools of occupational therapy required at least some college training and considerable arts and crafts background of their recruits. For the most part, only white urban women from upper-middle-class or upper-class backgrounds met such requirements. These privileged women seemed also to have family support in choosing occupational therapy, judging by the widespread backing that the schools and the clinics received from women's clubs and charity networks.

Such backing might not have been forthcoming had these women chosen to enter nursing. As an evolving profession, nursing had certainly begun to overcome its status as unskilled labor and was considered respectable skilled work for women. Among the leisured classes, however, nursing still lacked prestige. Most nursing practice took place in private homes, and this left nurses with the legacy of being seen as servants rather than as professionals. The fact that nursing training occurred in hospitals posed further risk to a daughter's respectability, for these institutions were still seen more as repositories for the working class than as citadels of medical science.[70]

Also worrisome to parents was exposure of their daughters to contagious disease. In other words, parents did not want their daughters to give up the physical protection of the home. Training for nursing required a period of living and working in a hospital with lower-class diseased patients. Once graduated, many nurses took on private duty, which often meant living in the patient's home; if the patient was suffering from a contagious disease, the nurse was at risk. According to Susan Barnes, member of a well-known medical family in St. Louis, nursing as a career choice was declared out of the question by her family. In the 1920s, when young Susan and her twin sister persisted in their wish to serve society, they became occupational therapists.[71]

Families of occupational therapists also feared that their daughters would be exposed to contagious diseases. In 1920, Thomas B. Kidner pleaded with members of the National Society for the Promotion of Occupational Therapy to work in institutions for the care of patients with tuberculosis. "There is no safer place on earth than in a sanitorium," he told them. According to physician H. A. Pattison and nurse Mary Marshall of the National Tuberculosis Association, many prospective practitioners who were willing to work with patients who had tuberculosis, were prevented from doing so by their mothers and fathers.[72]

Parents discouraged their occupational therapist daughters from working in psychiatric care as well. When Beatrice Wade, a student at the University of Iowa in the early 1920s, was sent to Chicago to gain clinical experience in psychiatry, she had to lie to her mother about the assignment. Wade's older sister and brother conspired with her in telling their mother that she was going to a hospital for nervous people for two months rather than to the state mental hospital for three months. At the end of the two months, Wade wrote to her mother and admitted that she had to stay for one more month. Mrs. Wade responded by sending Wade's uncle to Chicago to fetch her. Wade spent an evening with her uncle, telling him all about the exciting work in which she was involved in Chicago. Apparently she persuaded her uncle to take her side. During dinner he said, "Bea, I think you know what you are doing. Do you know why I am here?" Realizing that her mother had sent him, she replied yes. He responded, "I was to take you home with me. But I'll go home and tell your mother to leave you alone." Young Wade was thrilled that she "got to stay." Later she specialized in psychiatric occupational therapy.[73]

## Typical Career Tracks of the Reconstruction Aide Generation

Many leaders of the occupational therapy movement intended to devote themselves to the profession for a lifetime. They were members of the generation of pioneer professional women who had chosen to remain single in order to work professionally. Many of the younger women volunteering to become reconstruction aides during the war emergency did not necessarily ascribe to this life choice, however. Nor did they necessarily wish to follow the home-centered life of more traditional women.

Young and single during the war years, better educated than their late-Victorian-era mothers, and imbued with the middle- and upper-class values that called them to serve society, they seemed to embody many of the traits of the era's so-called new woman.[74] They stretched the boundaries of their mothers' home-centered lives by facing the challenges of traveling overseas or across the continental United States to work in military and civilian hospitals. They asserted their individuality by leaving home and striking out on their own. They self-confidently took on the responsibilities of health care practice, not only among patients of their own class and background but among patients of other classes and backgrounds. They made new friendships with women outside their own communities, friendships forged by the experience of working together during and following the war. The social bonds between practitioners and their mentors created a strong group identity, separate from their families and communities of origin. For years to come, former reconstruction aides kept in contact with one another in warm friendships and in more formalized organizations such as the Women's Overseas Service League and the World War Reconstruction Aides Association, organized in 1922. In 1929, reconstruction aides held a first national reunion in Chicago.[75]

Reconstruction aides did not completely fit into the lifestyle of the new woman, however. New women expected individuality, work, and a full family life as well. If reconstruction aides expected such completeness, little evidence exists that they accomplished it. Information about the personal and career lives of nearly 900 former occupational therapy reconstruction aides, compiled in 1933, nearly fifteen years after the reconstruction period ended, reveals the following major life and career tracks: Approximately 5 percent left occupational therapy to pursue fields as diverse as teaching, writing, painting, small business ownership, landscape architecture, missionary work, and professional golf. Only a few combined these pursuits with marriage. Another 5 percent were still working in occupational therapy in 1933. Generally, these women had assumed leadership roles in the profession by becoming supervisors of hospital departments or officers of the American Occupational Therapy Association. None reported marriage in combination with these career choices. The third and largest group consisted of roughly 50 percent who stayed in occupational therapy until the years 1922–25, after which they left to marry.[76] Unfortunately, without a follow-up compilation, which might show that some women returned to the field, little evidence remains to suggest such a trend.

What is certain is that family responsibilities, or what Joyce Antler calls the "family claim," often shaped the career tracks of first-generation occupational therapists.[77] Socialized to identify themselves primarily as dutiful wives, daughters, or sisters, these women often gave priority to family commitments or crises over career. Many women who otherwise seemed totally devoted to building the profession left work in the field, at least temporarily, to care for ailing or aging parents or to raise children of their own or of close relatives. Elizabeth Greene Upham married Carl Henry Davis in 1919, for example, and then spent the next seventeen years raising four children. During that time she continued "interest and assistance" in Milwaukee's Curative Workshop and also was a "regular lecturer" in the Department of Occupational Therapy at Milwaukee-Downer College, but her primary responsibilities centered on her family.[78]

In 1919 an exhausted Eleanor Clarke Slagle divided her time and energy between an active career and trips home to New York to care for her critically ill mother. Head of the Henry B. Favill School of Occupations in Chicago, Slagle also held the position of general superintendent of the Occupational Therapy Department for the State of Illinois, which required her to travel all over the state in order to assess the need for occupational therapy services in hospitals following the war. She did all this while recovering from a serious attack of influenza.[79] Privately Slagle was torn between professional demands and her role as daughter. In a letter to her friend and mentor William R. Dunton, Slagle explained that she would not be able to visit him during her planned two-week November vacation: "Mother will probably need every minute of my spare time, and if she does need it of course it manifestly is my duty to stay [with her] and not go gallivanting around the country." Slagle stayed much longer than two weeks because she was still at her mother's home in mid-December when her mother suffered an acute heart attack. In late spring 1920, Slagle turned in her resignation in Illinois to return east on account of the death of her mother.[80]

Beatrice Wade interrupted her career for two-and-one-half years and broke a marriage engagement in order to help her brother raise five children after the death of his wife. When her brother remarried, Wade prepared herself to return to occupational therapy, and helped herself get over her close attachment to her nieces and nephews, by taking a postgraduate course at the Bloomingdale Hospital in New York City.[81]

Several former reconstruction aides reporting in 1933 also felt the pressure of the family claim.[82] Lois Clifford complained that she was "at home" serving as "assistant housekeeper and chauffeur."[83] Henrietta Failing asserted that she had "had to stop [working] because of nerves" and that her "present occupation" was "daughter-of-the-house and family chauffeur, a real job . . . not recognized by the census takers."[84] Ellen Harvey managed both to work and to take care of her mother after her father's death.[85] Florence Hogoboom raised her sister's child after the sister's early demise.[86] Myrtle Hoffman also raised her sister's child.[87] Gracia Loehl worked until 1924, when both of her parents became ill. She married a former patient after her parents died in 1926, and thereafter stayed active in the World War Reconstruction Aides Association.[88] Lovina Earle explained, "Father died, leaving mother alone. This necessitated giving up work to remain with her."[89] Mildred Vander Vort hoped to return to "some branch of the Occupational [sic] work" after her four children grew up.[90]

Immediately following World War I, the budding occupational therapy profession teetered between the success of gaining acceptance and the difficulty of being able continuously to supply competent practitioners. Attracting women to occupational therapy during the war had gone smoothly; keeping competent practitioners in the field seemed not so straightforward. Susan Cox Johnson estimated that "eighty percent of the Teachers College students who entered occupational therapy training did not wish to take up the work as a profession but only as a war service."[91] Critical to the continued development of occupational therapy was to sustain a supply of competent practitioners and to promote the growth of institutions for education and practice. Slagle's return to New York helped ensure a supply of personnel and the promotion of institutional growth because there she could draw on her previous connections to women supporting occupational therapy's cause. In cities all over the nation and in the ranks of the American Occupational Therapy Association, men and women of the first generation cooperated to build on the gains of the World War I era.

## Notes

1. A. G. Crane, *The Medical Department of the United States Army in the World War*, vol. 13, pt. 1, *Physical Reconstruction and Vocational Education* (Washington, D.C.: U.S. Government Printing Office, n.d.), 60. The chart on page 60 shows a total of 124 reconstruction aides in October 1918. The Surgeon General's Office did not differentiate between occupational therapists and physical therapists. On the basis of my analysis of Laura Brackett Hoppin, ed., *History of the World War Reconstruction Aides* (Millbrook, N.Y.: William Tyldsley, 1933), I have assumed that approximately half were occupational therapists. Page 79 of Crane, *The Medical Department*, describes the differences between "ward" and "shop" occupations.

2. Norma Howat, "Annual Meetings of the Occupational Therapy Profession, 1917–1929," typescript, Official Archives of the American Occupational Therapy Association, Wilma L. West Library, American Occupational Therapy Foundation, Bethesda, Maryland (hereafter AOTA Archives).

3. "[Report on the] Afternoon Session, Monday, September 8, 1919, [Remarks by] Dr. W. R. Dunton, Jr.," in *Proceedings of the Third Annual Meeting of the National Society for the Promotion of Occupational Therapy* (Towson, Md.: NSPOT, 1919), 41.

4. "Side Remarks by President Slagle," in *Proceedings of the Fourth Annual Meeting of the National Society for the Promotion of Occupational Therapy* (Towson, Md.: NSPOT, 1920), 4.

5. Howat, "Annual Meetings"; "President's Report," in *Proceedings of the Fourth Annual Meeting of NSPOT*, 3; Myra L. McDaniel, "Forerunners of the *American Journal of Occupational Therapy*," *American Journal of Occupational Therapy* 25 (1971): 41–52.

6. "Presidents of the American Occupational Therapy Association (1917–1967)," *American Journal of Occupational Therapy* 21 (1967, Fiftieth Anniversary Issue): 290–98.

7. "[Report on the] Morning Session, Monday, September 8, 1919," in *Proceedings of the Third Annual Meeting of NSPOT*, 36.

8. Since at least 1917, Susan Cox Johnson had believed that a physician ought to lead the association. In a letter to William R. Dunton dated August 9, 1917, she wrote, "I think you should become president of the society because I think we should have a physician in that position" (AOTA Archives). Details of the election can be found in "[Report on the] Morning Session, Monday, September 8, 1919," in *Proceedings of the Third Annual Meeting of NSPOT*, 35–36.

9. "Experience of Eleanor Clarke Slagle," resumé, 1922, Papers of the American Occupational Therapy Association, AOTA Archives.

10. "[Report on the] Afternoon Session, Monday, September 8, 1919, [Remarks by] Miss Addams," in *Proceedings of the Third Annual Meeting of NSPOT*, 39–41.

11. "Report of the Nominating Committee," in *Proceedings of the Fourth Annual Meeting of NSPOT*, 25–26.

12. "Address by President-elect Dr. Herbert J. Hall," in *Proceedings of the Fourth Annual Meeting of NSPOT*, 39.

13. "Presidents," 290–91.

14. Letter, Helen Mansfield to Major M. E. Haggerty, 17 August 1918, Surgeon General's Office Correspondence, 1917–27, National Archives, Washington, D.C. Printed on the letterhead below the school's name is the phrase, "Organized with the Approval of the Surgeon General, United States Army."

15. Letter, Helen Mansfield to Major Henry R. Hayes, 29 March 1918, Surgeon General's Office Correspondence, 1917–27, National Archives.

16. Dozens of letters pertaining to the establishment of standards were exchanged between staff of the Surgeon General's Office and occupational therapy leaders between January and June 1918. Some participants in this exchange were Helen Mansfield, George E. Barton, William R. Dunton, Jessie Goldthwait, Susan Cox Johnson, Eleanor Clarke Slagle, and Martha Wadsworth (Surgeon General's Office Correspondence, 1917–27, National Archives).

17. Some of the letters exchanged between Martha Wadsworth and staff of the Surgeon General's Office asking for clarification of her position were written February 5 and 13, 1918; April 9, 13, and 25, 1918;

and May 14, 1918. The letters can be found in Surgeon General's Office Correspondence, 1917–27, National Archives.

18. Letter, Mansfield to Hayes, 29 March 1918, Surgeon General's Office Correspondence, 1917–27, National Archives. Colonel Frank Billings of the Surgeon General's Office wrote to Margaret A. Neall, the corresponding secretary of the Philadelphia School of Occupational Therapy, on June 18, 1918, to say that the surgeon general did not want schools to "use his department as an authority for the continuation of the schools." He did not want to be responsible for encouraging women to enter the field "lest there be no chance for them to engage in the service within a reasonable time" [Papers of the Philadelphia School of Occupational Therapy, Department of Occupational Therapy, University of Pennsylvania, Philadelphia (hereafter Papers of the Philadelphia School of Occupational Therapy)]. The surgeon general was likely under the influence of James E. Russell, formerly dean of Teachers College, Columbia University, who had recently been appointed as the head of the Educational Department of the Division of Special Hospitals and Physical Reconstruction in the Surgeon General's Office. Russell planned not to use women reconstruction aides in hospital work; he hoped to employ the soldiers with disabilities themselves to "aid their fellow soldiers."

19. Ibid.

20. "Interests of Women," published in a Boston newspaper, April 1918, and "Will Serve as Reconstruction Aides in Hospitals Both Here and Abroad," published in the *Boston Post* (n.d.), both mention Wadsworth's visit to Boston before the founding of the Boston School of Occupational Therapy. In "Memorandum Regarding the Early History of Occupational Therapy in the United States," an unpublished memoir by Arthur L. Williston of the Wentworth Institute in Boston, Wadsworth is described as "the wife of the Senator, [who] had come from Washington to explain just how the School was to operate—apparently with expectation of dominating it." Sarah Lake, acting director of the Boston School of Occupational Therapy in its founding period, on leave from Miss Windsor's Private School for Girls, also handled Wadsworth tactfully. Lake invited Wadsworth to the school and respectfully placed her in an armchair in the corner as Lake interviewed prospective students. According to Williston, Lake patronized Wadsworth, but never actually took any "advice or counsel." Scrapbooks, Papers of the Boston School of Occupational Therapy, Wessell Library, Tufts University, Medford, Massachusetts (hereafter Papers of the Boston School of Occupational Therapy).

21. John William Leonard, ed., *Women's Who's Who in America, 1914–1915* (New York: American Commonwealth Company, 1914), 538; "Mrs. Howard Mansfield," obituary, *New York Times*, 16 August 1957.

22. "Mrs. Cornelius J. Sullivan," obituary, *New York Times*, December 6, 1939.

23. "New York War Service Classes for Reconstruction Aides in Occupational Therapy," pamphlet, summer 1918, AOTA Archives.

24. Ibid.

25. Ibid.

26. Ibid.

27. Helen Mansfield, ms., n.d., Papers of the New York War Service Classes for Training Reconstruction Aides in Occupational Therapy, AOTA Archives, unprocessed materials (hereafter Papers of the New York War Service Classes).

28. Ibid. Other schools also carefully screened students. Geraldine R. L. Lermit reported in a letter to the American Occupational Therapy Association dated April 7, 1955, that in 1917 the Henry B. Favill School of Occupations had 165 applicants, from whom it selected 16 (AOTA Archives).

29. Surgeon General's Office, "Circular of Information Concerning the Employment of Reconstruction Aides," no. 2, Medical Department of the United States Army, 27 March 1918, Surgeon General's Office Correspondence, 1917–27, National Archives.

30. "New York War Service Classes for Reconstruction Aides in Occupational Therapy," pamphlet, summer 1918, AOTA Archives.

31. "Student Applications," ms., ca. 1918, AOTA Archives, unprocessed materials; "New York War Service Classes for Reconstruction Aides in Occupational Therapy," pamphlet, summer 1918, AOTA Archives.

32. Letter, Mrs. Cornelius J. Sullivan to Major Frankwood E. Williams, 2 October 1918, Surgeon General's Office Correspondence, 1917–27, National Archives.

33. Ibid.

34. Mansfield, for example, wrote to Margaret A. Neall of the National League for Women's Service, who represented organizers of the Philadelphia School of Occupational Therapy (letter, 22 August 1918, Papers of the Philadelphia School of Occupational Therapy).

35. Letter, Mansfield to Marguerite Sanderson, 17 June 1918, Surgeon General's Office Correspondence, 1917–27, National Archives.

36. Letter, Mansfield to General Ireland, 4 December 1918, AOTA Archives, unprocessed materials.

37. Letter, Everett S. Elwood to Mansfield, 1 November 1919, AOTA Archives; Letter, Charles H. Johnson to Mansfield, 3 November 1919, AOTA Archives; Letter, Pearce Bailey to Mansfield, 5 November 1919, AOTA Archives; Letter, Thomas W. Salmon to Mansfield, 7 November 1919, AOTA Archives.

38. Letter, Colonel Frank Billings to Margaret A. Neall (Philadelphia School of Occupational Therapy), 18 June 1918, Papers of the Philadelphia School of Occupational Therapy. In this letter, Billings warns Neall, "There is a danger of an over supply of people trained to administer occupational therapy . . . Therefore the Surgeon

General has requested [that] schools . . . engaged in teaching . . . no longer use his department as an authority for the continuation of the schools. His fear is that to encourage women to enter upon this work at this time should be considered very carefully lest there be no chance for them to engage in the service within a reasonable time." On August 21, 1918, Ellen Sabin of Milwaukee-Downer College received a telegram from James E. Russell in the Surgeon General's Office with a mixed message about whether or not to open the emergency course: "You may use circular material. No school is certified" [Papers of Milwaukee-Downer College, University of Wisconsin–Milwaukee (hereafter Papers of Milwaukee-Downer College)].

39. See, for example, *Milwaukee Journal*, 6 October 1918.

40. *Milwaukee Sentinel*, 29 September 1918.

41. "A New Call for Women's Service," flyer, Papers of the Philadelphia School of Occupational Therapy.

42. Student notebook, unidentified emergency school in Michigan, AOTA Archives, unprocessed materials.

43. Letters between Jessie Goldthwait and the Surgeon General's Office, 13 February 1918, 20 February 1918, 23 February 1918, 27 February 1918, 18 April 1918, Surgeon General's Office Correspondence, 1917–27, National Archives. By April 26, 1918, the Boston School of Occupational Therapy had been declared one of four officially recognized teaching centers.

44. Schools all over the nation published flyers to attract students. They also published articles in local papers, and their leaders gave talks at women's clubs and schools.

45. See Margaret A. Neall, "Philadelphia School of Occupational Therapy," *Annals of the American Academy of Political and Social Science* 80 (November 1918): 58–66, for a brief description of the Philadelphia School of Occupational Therapy. Organized in spring 1918 in cooperation with the Central Branch of the National League for Women's Service, this school also pulled together socially and medically prominent men and women. In St. Louis, representatives from several organizations supported the school: the St. Louis Woman's Committee, the Council of National Defense, the Barnes Hospital, the St. Louis Children's Hospital, the St. Louis School of Fine Arts, the medical departments of St. Louis and Washington universities, and the Junior League, to name just a few. Alice Dean, a graduate of the Henry B. Favill School of Occupations in Chicago, was the first director. The school opened in fall 1918 with a class of fifteen students.

46. Eleanor Clarke Slagle, "The Training of Teachers for Occupational Therapy," in *Proceedings of the Second Annual Meeting of the National Society for the Promotion of Occupational Therapy* (Towson, Md.: NSPOT, 1918), 53.

47. Susan C. Johnson, "The Training of Teachers for Occupational Therapy," in *Proceedings of the Second Annual Meeting of NSPOT*, 53.

48. Letter, Elizabeth Upham to Ellen Sabin, 11 January 1918, Papers of Milwaukee-Downer College.

49. Jacqueline L. Jones, "Looking Back—Early Occupational Therapy Education in Wisconsin: Elizabeth Upham Davis and Milwaukee-Downer College," *American Journal of Occupational Therapy* 42 (1988): 527–33.

50. Jones, "Looking Back."

51. Elizabeth Upham Davis, "Early History of the Development of the Department of Occupational Therapy, Milwaukee-Downer College," ms., Elizabeth Davis file, State Historical Society of Wisconsin, Madison.

52. Letter, Rachel Horner Slocumb [to unidentifiable recipient], n.d., Papers of the Wisconsin Occupational Therapy Association, State Historical Society of Wisconsin, Madison.

53. Jones, "Looking Back," 530.

54. Davis, "Early History"; letter, Elizabeth Upham to President Ellen Sabin, 29 October 1917, Papers of Milwaukee-Downer College.

55. Letters, Upham to Sabin, 29 October 1917, 11 November 1917, 11 January 1918, 29 March 1918, 17 June 1918, 22 June 1918, 13 July 1918, Papers of Milwaukee-Downer College.

56. Letter, Upham to Sabin, 22 June 1918, Papers of Milwaukee-Downer College.

57. "Elizabeth Upham Davis," resumé, ca. 1948, Elizabeth Davis file, State Historical Society of Wisconsin.

58. *Milwaukee-Downer College Bulletin*, series 1, no. 2, *Occupational Therapy* (Milwaukee, Wisc.: November 1918), Papers of Milwaukee-Downer College.

59. Bernice Sanborn, "Milwaukee-Downer College Offers Courses in Occupational Theraphy [sic]; A War Measure; Crippled Sick Will Be Benefited," *Milwaukee Sentinel*, 20 October 1918; *Milwaukee-Downer College Bulletin*, November 1918.

60. "Experience of Eleanor Clarke Slagle," resumé, 1922, Papers of the American Occupational Therapy Association, AOTA Archives.

61. Mary Virginia Stephenson, *The First Fifty Years of the Training School for Nurses of the Hospital of the University of Pennsylvania* (Philadelphia: J. B. Lippincott Company, 1940), 138–39.

62. *Fifty-first Annual Report of the Board of Managers of the Hospital of the University of Pennsylvania* (July 1, 1924, to June 30, 1925), p. 17, Archives of the Hospital of the University of Pennsylvania, Philadelphia.

63. "Extract from Annual Report, St. Louis City Hospital, April 1920," typescript, Papers of the St. Louis School of Occupational Therapy, School of Medicine Library, Washington University, St. Louis, Missouri (hereafter Papers of the St. Louis School of Occupational Therapy). Idelle Kidder, director of the Missouri Association for Occupational Therapy, stated in the first annual report that the asso-

ciation was supporting three hospitals: the Barnes Hospital, the St. Louis City Hospital, and the City Sanitarium ("First Annual Report of the Missouri Association for Occupational Therapy, 1919–1920," Papers of the St. Louis School of Occupational Therapy).

64. Following is a sample of articles that appeared in local newspapers based on the department's press releases: "Should Plan Now to Re-Educate the Disabled," *Milwaukee Free Press*, 13 September 1918; "Teach Disabled Soldiers: Women to Be Taught Important After-War Work at Downer," *Milwaukee Journal*, 15 September 1918; "Fit Selves to Aid Maimed: Lectures for Students in War Work Study at Downer," 29 September 1918 (Papers of Milwaukee-Downer College).

65. "Society Here Takes Up New Study to Aid the Wounded," *Milwaukee Journal*, 26 January 1919; "Cure Soldiers by Work: Hospital Workshop for Disabled Army Men Is League Plan; Women to Study Occupational Therapy and Give Services to Hospitals; Plan Theater Benefit to Finance Move," *Milwaukee Journal*, 13 October 1918; Papers of Milwaukee-Downer College.

66. Anna Wheelright Codman, interview by Nedra Gillette, 6 August 1986, Oral History Collection, American Occupational Therapy Foundation, Bethesda, Maryland (hereafter Oral History Collection).

67. Elizabeth Upham Davis, interview by Nedra Gillette, 12 October 1983, Oral History Collection.

68. Lois Clifford, interview by Helen Hopkins, May 1986, Oral History Collection.

69. The following newspaper articles are contained in scrapbooks among the Papers of the Boston School of Occupational Therapy: "34 Society Girls Taking an Intensive Course of Training; Will Serve as Reconstruction Aides in Hospitals Both Here and Abroad," *Boston Journal*, 10 May 1918; "Teach Wounded Men Bedside Occupations: Society Girls to Teach Bedside Occupations," *Boston Post*, 30 June 1918; "Girls Learn to Carve to Teach Wounded: Society Girl Members of Wood Carving Class," *Boston Post*, n.d.

70. Susan M. Reverby, *Ordered to Care: The Dilemma of American Nursing, 1850–1945* (Cambridge: Cambridge University Press, 1987), 95–117.

71. Susan Barnes, personal conversation with author, St. Louis, Missouri, March 1990.

72. "Report of the Committee on Research and Efficiency," in *Proceedings of the Fourth Annual Meeting of NSPOT*, 6.

73. Beatrice Wade, interview by Nedra Gillette, Chicago, 1983, Oral History Collection.

74. Discussions of the new woman can be found in Nancy Cott, *The Grounding of Modern Feminism* (New Haven, Conn.: Yale University Press, 1982); Carroll Smith-Rosenberg, *Disorderly Conduct: Visions of Gender in Victorian America* (New York: Oxford University Press, 1985); and Lois Rudnick, "The New Woman," in *1915: The Cultural*

*Moment*, ed. Adele Heller and Lois Rudnick (New Brunswick, N.J.: Rutgers University Press, 1991), 69–81.

75. Newspaper announcement, Papers of the New York War Service Classes, AOTA Archives, unprocessed materials.

76. The comments in this and later paragraphs are based on my analysis of Laura Brackett Hoppin, ed., *History of the World War Reconstruction Aides* (Millbrook, N.Y.: William Tyldsley, 1933). The book is a compilation of raw information about 1,844 former reconstruction aides who were alive in 1933. The information included, in most cases, is name (in alphabetical order), current address, place of service (Fort Snelling, Fort McHenry, etc.), present place of employment, marital status, and number of children. Often entries hold greetings to others and further information about personal and professional life. Because the editor gives no explanation about how the information was gathered, interpreting certain aspects of it is difficult. For example, how the former reconstruction aides were identified as either occupational therapists or physical therapists is not explained. Therefore, what is the significance of the fact that nearly half of the women, or 877, were clearly identified as occupational therapists; 513 were labeled physical therapists; and the remaining 454 were not categorized at all? Does it mean that many of the women identified themselves more as reconstruction aides than as anything else?

77. Discussions of the family claim can be found in Joyce Antler, "'After College, What?': New Graduates and the Family Claim," *American Quarterly* 32 (Fall 1980): 409–34; and Antler, "Was She a Good Mother?" in *Women and Social Structure*, ed. Barbara Harris and Jo Ann McNamara (Durham, N.C.: Duke University Press, 1984), 57.

78. "Elizabeth Upham Davis," resumé, ca. 1948, Elizabeth Davis file, State Historical Society of Wisconsin; as cited in Jones, "Looking Back," passim.

79. "Experience of Eleanor Clarke Slagle," resumé, 1922, Papers of the American Occupational Therapy Association, AOTA Archives.

80. Letters, Eleanor Clarke Slagle to William R. Dunton, January 1920; Dunton to Slagle, 29 March 1920, AOTA Archives.

81. Beatrice Wade, interview by author, Chicago, March 1990.

82. Hoppin, *History of the Reconstruction Aides*.

83. Ibid., 26.

84. Ibid., 37.

85. Ibid., 46.

86. Ibid., 52.

87. Ibid.

88. Ibid., 64.

89. Ibid., 34.

90. Ibid., 100.

91. Susan C. Johnson, ms., ca. 1920, History of Nursing Collection, microfiche 0513, Milbank Memorial Library, Teachers College, Columbia University. See pages 1–4 for positions occupied by former occupational therapy students.

# Part III

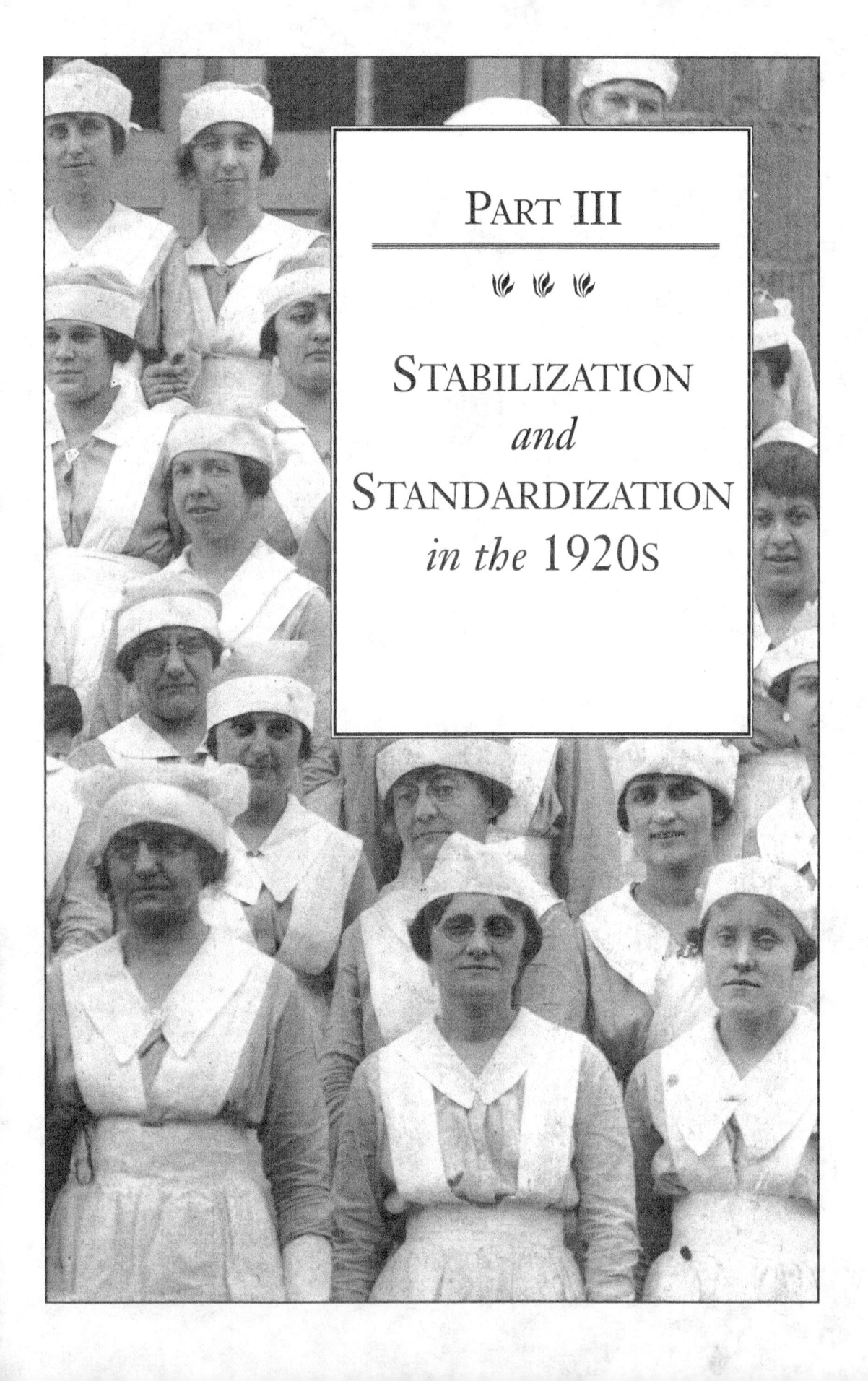

## Stabilization *and* Standardization *in the* 1920s

## Introduction

> The Philadelphia School of Occupational Therapy was founded by the National League for Women's Service ... One of the notable features which has characterized the work in Philadelphia from the first has been the splendid co-operation of big men and women,—busy people who saw the need and opportunity. Not only did they support the movement in its beginning, connected as it was with war work, but are now standing squarely behind the movement to enlarge the work and make it permanent.
>
> *Dr. Arthur J. Jones, professor of secondary education, in a speech given at the Third Annual Meeting of the National Society for the Promotion of Occupational Therapy, Chicago, 1919*

> It is unfortunate that the 250,000 or more patients in the hospitals today cannot have advantage of occupational therapy; but, instead of supplying such workers, I would rather go slowly, build up a good organization of well-trained people and put them in hospitals, and then it will be permanent. Otherwise it will be forgotten inside of a few years.
>
> *Frankwood E. Williams, associate medical director, National Committee for Mental Hygiene, in a speech given at the Third Annual Meeting of the National Society for the Promotion of Occupational Therapy, Chicago, 1919*

In the decade following World War I, many emergency schools and clinics remained open and continued to attract practitioners to "the new profession for women," although not at the boom pace so characteristic of the war years. As the 1920s unfolded, leaders and many practitioners began to realize the necessity of establishing national standards for practice and training, even in the context of vast expansion occurring in American health care in general. The existing heterogeneous work force, made up of arts and crafts instructors (mainly working in mental hospitals), emergency-trained reconstruction aides, and a few college-educated practitioners, had to be made uniform in order to advance occupational therapy on the continuum of professionalization. Resisting pressure from the larger world of medicine, which demanded greater numbers of health care workers, the American Occupational Therapy Association put quality before quantity in 1923 by adopting minimum standards for the training of practitioners. In 1929 the association followed the example of the American Nursing Association by establishing a national registry that defined a hierarchy of practitioners.

Even more critical to sustaining occupational therapy as a profession was the necessity for practitioners clearly to identify themselves as occupational therapists, not reconstruction aides. In other words, practitioners had to transform their self-identity from altruistic volunteer to professional with career aspirations. This was no easy task, given that so many of the women had entered the field because of the crisis atmosphere. As the crisis waned, leaders in the occupational therapy movement had to shift the ideology of recruitment from "Do your bit" to the financial, professional, and personal satisfaction of being an occupational therapist. To do so, the leadership had to continue building and stabilizing the profession's educational and practice institutions, and create more inroads into the care of patients with chronic illness.

To ensure the profession's growth, occupational therapy leadership leaned heavily on the tradition of women's charity and club networks. Yet the very tradition that provided moral and financial support often prevented practitioners from seeing themselves as professionals. In the early 1920s, only a few occupational therapists saw any reason to change the tradition of volunteer charity worker for a model of paid medical professional. Women such as Eleanor Clarke Slagle, Susan Cox Johnson, and Elizabeth Upham Davis worked with the men connected to the American Occupational Therapy Association to shape the field into a health profession. As they took on different areas of activity to help occupational therapy progress, the characteristic division of labor by gender carried on into the 1920s.

For the women who had experienced the heady days of helping reconstruct soldiers, sailors, and other patients with chronic illness, the top priority became strengthening existing local institutions for training and practice. Loyalty to peers, mentors, school, and workplace undergirded their activities. Volunteerism, social connections, female camaraderie, fundraising, public relations efforts, and sheer will kept many an institution afloat during this pivotal period in occupational therapy's history. Slowly, however, leaders realized that they had to transcend such a local focus to ensure the profession's growth and development; isolated practitioners had to be persuaded to identify with the aims of the profession at large. Eventually members of the occupational therapy movement organized on the state or regional level. Some even concerned themselves with national issues, overcoming a widespread indifference toward the American Occupational Therapy Association.

While the women spent most of their energy building the profession from the inside, the men involved in the movement concentrated on convincing outsiders of the value of occupational therapy. Herbert James Hall, Thomas B. Kidner, and C. Floyd Haviland held the presidency of the American

Occupational Therapy Association during the 1920s. These men moved in prominent circles of psychiatry, rehabilitation, and care of persons with tuberculosis, respectively, and were key to making sure that occupational therapy played important roles in these medical specialties.

This section examines the crucial decade of the 1920s, in which occupational therapy stabilized its professional identity. To accomplish this goal, occupational therapy gained control over practice and practitioners by standardizing practice and curriculum, establishing entry and exit criteria for schools, and expanding opportunities in the care of persons with chronic illness. Further, the profession created and nurtured a well-trained elite corps of leaders. Also crucial in this period was the strengthening of communication between the American Occupational Therapy Association and other organized medical groups—the American Hospital Association, the American Medical Association, the National Tuberculosis Association, and more. Using such linkages, the first generation of occupational therapists, allied with their male supporters, set the profession squarely in a medical model.

# Chapter 8

❦ ❦ ❦

# Professional Culture *and* Education *in* Occupational Therapy *in the* 1920s

*Professional Culture and Education in Occupational Therapy in the 1920s*

Beatrice Wade was in her sophomore year at the University of Iowa in 1922 when she met Professor Jenny Kaye Allen, a former reconstruction aide who was aggressively recruiting liberal arts students into occupational therapy. Allen directed the last two years of Wade's bachelor's program, sending her to a nearby children's hospital to work with orthopedic patients and to Chicago to a clinic founded by Eleanor Clarke Slagle for psychiatric clinical experience. Wade was smitten, and when she graduated in 1924, her greatest concern was whether she would be able to find work in this exciting new field. She asked her mentor where to inquire. Allen replied that she had twice tried to persuade local neuropsychiatrist Samuel T. Orton to create a position for an occupational therapist, but he had refused. Even though he had come to Iowa from Boston, where occupational therapy was well-known, he was not convinced that it would help his patients. On Allen's advice Wade went to Orton and asked if she might spend the summer caring for a few patients on a volunteer basis. Orton agreed, telling her that he was "promising nothing." By the end of the summer, Wade had secured full-time employment, probably, she said later, because she individualized programs for the patients. In Boston, she surmised, Orton had seen only groups of patients working in "classes," which would not have been as effective.[1]

Wade never felt that she had continuously to prove herself to the skeptical psychiatrist; she was quite confident in her own abilities. She just "went along with [her] job in the way Miss Allen had instilled" in her. Wade evaluated herself by the standards of her mentor, with whom she shared social values that stressed service to the community. She did not see herself as a joiner of organizations or as a builder of a profession. Looking back during a 1990 interview in Chicago, she commented that she had thought proving the value of the work was the concern of the American Occupational Therapy Association, which was not out in the Midwest yet.[2]

Later in the 1990 interview Wade said that the association had not made it "over the Appalachians" until the late 1920s. She was articulating a common complaint among midwestern and western practitioners of that era. In Wade's case, however, a more accurate version of her connection with the American Occupational Therapy Association would be that she went to the association rather than the association's going to her. In 1929, Wade took a postgraduate course at one of the best psychiatric facilities in the United States, New York City's Bloomingdale Hospital. There she worked with occupational therapists Paula Gunderson, who oversaw the women patients, and Louis Haas, one of the very few male practitioners in the field, who ran the men's section. Louis Sprague was the psychiatrist in charge. After the experience of being at the Bloomingdale Hospital, Wade found it difficult to work in settings such as the Occupational Therapy Department at Chicago's Michael Reese Hospital, where her work involved "taking crafts to the bedside, . . . making stuffed animals and selling them." The women's auxiliary ran and financed the program. Wade found that she could not agree with "their theory," or rather their lack of one. The department's emphasis on crafts did not satisfy Wade, who had begun to internalize a medical model of occupational therapy.[3]

She could not continue in occupational therapy "at that level," Wade explained, and thereafter she became involved in the national association. She began this involvement when Eleanor Clarke Slagle recruited her to speak in roundtable discussions on psychiatric topics at several national conferences.[4] Wade followed in the footsteps of Slagle, who skillfully embodied the continuum from individual service to professional career.

## Professional Culture: Recruitment, Mentoring, and Networking

Wade's initial attraction to occupational therapy, characterized by the personal relationship that she shared with Jenny Kaye Allen (which incidentally preceded her intellectual interest in the work), exemplifies a grass-roots recruiting system devised and practiced by the first generation of occupational therapists. Certainly Helen Mansfield of the New York War Service Classes for Training Reconstruction Aides in Occupational Therapy, who was well placed in the world of organized womanhood in New York City, used her personality to attract women to reconstruction aide work during the war mobilization. Women like Mansfield and Allen, who had internalized the social and civic duty to serve, spoke to the ready ears of many young women with similar values who were ripe for calling to a meaningful vocation such as occupational therapy.

Many recruits developed strong bonds with, and in some cases a nearly religious reverence toward, mentors who had converted them to occupational therapy. Allen, according to Wade, "idolized" her own mentor, Eleanor Clarke Slagle, whom she had known since her training at the Henry B. Favill School of Occupations in Chicago. On occasion Slagle used the religious language of the Progressive Era's so-called social gospel in exhorting her colleagues to remain loyal and devoted to the cause of occupational therapy. For example, in 1920 she promised that they would "see in [their] own day . . . [their] work ministering to the highest needs of man."[5] As Allen had idolized Slagle, so did Wade look up to both women influencing her to devote her life to the cause. Wade shaped her ever-evolving professional self-image by modeling herself after them. Moreover, these relationships sustained her own determination to go on in a field whose status at the time was at best questionable.

During the 1920s the bonds created between recruiters and recruits often continued in long-term mentor-protegé relationships. Typically operating on the local level, the relationships effectively distracted many practitioners from attending to the formal trappings of the profession, especially a national association. Yet some became interested in developing the national association, ironically because of the organizational experience that women had gained from traditional club work. Observation showed them that much more could be accomplished by joining small, local groups into a national network. (The suffrage campaign was an excellent example of the power of women's organizing to accomplish a goal.) Thus the first generation of occupational therapists took the best traditions of women's organizations and reshaped them to make the new profession.

Slagle had exercised skills in grass-roots recruiting, mentoring, and networking while she lived and worked in the Midwest. When she returned to New York during the early 1920s, she perfected the skills into a system. More than interacting with individual colleagues or serving as a mentor to new recruits, she networked with club women to promote the field. Slagle understood the crucial role that women's clubs had played during the war years, and she planned to continue cooperative relationships with organized womanhood in the years to come. She nurtured relationships with Helen Mansfield and Mrs. Cornelius J. Sullivan of the New York War Service Classes for Training Reconstruction Aides in Occupational Therapy, for example, by involving them in both the national association and the New York State Occupational Therapy Association.

She also invited collaboration from women club leaders whom she knew through her family's earlier philanthropic activities. President Hewitt of the New York State Federation of Women's Clubs, according to Slagle, had known her before she identified herself as a professional woman. Hewitt worked with Slagle because she believed that the National Society for the Promotion of Occupational Therapy and the New York State Federation of Women's Clubs shared aims. Hewitt and her 275,000 members were committed to tackling problems in child welfare, public health, education, and what she called "humanity," or promoting "better ways and means for the betterment of . . . defectives, misfits, and unfortunates." At the annual meeting of the National Society for the Promotion of Occupational Therapy in 1920, Hewitt told members that the General Federation of Women's Clubs, with its two million enfranchised women, would bring "spiritual" and political power to the movement. She pledged the club women's vote to help pass federal bills to provide funding for the "humanitarian" and "good business" aims of bringing "human souls" back "to the plane of independent action."[6]

Slagle followed up immediately on the offer of collaboration with the General Federation of Women's Clubs. In late fall 1920 she took the position of chair of the Committee on Occupational Therapy, Division of Health, General Federation of Women's Clubs. Her duties involved educating women to use occupational therapy in hospital and community activities across the nation, which dovetailed with her duties as chair of the Committee on Installations and Advice of the National Society for the Promotion of Occupational Therapy. For the latter committee, Slagle used her influence to organize new clinics and workshops all over the United States; her role with the General Federation of Women's Clubs committee was nearly identical. During her first year Slagle appointed twenty-four chairs of occupational therapy committees in state federation chapters. She then sent recommendations for initiating occupational therapy projects to each of these chapters. In 1921, Slagle brainstormed with the members of the National Society for the Promotion of Occupational Therapy, asking them to generate more recommendations to pass on to federation members at the biennial meeting to be held at Chautauqua, New York, in June 1922. Realizing the opportunity for publicity that the Chautauqua meeting offered, she arranged for occupational therapy schools to prepare exhibitions. Slagle also urged each school to send a representative to talk "scholarships, local programmes [sic], state program legislation, the particular problem of the home-bound, and how club women can help intelligently." She underscored the importance of participating in the Chautauqua events by saying, "We have this chance with the largest organized group of women in the *world* [emphasis in original]—what will you do with it?"[7]

In 1921, Slagle interacted with several Junior League and General Federation of Women's Clubs state chapters, using grass-roots organizing methods. She advised Junior League groups setting up workshops in Detroit, Michigan; Bridgeport and Stamford, Connecticut; and the Oranges, New Jersey. She gathered lecture fees for club talks and donated them to build a state organization of occupational therapists in New York. At Ogdensburg, New York, she urged Northern New York Federation of Women's Club members to study their own communities and then raise funds to send students to training schools, with scholarships when appropriate.[8]

Slagle was as comfortable in speaking at various medical profession meetings as she was in working with the women's clubs. In 1921 she organized a group of speakers and an exhibition for the annual meeting of the National Tuberculosis Association. Male associates Philip King Brown, Herbert James Hall, and H. A. Pattison supported the cause by giving talks on occupational therapy at the meeting. Slagle recalled delightedly that the physicians spoke not about "what occupational therapy is . . . but how it is given!" Hall and she both appeared at the annual meeting of the American Psychiatric Association, he speaking on financial considerations and she on starting new departments of occupational therapy, from the viewpoint of the practitioner. That year Slagle wrote plans for two large tuber-

*Professional Culture and Education in Occupational Therapy in the 1920s*

culosis sanatoriums in Tennessee and Indiana. She also toured the country to give keynote talks at the launchings of at least six state associations and training schools.[9] During 1922, Slagle continued her networking by visiting several state occupational therapy associations, other medical associations, schools, women's clubs, and hospitals in Wisconsin, Illinois, Indiana, Ohio, the District of Columbia, and Minnesota, where according to a later comment, she met William Mayo of the famous Mayo Clinic.[10]

Slagle attended to the association's locating its offices physically with other organizations representing health professions. After obtaining the approval of the board of the American Occupational Therapy Association at its mid-year meeting in February 1922, Slagle rented a room from the National Health Council to serve as headquarters for the association. (Previously Slagle, in her role as secretary-treasurer, had conducted most association business from her own apartment, keeping all official files in a packing box in the kitchen.) The association shared its prestigious midtown-Manhattan address in a modern office building with other nursing and health organizations, including the National Committee for Mental Hygiene and the National Tuberculosis Association. Aside from sharing the rent and other overhead costs, the organizations collectively hired clerical staff to provide basic office services. Association office work became so heavy in 1922 that Slagle tried to persuade the board to hire a half-time stenographer-clerk. She regularly corresponded with medical authorities all over the country; she singlehandedly conducted a placement service for therapists, naming sixty-seven candidates for positions that year; and she received dues and sent routine correspondence to the association members. In another gesture tying occupational therapy to the larger world of medicine, she sent 3,805 invitations to the planned Sixth Annual Meeting of the American Occupational Therapy Association in Atlantic City, New Jersey, where the American Hospital Association was scheduled to meet concurrently.[11]

Meeting in Atlantic City was a hotly contested issue among American Occupational Therapy Association members, not because of opposition to the idea of meeting with another medical organization, but because of the proposed East Coast location. Only one previous annual meeting had taken place elsewhere than on the East Coast (the 1919 meeting, in Chicago; the 1917 and 1918 meetings had taken place in New York, the 1920 meeting in Philadelphia, and the 1921 meeting in Baltimore.) To members residing and working all over the

United States, such an East Coast bias made the national association and its meetings inaccessible. At the 1921 meeting, several midwestern representatives tried to take the 1922 meeting to Milwaukee, Wisconsin, but in the voting, Milwaukee came in second, behind Boston, which was favored by the stronger eastern contingent.[12]

Midwestern representatives confronted the issue of the association's East Coast power monopoly at the mid-year meeting of the board. Elizabeth Upham Davis from Milwaukee and Idelle Kidder from St. Louis described a variety of sentiments expressed by practitioners in Wisconsin, Missouri, and Illinois. Davis herself was conflicted. She was one of the few occupational therapists in the Midwest with strong personal and professional ties to association leaders in the East; therefore she saw value in organizing nationally. Her midwestern colleagues resisted the idea, however. Most preferred strengthening their own state and local groups to expending the time, the energy, and the money to associate themselves with the East. Davis quoted them as saying, "What is the national association to us? . . . It is represented by a few people in the East who are very courteous, but . . . it doesn't mean anything to us. Let us support our locals."[13]

Kidder's contingent was more than indifferent toward the national association; it was antagonistic. Kidder went so far as to suggest that the eastern contingent was elitist and possibly did not appreciate the accomplishments of the reconstruction aides in her region and beyond. She quoted her group as saying, "The East must realize that Illinois, Wisconsin, Michigan and Missouri are east to the many aides far west of us who did very conscientious work during the war—and some of them are at the present time little interested in the American Occupational Therapy Association . . . When one sees the vast numbers of invalids along our western coast it is hard not to feel almost resentful that more publicity and education from the national association is not gotten out to them."[14]

The association finally decided to put aside this regional rivalry and make a decision that was better for the profession at large. Meeting with other medical groups offered networking opportunities that were essential to the growth of occupational therapy. The possibility of national attention overcame local loyalties and petty differences; over 1,000 people were expected to attend the proposed Atlantic City meeting. Participants would include members of the Social Hygiene Association and the American Dietitians Association as well as physicians from all fields. American Occupational Therapy Association members hoped that by meeting with these other organizations, they could "put the message over to the physicians" or "divert some [of the other health professionals] to [their] meetings." From 1922 through 1929 the annual meetings were held jointly with the American Hospital Association, making the location of the annual meeting a moot issue. No longer did the American Occupational Therapy Association have the responsibility of deciding where to meet; that was assumed by the American Hospital Association.[15]

## THE BEGINNINGS OF EDUCATION REFORM

During the pivotal early 1920s, as some members of the association found ways to enlarge occupational therapy's circle nationally, others focused on strengthening the profession from the center. Susan Cox Johnson and Elizabeth Upham Davis served on the Committee on Admissions and Positions, which they defined as having the following duties: to standardize education requirements, to establish a hierarchy of practitioners, and to conduct studies to gather information about the actual conditions under which occupational therapy practitioners worked.[16]

Because this committee pushed for self-regulation, there was potential for conflict with the general membership and the community of club women. The committee's recommendation to raise education standards threatened to alienate many practitioners who had received their training in the war emergency schools. Johnson wanted to hold a high standard for the education of practitioners. Her position subtly implied that the emergency schools, many of which had been set up by women's charity networks, were inferior. Although she acknowledged that the emergency schools had served a useful purpose during the war, she openly expressed fear for the success of the new profession if underqualified practitioners entered the field. Referring to the important role that the individual practitioner played in ensuring occupational therapy's future, Johnson bluntly said, "If she fails, all else will fail." Johnson recommended adopting some kind of certification system and also eventually eliminating many of the independent emergency schools founded during the war. She favored placing the training schools in already established educational institutions, such as Teachers College, with which she was affiliated, or Milwaukee-Downer College, with which her colleague Davis was associated. Johnson argued that the status already held by colleges would make it easier for occupational therapy to establish itself. She wanted future occupational therapists to hold college degrees so that occupational therapy would "gain . . . all the more quickly a recognized place among other professions."[17] At the fifth annual meeting, held in late 1921, Johnson called for the establishment of a standing committee specifically devoted to education issues.[18] Herbert J. Hall, president of the association, created the Committee on Education and named Johnson its chair.

Johnson's anxieties were shared by many members of the occupational therapy education community, judging from the protracted discussions that took place at the national meetings throughout the early 1920s. Individual schools looked to the national association for guidance. The director of the Philadelphia School of Occupational Therapy, Mrs. Frederick Rockwell, expressed the expectations this way: "Those of us who are interested in the schools and educational side of occupational therapy want to keep in touch and be sure the society is holding something above us constantly. We have always felt that the society held the standard higher than we have all reached." Idelle Kidder of St. Louis, despite her resentment of the East Coast monopoly on power, looked to the national association for help in establishing high standards and promoting excellent training. She succinctly articulated the problem that occupational therapy faced when she said, "We believe courses should not be lengthened too rapidly to seriously hinder hospitals in being able to open occupational therapy departments, nor the standards be lowered by shortening courses so that existing and future departments cannot continue with well-trained aides."[19]

With this consensus backing them, Johnson and the Committee on Education started their formidable task by evaluating the status of the profession. Johnson was under considerable pressure from Teachers College to prove that occupational therapy was a viable field for the college's students. In 1919, after receiving replies to a questionnaire from 133 mental hospitals and tuberculosis sanatoriums, she had been able to justify continuing to train practitioners by demonstrating to the head of the Department of Nursing and Health, Adelaide Nutting, how many hospitals had organized occupational therapy departments during and immediately following the war, how many practitioners they employed, and how many practitioners they estimated would be needed in the future. The demand far exceeded the supply. Not only had Teachers College's own list of eligible candidates for placement "long . . . been exhausted," but according to a communication from Slagle, all of her students from the Henry B. Favill School of Occupations had "received civil or military appointments."[20]

The Teachers College program reached its greatest heights in the late 1910s in turning out large numbers of highly qualified practitioners. Many went on to do volunteer work at several military and civilian hospitals in the New York City area and in other parts of the country. Some became leaders in the field by taking supervisory positions in hospitals or working for state and national associations. Johnson's program, which included several liberal arts, nursing, and craft courses, and an outstanding practical stint at the Montefiore Home and Hospital for Chronic Diseases, had no equal in the New York metropolitan area.[21]

In just a few years, however, enrollment in the Teachers College program plummeted, even though Johnson had demonstrated a need to her own administration and offered excellent training.[22] Johnson realized that if occupational therapy hoped to continue recruiting high-quality candidates, it had to provide steady employment, a respectable salary range, and decent working conditions. In reality the field held no such promise in the 1920s, according to the 1922 study by the Committee on Education. After receiving 108 completed questionnaires from medical superintendents all over the United States, Johnson concluded that conditions for service and salary ranged so widely that "no standard exist[ed]." Salaries of so-called head aides ranged from $510 to $2,500 a year. Some practitioners had two weeks of vacation per year while others had thirty days. Educational background was the most diverse category: "recently established centers" employed practitioners who had received their training in college art schools; "older centers, especially public hospitals," employed practitioners who had "received their training only through experience in the hospital"; a mere handful of practitioners had graduated from schools of occupational therapy. Practitioners did not even have a common name: although some were called "occupation aide" or "occupation therapist," others held the title of "industrial supervisor," "industrial aide," "industrial teacher," "reconstruction aide," "attendant," "craft teacher," "manual training teacher," or finally, "teacher."[23]

In spite of all Johnson's efforts, the training of occupational therapists at Teachers College, under the direction of the Department of Nursing and Health, ceased by 1924 for many reasons. Lack of sufficient enrollment was the obvious problem, but also important was the fact that occupational therapy did not really belong in the nursing department. Occupational therapy and nursing had to sever ties completely to ensure their independence; terminating a joint academic department was a necessary step in that direction. Further evidence of dissolving ties between nursing and occupational therapy appears in nurse Susan E. Tracy's evolving relationship with the American Occupational Therapy Association. Tracy discontinued active involvement in the association in 1923, when she dropped her role as chair of the Committee on Teaching Methods. Ruth Wigglesworth from the Boston School of Occupational Therapy, an institution that would rapidly take a leadership role in reforming occupational therapy education, appropriately took over the position. Wigglesworth tried to make her colleagues understand that their duty was to train "medical workers," not "teachers of occupational therapy" or nurses who taught crafts. Such a distinct medical identity, separate from nursing and teaching, she argued, was vital to practitioners who had to win the cooperation of physicians.[24]

Susan Cox Johnson lost her central role in reforming occupational therapy education when her institutional affiliation with Teachers College terminated. She remained active as a practitioner, however, taking important positions in several of New York's charity-based institutions for the care of persons with chronic illness. By 1923 she had left the occupational therapy department that she had helped establish at the Montefiore Home and Hospital for Chronic Diseases to direct the Jefferson Needle-Craft Shop, a center for women with tuberculosis. From 1925 until her death from pneumonia in 1932, she directed the Convalescent Workshop in New York City, which was under the authority of the Visiting Committee of the State Charities Aid Association.[25]

Johnson's career was distinguished; certainly her leadership in the development of the association and the profession in general was an important legacy. However, she did not realize her ambition to see the training of occupational therapists take place mainly in college settings. Occupational therapy still could not claim a professional status equal to that of other women's fields such as teaching and nursing.

The other New York school that had been so crucial to the development of the profession during the war also ceased to exist in the postwar period. The New York War Service Classes for Training Reconstruction Aides in Occupational Therapy closed because the leaders, Helen Mansfield and Mrs. Cornelius J. Sullivan, both from the art world rather than from a specifically medical orientation, decided to direct their energy into other projects. Mansfield and Sullivan helped Eleanor Clarke Slagle set up a special summer school program in a rural community in upstate New York. In 1921, at the short-lived Byrdcliffe School, Sullivan tapped well-used women's charity and art networks to bring outstanding artists to the idyllic setting (near the New York art mecca Woodstock), where at least twenty-one occupational therapists had the opportunity to advance their craft skills. Many of the instructors, and Slagle acting as the director, volunteered their services.

Slagle and Sullivan called the program a "post-graduate" course, and they tried to persuade association members both to provide financial support and to designate the Byrdcliffe School as the organization's official graduate program. They succeeded in convincing the membership of the need for postgraduate education, but they failed to establish the Byrdcliffe School as the official location for it. Susan Cox Johnson, for one, argued that the association ought to support already existing schools instead of starting new ones. Others found the East Coast location to be inconvenient if not inaccessible to most of the national membership. Finally, Slagle and Sullivan dropped the idea.[26]

As the doors of the Teachers College program and the New York War Service Classes for Training Reconstruction Aides in Occupational Therapy closed, and as the Byrdcliffe School's future dimmed, New York's centrality in occupational therapy's educational development ended. In the meantime the Boston, Milwaukee, Philadelphia, and St. Louis training schools pushed forward into leadership positions in the effort to provide high-quality training for practitioners. Representatives of these schools conducted committee work for the American Occupational Therapy Association, continuing the effort that Johnson had started. By 1923 they had gathered enough information to set up national education standards for the profession of occupational therapy.

# Minimum Standards for Courses of Training in Occupational Therapy

In the academic year 1922–23, national association personnel knew of a mere eight schools of occupational therapy operating in the United States, which would produce only 103 students that year.[27] The eight schools consisted of four types: four were independent schools of occupational therapy, three of which were founded during the war emergency; one was a college program; two were courses given in mental hospitals; and one was an innovative high school program conducted under the auspices of a city board of education in cooperation with the Red Cross. This small number of schools seemed to make the job of the Committee on Teaching Methods of the American Occupational Therapy Association a relatively simple one, especially if compared with that of nursing education reformers, who had to study hundreds of established schools during the 1920s in a similar period of self-assessment.[28]

Nonetheless, the committee faced no small task. It had to determine what good training entailed, and that was quite a challenge because so many variables were involved in the actual practice of occupational therapy. Occupational therapists realized that practitioners had to possess sophisticated technical and teaching skills as well as sufficient medical knowledge if they were to deliver high-quality care of patients. Moreover, because occupational therapy as a profession still had to prove its efficacy, the success of practitioners was crucial not only to patients, but to the profession itself. Taking slow, deliberate steps to build a pool of high-quality professionals was more important than flooding the market with mediocre practitioners. As committee chair Ruth Wigglesworth expressed it, even though the schools produced only 103 practitioners in 1923, those practitioners would probably touch the lives of at least 20,000 patients per year, and the fate of those patients would be observed by physicians and other medical professionals. Therefore, she said, the "question of training must receive serious thought."[29]

Wigglesworth, a graduate of the first class of the Boston School of Occupational Therapy and formerly the head reconstruction aide at the Walter Reed Hospital, collected information with her committee, then analyzed and debated it. The committee studied reports of existing training programs and solicited letters from hospital administrators and physicians on the qualities that they sought in occupational therapy practitioners. The letters were read aloud at national meetings and later published as a series called "The Aide I Want."[30] After much discussion the committee finally presented a document titled "Minimum Standards for Courses of Training in Occupational Therapy" to the membership of the American Occupational Therapy Association. In late 1923 the membership adopted it by a unanimous vote.[31]

The document covered three major areas in the training of occupational therapists: prerequisites for admission into training programs; the length of courses; and the content of courses. Students admitted to training had to be of such an age that they would be at least twenty years old when they graduated from the program. Among the many criteria on which the committee totally agreed was that practitioners had to be mature, tactful, and patient. Having a minimum-age policy had paid off during the war years, and there was no reason to believe that there would be fewer pressures on practitioners in the future. The committee also set a minimum educational background: students had to be high school graduates, and candidates with more education in arts and crafts or social service, or with advanced academic work, were preferred. The minimum length of a course of study was one year, with eight or nine months of medical and craft training and four or three months, correspondingly, of clinical work in hospitals. The idea of setting the standard at one year of training met with almost immediate consensus; there was, however, some debate over the relative amount of time to be spent on medical course work, craft training, and clinical experience. Therefore the committee left the particulars to the judgment of the decision makers at individual schools.[32]

When the committee set out to write the minimum standards, it had little authority to enforce them. That is, the American Occupational Therapy Association did not have the direct power to close poor-quality schools. This lack of legal clout did not dampen enthusiasm, however, because the document did give the association the power to endorse schools of occupational therapy or to use the criteria to discourage would-be students from attending lesser-quality schools. Eleanor Clarke Slagle, as secretary-treasurer of the association, had already informally taken on the role of advisor to prospective students of occupational therapy. She reported in 1921 that "requests for advice literally poured in from Maine to California and from Minnesota to Louisiana."[33] Once the minimum standards were set, her job was substantially simplified.

She started sending out a list of endorsed schools in response to letters of inquiry. Thus the American Occupational Therapy Association employed an indirect but nonetheless effective method to enforce a minimum standard of training. In addition, Slagle used the criteria set out in the document to reject candidates applying for work, telling them that they could not be recommended for jobs if they had not graduated from one of the accepted schools.[34]

The passage of the minimum standards affected existing schools. Most of them already met or exceeded the minimum standards; therefore the document legitimized them in the educational marketplace and protected them from competition from emerging schools of lesser quality. When schools received endorsement from the association, they immediately used it in their public relations materials and school brochures as a magnet to attract students.[35] The passage of the standards worked against some existing schools, however. In the late 1920s, for example, the American Occupational Therapy Association declined to endorse the Maryland Institute School of Applied and Fine Arts in Baltimore because the training that the institute offered lacked a clinical component. Director Hans Schuler proposed setting up a hospital experience for students once they graduated, but this suggestion did not meet with the approval of President Thomas B. Kidner or Secretary-Treasurer Eleanor Clarke Slagle. They responded to Schuler's request for endorsement by saying that the leading training schools were extending the minimum hospital experience to nine months, and that students needed to be assigned to institutions "in which departments of occupational therapy are organized and functioning under trained occupational therapists who supervise the entire period of practice training." Schuler could meet neither of these association standards.[36]

The American Occupational Therapy Association twice revised the document during the 1920s, gradually raising the minimum standards. By 1930 the age requirement was twenty-one years at graduation, and students with at least two years of training in arts and crafts, education, nursing, or social service were being actively sought. The minimum length of courses of study was extended to fifteen months in 1927 and then to eighteen months in 1930, reflecting the growing realization that practitioners needed much more background in medical subjects and clinical training than had first been anticipated. Required time for medical lectures more than doubled between 1923 and 1930, from 75 to 165 hours. Similarly, the necessary investment in craft training and hospital practice lengthened; whereas in 1923, minimum standards required 1,080 hours for craft instruction and hospital practice combined, by 1930, the standards called for 1,000 hours of craft training and 1,300 hours of practice training in the hospital.[37] Figure 2 presents the standards as they were adopted in 1930.

The first minimum standards document also announced that the American Occupational Therapy Association anticipated setting standards for individuals through a national register of qualified practitioners, in order to protect "hospitals and institutions from unqualified persons posing as occupational therapists."[38] On the register would be practitioners who had graduated from one of the endorsed schools and had demonstrated successful practice in the field. Whether or not standards would be waived for practitioners who had entered the field before or during the war was ambiguous. How these practitioners would be assessed presented a difficult problem. Moreover, their very existence posed a serious issue for members of the association who valued stabilizing the workforce.

To the practitioners who had not received the newly standardized training, the American Occupational Therapy Association seemed more like a threatening enemy than a protective friend. Without a doubt, all the talk about a register brought into question the status of emergency-trained occupational therapists and their predecessors who had received little formal training at all. It is no wonder that many of those who had established the profession in the first place felt alienated from the association.

The attempt to standardize the training of occupational therapists and to create a register of qualified practitioners reflected the normal course of development of a profession in the making. Setting boundaries establishes gateways through which only full-fledged members of the profession may enter. Wendy Colman has argued that in occupational therapy's case such a system was elitist.[39] This book contends, however, that requiring high standards for the preparation of practitioners was a necessity. Caring for patients with chronic illness presented practitioners with myriad challenges. The next chapter addresses experiences that occupational therapists faced in practice during the 1920s, the ways in which they tried to share their knowledge, and the methods by which the men associated with the field supported their efforts.

# FIGURE 2.

## AMERICAN OCCUPATIONAL THERAPY ASSOCIATION
An Association Incorporated Under the Laws of the District of Columbia
175 Fifth Avenue
New York, N. Y.

## MINIMUM STANDARDS FOR COURSES OF TRAINING IN OCCUPATIONAL THERAPY

### FOREWORD

Although Occupational Therapy was in use before the World War in many hospitals in this country—in particular, in hospitals for mental diseases—the training of Occupational Therapists had received little attention. In fact, only one definite course of training was in existence at the time of the entry of the United States into the War; namely, the Henry Favill School, of Chicago, Ill., which had established a training course in 1915.

When, however, the great value of Occupational Therapy as an important factor in the rehabilitation of soldiers and sailors disabled in the World War was officially recognized by the U. S. Army medical authorities, many emergency training courses were established to meet the demand for "Reconstruction Aides", as the Occupational Therapists were termed in the Army hospitals.

After the World War, a great increase of interest in Occupational Therapy was manifested in civilian hospitals, and to meet the growing demand for Occupational Therapists a few of the training schools which had been established to meet the War emergency were continued, and developed more thorough courses.

In the year 1921, the attention of the American Occupational Therapy Association was called to the need that was beginning to be felt by some hospital authorities for a National Register or Directory, of qualified Occupational Therapists; in particular, for the purpose of maintaining high standards, and for the protection of hospitals and institutions from unqualified persons posing as Occupational Therapists.

The Association had already taken cognizance of the fact that the training courses then being given varied considerably in the content of their courses. The need of minimum standards of training was, therefore, evident; alike for the development of Occupational Therapy on proper lines, and for the eventual establishment of a National Register or Directory, of qualified Occupational Therapists.

A careful study was therefore made by the Association's Standing Committee on Teaching Methods; with the result that a schedule of Minimum Standards of Training was adopted by unanimous vote of the members at the Association's annual meeting in 1923. Later, at the annual meeting in 1927, the members voted to increase the length of practice-training from the minimum standard of three months, as approved in 1923, to a minimum period of six months. At the annual meeting of the Association in October 1930, the Standing Committee on Teaching Methods presented a comprehensive report, recommending a further increase in the Minimum Standards of Training. The report was unanimously adopted and the new Standards are set forth below.

At the annual meeting in 1929, the Association also decided to establish a National Register or Directory, as soon as funds were available, and registration was begun on January 1, 1931.

### TRAINING SCHOOLS

Three types of training schools are available for persons who desire to become registered Occupational Therapists.

I. Special Occupational Therapy Schools.
II. Courses in Colleges and Universities.
III. Courses given in hospitals.

Post-graduate courses are also offered in some hospitals and are planned for two types of students: (a) Those who desire to specialize in the application of curative occupations in some particular type of illness or disability. (b) Those who have been in the field for some years and desire to refresh their knowledge and skill.

### COURSES IN COLLEGES AND UNIVERSITIES

These courses are usually combined with work for a bachelor's degree, but comprise all the work given in the courses in the special Occupational Therapy Training Schools; including the required period of practice-training in hospitals. Some colleges, however, also offer a short course as given in the Special Schools, without relation to other college courses.

### Figure 2 (cont.).

### NEW MINIMUM STANDARDS OF TRAINING FOR OCCUPATIONAL THERAPISTS WHO DESIRE TO QUALIFY FOR REGISTRATION. (Adopted October, 1930)

1. Pre-requisites for Admission.

   (a) Age.

   Candidates for admission to training courses shall be of such an age that they will be not less than twenty-one years old at graduation.

   (b) Education.

   All candidates for special schools must furnish proof of having completed a high school education or its equivalent. In addition it is desirable that all candidates, except those for the degree course, shall have had at least one year, and preferably two years, of further education or successful experience in college, art school, social service, nurse's training or the commercial field.
   Candidates for admission to a training course in a College or University which is combined with work leading to a bachelor's degree will, of course, only be required to comply with the regular entrance requirements of the institution concerned.

   (c) Character.

   All candidates will be required to present evidence of good character and general fitness; the evidence of which will be investigated and duly weighed by the school concerned.

   (d) Health.

   A medical certificate of good mental and physical health will be required, and verified by the school concerned.

   (e) Probationary Period.

   All training schools reserve the right to drop a student at any time for any cause which the school authorities deem sufficient.

   (f) Credits.

   The allowance of credits for previous special training is properly a matter for which individual training schools will make suitable regulations.

2. The Course of Training.

   (a) Length of course.

   The minimum length of the course shall be eighteen calendar months of full-time training; i.e., 72 weeks, exclusive of holidays, or 2500 net working hours. The course shall include not less than NINE months (36 weeks) of theoretical and technical work, and not less than NINE months (36 weeks) hospital practice-training under COMPETENT SUPERVISION; all as set forth in detail in succeeding sections.

   (b) Distribution of Time.

   A. Lectures on theory and technical training in Occupations......1200 hours
   B. Practice-Training in Hospitals..............................1300 hours

   Distribution of Time in "A".

   Lectures ................................................... 165 hours
   Training in Occupations.....................................1000 hours
   Electives .................................................... 35 hours

   Total .......................................................1200 hours

   Distribution of Time in "B"

   The time devoted to hospital practice-training shall be spent in the following types of hospitals or services:

   Mental Hospitals—Not less than 2 months (8 weeks at 40 or 320 working hours)

   Tuberculosis Hospitals or Sanatoriums  
   General Hospitals (General Medical and Surgical Cases)  
   Children's Hospitals  
   Orthopedic Hospitals or Services  
   } One month shall be the minimum requirement on each of these services.

## Figure 2 (cont.).

NOTE: The time devoted to practice-training in the treatment of mental cases must be spent in hospitals for mental and nervous diseases and disorders. Where, however, as in some cities, there is available a large general hospital in which all types of illness and disability are treated, and in which a properly organized department of Occupational Therapy is maintained, practice-training with other than mental cases may be taken in such an institution. Practice-training in certain types of disability may also be taken in special institutions; such as approved curative workshops apart from hospitals.

(c) In the School.

The time given to work and lectures in the school shall be not less than six hours daily.

NOTE: Throughout the technical training in occupations, a properly qualified person shall interpret each subject in terms of its therapeutic application in different types of mental and physical conditions. (See later, "Occupations".)

3. Content of Course.
    Lectures on Theory, etc.

    | | Minimum number of hours |
    |---|---|
    | (a) Mental Sciences, shall include: | |
    |     Neurology | |
    |     Psychology | |
    |     Abnormal Psychology | |
    |     Psychiatry | 35 hours |
    |     Mental Hygiene | |
    |     Epilepsy | |
    |     Feeble-mindedness | |
    | (b) Physical Sciences, shall include: | |
    |     Personal and social hygiene | |
    |     Physiology and anatomy | |
    |     Kinesiology and joint motion | 50 hours |
    |     Physical therapy | |
    |     American Red Cross First Aid | |
    | (c) Medical Lectures, shall include: | |
    |     Blindness and Deafness | |
    |     Tuberculosis | |
    |     Cardiac diseases | |
    |     Orthopedics | 25 hours |
    |     General medical condition | |
    |     Surgical conditions | |
    |     Contagious diseases | |
    | (d) Occupational Therapy, shall include: | |
    |     History of Occupational Therapy | |
    |     Theory of Occupational Therapy | |
    |     Occupational Therapy in various types of institutions | |
    |     Occupational Therapy as applied in various diseases | |
    |     Occupational Therapy and its relation to Vocational and Industrial Rehabilitation. (Federal Industrial Rehabilitation Act, 1920) | 45 hours |
    |     Occupational Therapy in its relation to other social agencies | |
    |     Organization of Departments and Records | |
    |     Hospital etiquette and ethics | |
    |     Miscellaneous general lectures | |
    |     Observation; including directed visits to institutions and clinics | |
    | (e) Electives | 10 hours |
    | Total | 165 hours |

Training in Occupations

Craft analyses, and notes on the adaptation and suitability of the various occupations to different types of illness and disability, must be presented by an experienced Occupational Therapist as an integral part of the study of each occupation. Training must be given in the following occupations:

## Figure 2 (cont.).

| | Minimum number of hours |
|---|---|
| Design, shall include:<br>  Theory and appreciation<br>  Applied Design<br>  Mechanical Drawing | 150 hours |
| Textiles, shall include:<br>  Weaving<br>  Rake knitting<br>  Needle crafts<br>  Dyeing, block printing, stencilling<br>  Knotting and netting<br>  Miscellaneous; such as, jute, knitting, crocheting, rugs, colonial mats, mops, etc., including use of waste materials<br>  O. T. analysis and adaptation | 210 hours |
| Basketry, shall include:<br>  Raffia<br>  Willow<br>  Fibre<br>  Chair-seating (reed, cane, rush)<br>  O. T. analysis and adaptation | 85 hours |
| Woodwork, shall include:<br>  Bench work<br>  Carving<br>  Toy making<br>  O. T. analysis and adaptation | 175 hours |
| Metal Work, shall include:<br>  Jewelry<br>  Miscellaneous<br>  O. T. analysis and adaptation | 65 hours |
| Bookbinding and Leather Work, shall include:<br>  O. T. analysis and adaptation | 90 hours |
| Plastic Arts, shall include:<br>  Clay modeling<br>  Pottery<br>  O. T. analysis and adaptation | 15 hours |
| Minor Crafts and use of Waste Materials:<br>  Beadwork, the making of tin toys, brush-making, marionettes, etc.:<br>  O. T. analysis and adaptation. | 50 hours |
| NOTE: This list is merely suggestive and other minor crafts may be selected at the discretion of the individual training school | |
| Miscellaneous:<br>  Recreation and remedial games and plays; including music, story telling, library work.<br>  Crafts for children<br>  Calisthenics<br>  Remedial gymnastics<br>  Horticulture<br>  O. T. analysis and adaptation of the above-named activities | 160 hours |
| | 1,000 hours |

NOTE: Emphasis must be placed on the importance of recreation and physical exercises in a program of therapeutic activities.

4. Practice Training.
  (a) Length of Time
  (b) Distribution of Time
  (c) Supervision
See Section 2 (b), above

    The hospital-practice training of students must be supervised by a properly qualified, registered occupational therapist, who is not only competent in her department, but has shown ability to handle students-in-training. (Wherever a teaching hospital with a well-organized department of occupational therapy is available, training schools should endeavor to arrange for the admission of their students to the hospital for practice-training.)

January 10, 1931

Note: This is a duplication of the original document.

# NOTES

1. Beatrice Wade, interview by the author, Chicago, March 1990.
2. Ibid.
3. Ibid.
4. Ibid.
5. "Report of the President," in *Proceedings of the Fourth Annual Meeting of the National Society for the Promotion of Occupational Therapy* (Towson, Md.: NSPOT, 1920), 3. The term "social gospel" has been used by historians of the Progressive Era to describe the quasi-religious/quasi-secular ideology and rhetoric of the reformers of the period. See, for example, Ronald C. White, Jr., and C. Howard Hopkins, *The Social Gospel* (Philadelphia: Temple University Press, 1976); and Shailer Mathews, "Social Gospel," in *A Dictionary of Religion and Ethics*, ed. Shailer Mathews and Gerald Birney Smith (New York: Macmillan Company, 1923), 416–17.
6. Mrs. Hewitt, "Address of Welcome," in *Proceedings of the Fourth Annual Meeting of NSPOT*, 32–33.
7. "The Fifth Annual Meeting of the National Society for the Promotion of Occupational Therapy," *Archives of Occupational Therapy* 1 (1922): 81.
8. Ibid., 83.
9. Ibid., 82.
10. "The Sixth Annual Meeting of the American Occupational Therapy Association, September 1922," *Archives of Occupational Therapy* 2 (1923): 53–56.
11. "Meeting of the Board and Members of the House of Delegates of the American Occupational Therapy Association," *Archives of Occupational Therapy* 1 (1922): 337–38.
12. "Minutes of the Fifth Annual Meeting," *Archives of Occupational Therapy* 1 (1922): 151. After two letters were read, one inviting the membership to Colorado Springs and the other to Milwaukee, the vote took place. Boston was first with 36 votes; Milwaukee second with 28; Colorado Springs third with 20; and Washington, D.C., fourth with 13.
13. "Meeting of the Board and Members of the House of Delegates of the American Occupational Therapy Association," 341–43.
14. Ibid.
15. The American Occupational Therapy Association met with the American Hospital Association in the following cities during the 1920s: Atlantic City, 1922, 1926, 1929; Milwaukee, 1923; Buffalo, New York, 1924; Louisville, Kentucky, 1925; Minneapolis, Minnesota, 1927; and San Francisco, 1928.
16. "[General Discussion of] the Training of Teachers, [Remarks by] Susan C. Johnson," in *Proceedings of the Fourth Annual Meeting of NSPOT*, 51–55.
17. Ibid, 53.
18. "The Fifth Annual Meeting of NSPOT," 76.
19. Ibid., 227–28.
20. Letter, Susan C. Johnson to Adelaide Nutting, 17 June 1919, History of Nursing Collection, microfiche 0513, Milbank Memorial Library, Teachers College, Columbia University (hereafter History of Nursing Collection).
21. Susan C. Johnson, ms., ca. 1920, History of Nursing Collection, microfiche 0513. See pages 1–4 for positions occupied by former occupational therapy students under the categories of "volunteers," "positions in civil hospitals," "U.S. Public Health Hospitals," and "Army Service."

22. Ibid. The number of students enrolled in "occupation therapy" from summer 1917 to summer 1920 was reported to be as follows: summer 1917, records incomplete, probably 10; fall 1917, 12; spring 1918, nursing and health department 35, vocational education department 51; fall 1918, 71; spring 1919, 14; fall 1919, 10 (2 dropped); spring 1920, new—2, carried over—7, for a total of 9. Total: 212 (nursing and health department 161; vocational education department 51).

23. "Report of Committee on Education," *Archives of Occupational Therapy* 2 (1923): 69–72.

24. "The Sixth Annual Meeting of the American Occupational Therapy Association," *Archives of Occupational Therapy* 2 (1923): 64. Ruth Wigglesworth led a roundtable on training courses at the 1922 annual meeting [*Archives of Occupational Therapy* 2 (1923): 119–31]. She is listed as chair of the Committee on Education at the following year's meeting [Archives of Occupational Therapy 3 (1924): 54].

25. "Susan Johnson," obituary, *Occupational Therapy and Rehabilitation* 11 (1932): 152–53.

26. "Meeting of the Board and Members of the House of Delegates of the American Occupational Therapy Association," 329–37.

27. "Report of the Committee on Teaching," *Archives of Occupational Therapy* 2 (1923): 35–37.

28. Susan M. Reverby, *Ordered to Care: The Dilemma of American Nursing, 1850–1945* (Cambridge: Cambridge University Press, 1987), 151–79.

29. "Roundtable on Training Courses Conducted by Miss Ruth Wigglesworth," *Archives of Occupational Therapy* 2 (1923): 119–31.

30. See, for example, five letters titled "The Aide I Want" by John B. Hawes, Harvey Cushing, C. Macfie Campbell, Arthur Steindler, and C. D. Mitchell, all written in 1922 and published in *Archives of Occupational Therapy* 2 (1923): 133–38.

31. Adoption of "Minimum Standards for Courses of Training in Occupational Therapy" took place at the 1923 annual meeting of the American Occupational Therapy Association [*Archives of Occupational Therapy* 3 (1924): 477].

32. "Minimum Standards for Courses of Training in Occupational Therapy," *Archives of Occupational Therapy* 3 (1924): 295–98.

33. "The Fifth Annual Meeting of NSPOT," 83.

34. "Minutes of the Eighth Annual Meeting," *Archives of Occupational Therapy* 4 (1925): 478.

35. See, for example, a 1923 brochure of the Boston School of Occupational Therapy, which says on page 3: "This is the only school in New England endorsed by the American Occupational Therapy Association." (Papers of the Boston School of Occupational Therapy, Wessell Library, Tufts University, Medford, Massachusetts).

36. Letters between Hans Schuler and Thomas B. Kidner and Eleanor Clarke Slagle, September 1927–May 1931, Official Archives of the American Occupational Therapy Association, Wilma L. West Library, American Occupational Therapy Foundation, Bethesda, Maryland (hereafter AOTA Archives).

37. "Minimum Standards for Courses of Training in Occupational Therapy," adopted 1 November 1923, and "New Minimum Standards of Training for Occupational Therapists Who Desire to Qualify for Registration," adopted October 1930, AOTA Archives.

38. "Minimum Standards for Courses of Training in Occupational Therapy," *Archives of Occupational Therapy* 3 (1924): 295–98.

39. Wendy Colman, "A Study of Educational Policy Setting in Occupational Therapy, 1918–1981," (Ph.D. diss., New York University, 1984).

# Chapter 9

## Men, Medical Identity, *and* Survival *in the* 1920s

**Principles of Occupational Therapy**

1. Occupational therapy is a method of treatment of the sick and disabled by means of scientifically applied activity.
2. Its purpose is to arouse interest, courage and confidence; to exercise mind and body in healthy activity; to overcome disability; and to reestablish capacity for industrial and social usefulness.
3. The treatment should be prescribed by a physician for definite mental, physical and social results.
4. The selection and direction of the appropriate occupations to fill the prescription should be carried out only by a trained occupational therapist.
5. Quality and quantity of products may prove beneficial by satisfying and stimulating the patient but should always be kept secondary.
6. The real product of occupational therapy and the only reliable measure of treatment is the effect upon the patient.

*Presented by William R. Dunton at the Second Annual Meeting of the National Society for the Promotion of Occupational Therapy, New York, 1918*

In 1921, at the annual meeting of the national association, President Herbert James Hall chaired a discussion with the membership about the administration of occupational therapy in hospital settings. Given that occupational therapists were, in his words, "a new type of assistant," surely issues abounded pertaining to the establishment of secure positions for occupational therapists in the hospital hierarchy.[1]

Eleanor Clarke Slagle told the membership that one of the most important issues facing occupational therapists was the need for cooperation from physicians, symbolized by the giving of prescriptions for occupational therapy. Practitioners and patients, she said, "*must* have the protection of the prescription [emphasis in original]." With prescriptions from physicians, occupational therapists could take on the role of modern health care professionals. Procuring such a legitimate place in medicine would distance them from the do-gooder image of the pre-war period, when practitioners came to the hospital under the auspices of women's volunteer charity programs, often only providing diversional activities. Slagle recounted a story to the membership, describing how she had insisted that every patient sent to occupational therapy come by prescription. "I know," she said, "that you can get the cooperation of physicians in hospitals if you are sufficiently persistent, and if they are brought to realize the importance of our work, particularly the younger physicians who are coming in."[2]

Her colleague Mary M. Atwater, from Seattle, Washington, confirmed Slagle's view of the importance of occupational therapy's taking on a clear medical identity. At the same meeting, Atwater spoke of the need to make occupational therapy's therapeutic aim a priority, and the need to minimize its traditional diversional and utilitarian purposes. Too many people, in her opinion, sentimentally viewed occupational therapy as only providing entertainment for the person who was ill; or they saw occupational therapy in terms of its nineteenth-century predecessor, moral therapy, which not only taught patients right living habits, but also saved the hospital money through the labor provided by patients. In the 1920s occupational therapists fought these persistent misconceptions of the purposes of their work. "No one," Atwater said, "sentimentalizes over giving a patient a pill for a headache, or a specially constructed shoe for a flat foot—why [do they continue to] sentimentalize over giving him a job of work for the purpose of stimulating him out of a depression, or of giving exercise to a weakened arm?" The point of occupational therapy, she continued, is "not to produce a good basket [or] rag rug . . . but a cured patient."[3]

Idelle Kidder, from St. Louis, bluntly stated that prescriptions were often "not forthcoming." Many physicians seemed reluctant to prescribe occupational therapy, partly because they did not know "what to do or how to go about it." She suggested that the association "give a little publicity to the medical profession" so that physicians would realize that they were expected to be involved in providing occupational therapy, and so that future hospital departments of occupational therapy would be set up under medical authority.[4]

During the 1920s the men and the women of occupational therapy took the risk of moving the profession closer to medicine and further from women's volunteer work and reconstruction. They did so with ambivalence, understanding that the latter two traditions had provided a strong foundation on which to build the profession. The women's volunteer tradition had given occupational therapy a workforce and institutions of teaching and practice; it never occurred to the leaders to purge the field totally of that tradition. Restoring the wounded to productivity during the war years had helped occupational therapy gain prestige with the American public; to eliminate this emphasis completely would have been professional suicide.

The war was over, however, and to survive, occupational therapy had to adjust its aims and emphasis to meet new conditions. Occupational therapists had to show the American public that they could contribute to the care of all persons with chronic illness, not just persons wounded in the war, and that such work was vital to the nation's well-being. Occupational therapists had to convince physicians, many of whom were geared to acute care, that their duty encompassed restoring patients to a full healthy life, which included being a productive citizen in society. Occupational therapists also had to continue to increase the size of their workforce and the number of their institutions while maintaining the independence that women's networks had provided. The established schools were self-regulating, with little interference from male physicians; and in the many workplaces organized and supported by women's clubs, even those within hospital walls, physicians rarely tampered with decisions about when, how, and why patients were received, treated, and discharged. Thus occupational therapy had to perform a delicate balancing act: to continue stressing the utilitarian value of occupational therapy without encroaching on the domain of vocational rehabilitation; to obtain the approval and the support of male physicians, for purposes of legitimizing the field as a medical profession, but not at the price of losing autonomy; to sustain decision-making power over the care of individual patients; and to maintain the social and financial support provided by women's networks.

This chapter examines the ways in which male supporters in the 1920s helped occupational therapy continue to establish itself in the world of medicine by educating their colleagues and by encouraging occupational therapists to accept the increasingly rationalized procedures of medical care. These men published promotional literature in books and in mainstream medical journals such as *Mental Hygiene, Modern Hospital*, and (occasionally) the *Journal of the American Medical Association*, in order to convince physicians that occupational therapy was a useful tool in the care of patients with chronic illness. Realizing that hospitals were growing in importance as the ideal location for treatment and that occupational therapists had to become part of the growing number of health care professionals who would provide the new services, the men nurtured the American Occupational Therapy Association's relationship with the American Hospital Association because of the latter's influence on hospital policies and structure. In the mid-1920s the physicians connected to the American Occupational Therapy Association pushed for occupational therapy to be included in medical school curricula so that new physicians would learn the principles of occupational therapy and the application of those principles in practice. They promoted the gathering of statistics and the keeping of medical records so that generalizations could be drawn from studying occupational therapy practice and its accomplishments. Physicians wanted occupational therapists to be able to measure what would today be called "patient outcomes," thereby bringing occupational therapy in line with other fields of medicine. Eventually the profession won the approbation of the American Medical Association, a goal sought by both men and women in the field.

During the 1920s, occupational therapists sought and obtained medical legitimacy. They won the cooperation of physicians, convinced physicians to write prescriptions for patients, and adopted mainstream medicine's record-keeping systems. This apparent capitulation to medical routines did not mean that practitioners lost ground in their area of authority; if anything, they held and widened it. Such routines helped them gather evidence that proved the importance of their role in the care of patients with chronic illness. Case records, in other words, helped them assert that each patient's condition had its uniqueness, and therefore needed careful attention that could only be given by skilled, educated occupational therapists. They learned to argue that only their professional expertise could properly initiate, execute, monitor, and complete patients' cases, and they thereby kept physicians and other medical personnel outside their area of authority. By the end of the 1920s, the new profession had well established the notion that the relationship between the patient, the therapist, and the cure was sacred ground on which only well-trained occupational therapists could tread.

## HERBERT JAMES HALL, HORATIO M. POLLACK, AND RECORD KEEPING

Between the association's sixth and seventh annual meetings, Herbert James Hall died at only fifty-three years of age, but not before he set the men's agenda for their work in the 1920s.[5] Hall felt that the most important task for occupational therapy to accomplish was to standardize its record-keeping systems, in order to facilitate its acceptance among his medical colleagues. "It does not do a single thing to say that the patient was very sick and got better," he lamented. He wanted to be able to "measure in some way the actual benefit and effect of occupational therapy upon the patient." Hall suggested that practitioners record exactly how long patients could work, in the same way that nurses recorded temperatures on charts. "When we show a patient is able to work one day for an hour and at the end of a week for two hours and at the end of the third week for three hours," occupational therapy could take at least part of the credit for such progress. Most important, Hall wanted the records to be able to show in a simple way that a patient could "take and do his work in life after having been disorganized . . . and idle for quite a length of time." He wanted "the medical mind" (other physicians) to be able to glance at a patient's record and understand immediately the important role that occupational therapy had played in the restoration of the patient's health.[6]

Horatio M. Pollack, Ph.D., a statistician for New York State's Hospital Commission, a mental hygiene advocate, and a supporter of occupational therapy, took up the challenge. In the same year that Ruth Wigglesworth held the roundtable on training courses, Pollack held a roundtable on records. For Pollack, keeping records meant that occupational therapy would enter the realm of efficiency and science. Records, he argued, guided practitioners, allowing them to compare progress made from one year to the next. Records also gave practitioners the advantage of being able to compare their department's work with the work of other departments. Further, records assisted physicians, hospital administrators, state board members, and legislators in planning and distributing resources for occupational therapy programs.[7]

According to Pollack, state mental hospitals all over the United States had adopted uniform systems of gathering statistics regarding diagnoses, admissions, discharges, and deaths;[8] occupational therapy, he insisted, ought to do the same. He recommended four forms for record-keeping purposes: prescription forms, administrative cards, class-attendance registers, and yearly statistics cards. Pollack expected physicians to share authority over patients with occupational therapists. He believed that a physician, "the superior officer," ought to write prescriptions, but only "after a consult with the head teacher of occupational therapy." Further, he expected physicians and occupational therapists to discuss patients' progress so that the prescription could be adjusted accordingly.[9]

Pollack envisioned the department of occupational therapy as a school that helped transform the hospital "from a more or less passive institution to an active one." He charged hospital physicians with a number of duties: they should provide for classrooms and workshops, buy supplies, sell finished products, confer with other physicians, and obtain other physicians' cooperation. The "chief occupational therapist" held a managerial role and therefore had to have professional and personal qualities such as excellent training in the arts and crafts, experience in dealing with patients, "enthusiasm, vision, initiative, and tact." As "head of the teaching front," the chief occupational therapist organized the "school," supervised "assistant teachers," kept records, received patients and assigned them to "proper classes," "promoted and transferred" patients, held "teacher" meetings, and finally, promoted "efficiency" in the school. The "therapists" or "assistant teachers," placed below the chief occupational therapist in the hospital hierarchy, needed to be well trained in a school of arts and crafts or occupational therapy, and also must have had "practice work" or clinical training "before being engaged."[10]

In short, Pollack advised hospital administrators of "six 'musts' for occupational therapy" departments if they were to meet modern medicine's standards. Institutions had to provide (1) suitable space and equipment; (2) a trained teacher; (3) a systematic progressive course of instruction, outlined and followed; (4) an adequate system of records; (5) a revolving capital fund; and (6) full cooperation among physicians, nurses, and teachers of occupational therapy.[11]

Pollack hoped to win the support of hospital administrators when he explicitly contended in a *Modern Hospital* article that occupational therapy saved the hospital money and served a distinct utilitarian purpose. "Fewer attendants will be needed" in mental hospitals, he wrote, because the patients will be "better behaved." Furthermore, the "increased productivity" of patients will "more than compensate for the added expense of maintaining the school." Properly individualized "instruction," Pollack continued, will improve the patient's condition and make the patient a "contented and effective member of the hospital community" and "fit for usefulness outside of the hospital."[12]

Pollack's characterization of the hospital as a school echoed a major tenet of the mental hygiene movement, of which he was an active member. Persons who were mentally ill had to learn new life habits in order to cure their illness and prevent its recurrence. Occupational therapists not only shared such thinking, but saw the hospital as the ideal setting in which to transform patients' lives through closely supervised treatments.

Pollack's reference to "classes," moreover, dovetailed with the well-established methods of antituberculosis activists, who had also begun to see hospital care as crucial to the treatment of infected patients. G. L. Bellis, superintendent of the Muirdale Sanatorium in Wisconsin, for example, explicitly stated that the purposes of tuberculosis sanatoriums were to provide patients with the best possible chance for recovery, to teach patients the "principles and practice of personal hygiene and sanitation," and to return them to the community as self-supporting citizens.[13] Thus by the 1920s, the mental hygiene, antituberculosis, and occupational therapy movements shared much ground.

Since the early twentieth century, public health advocates, lay reformers, physicians, nurses, patients, and members of the new professions of social work, occupational therapy, and psychiatric social work, to name just a few, had been trying to eradicate mental illness and tuberculosis in America. Both the mental hygiene movement and the antituberculosis movement sought to educate the general public about healthful behaviors to prevent these dreaded illnesses. If preventive measures failed, mental hygiene and tuberculosis activists promoted removing patients from their environment when possible and placing them in long-term therapeutic settings, such as Philip King Brown's rural tuberculosis sanatorium Arequipa, Herbert J. Hall's Devereux Mansion, and the many large-scale private and state hospitals that had recently been built all over the nation. By the 1920s, in other words, leaders within both movements were increasingly depending on the hospital as the ideal treatment center.

In addition, activists in both movements feared the economic dependency that attended mental illness and tuberculosis. As a mental hygiene advocate, Pollack certainly took it for granted that occupational therapists would be part of the hospital team responsible for putting patients with mental illness back on the road to self-support. Similarly, leaders of the antituberculosis movement saw a crucial role for occupational therapy in the care of patients. Just as patients' rest, diet, and fresh air had to be regimented, so did their work activities have to be closely monitored. As a result, superintendents of tuberculosis sanatoriums all over the country employed occupational therapists. According to Thomas B. Kidner, caring for patients with tuberculosis was an important growth area for occupational therapy, second only to mental health care.[14]

*Part III: Stabilization and Standardization in the 1920s*

THOMAS B. KIDNER, REHABILITATION, AND TUBERCULOSIS

If Herbert J. Hall and William R. Dunton helped the field of occupational therapy gain professional recognition in psychiatry, then Thomas B. Kidner used his influence to establish a foothold for occupational therapy in rehabilitation and tuberculosis care. An architect by training and well-known in Canada, Europe, and the United States as a specialist in constructing institutions for persons with physical disabilities, Kidner first advocated occupational therapy in the wartime reconstruction movement. Concerned with reeducating wounded soldiers, he always included workshop spaces for occupational therapy in his hospital plans. Kidner became particularly interested in tuberculosis when along with other reconstructionists, he noticed that a large percentage of the men disabled during the war suffered from the disease.[15] Following the war, Kidner helped fuel the trend to hospitalize persons who had tuberculosis. He served as the institutional secretary of the National Tuberculosis Association, designing many Canadian and United States hospitals for the care of patients with tuberculosis.[16]

Kidner wanted occupational therapy to capitalize on opportunities offered by postwar reconstruction work, by then more commonly called "rehabilitation." In June 1920, Congress had passed the Industrial Rehabilitation Act, which provided funding for "vocational rehabilitation for persons disabled in industry, or otherwise, and their return to civic employment." The act encouraged cooperation between the federal and state governments by setting up a matching fund; Washington would match every dollar that the states spent on rehabilitation. By 1923, at least thirty-eight states had already used the funding by setting up vocational rehabilitation services.[17]

Kidner wanted occupational therapy to dip into the rehabilitation pork barrel, even though the services to be provided by the act were slated to be more vocational than medical. Section II of the act stated, "The term 'rehabilitation' shall be construed to mean the rendering of a person disabled fit to engage in remunerative occupation."[18] However, that did not stop Kidner from seeing potential development for occupational therapy in rehabilitation. In a letter to William R. Dunton, Kidner wrote, "There is a great zone . . . between pure occupational therapy and vocational rehabilitation which in my judgement can best be occupied and covered by occupational therapists who have the vision."[19]

Kidner was not alone in wanting to see occupational therapy obtain rehabilitation funds. When leaders of the profession published in *Modern Hospital* during the 1920s, they titled their section of the journal "Occupational Therapy and Rehabilitation." In 1924, heralding the rehabilitation theme even more blatantly, they changed the name of the association's journal from *Archives of Occupational Therapy* to *Occupational Therapy and Rehabilitation*.

These leaders were careful to maintain an identity separate from rehabilitation, though. Throughout the 1920s, articles abounded in *Modern Hospital* and *Occupational Therapy and Rehabilitation* asserting that occupational therapy had a rightful place in preparing various kinds of patients for vocational training. Just as they had done during the war, occupational therapists claimed that their area of expertise was the medical prerequisite to vocational rehabilitation.

In this context it is clear why occupational therapists insisted on physicians' prescriptions during the postwar era; prescriptions represented another way to identify their work as medical, not vocational. In their view, keeping occupational therapy within medicine was absolutely a necessity, especially for patients with chronic or disabling diseases. Patients with tuberculosis, for example, needed very close medical supervision, they argued, because the physical conditions of such patients were often precarious. An improperly trained worker, or one without a medical background, might suggest activities for patients that would cause fatigue, bringing them more danger than help.[20]

In 1922, speaking in Brussels, Belgium, at the meeting of the International Union against Tuberculosis, Kidner proclaimed the importance of medical supervision of work for patients with tuberculosis and clearly delineated the complementary roles to be played by the physician and the trained occupational therapist. The physician, he said, was "the proper person to decide on the suitability, or otherwise, of any work or occupation to be used as a therapeutic measure." Because "exercise in tuberculosis may be 'vastly more dangerous,'" he argued, that was all the more reason why it had to be "under the control of the physician." Then, supporting occupational therapists' authority in caring for patients, he said that physicians had to ensure that "the proper person will see that [the prescription] is applied."[21]

## Occupational Therapy and the Problem of Commercialism

Related to occupational therapy's struggle with maintaining a medical identity on the rehabilitation continuum was the problem of resisting the trend toward commercialism. Hospital superintendents too frequently saw occupational therapy as an opportunity for the institution or the patients to earn money. Occupational therapists saw such thinking as crass commercialism, having little to do with their self-perceived role in health care. They increasingly found themselves at odds with those who saw a medical and an economic aspect to their work.

Among those whom occupational therapists had to fight on this issue were lay and medical wartime reconstructionists, orthopedic specialists, and physicians specializing in the care of patients with heart disease or tuberculosis, who nearly unanimously agreed that patients had to find a means to earn a living in spite of disability. In fear of widespread dependency, they wanted patients working and earning money during treatment. Moreover, these lay persons and medical professionals wanted patients to be taught new vocational skills appropriate to the patients' disabilities so that they could support themselves on discharge from the hospital. The lay persons and medical professionals had achieved self-sufficiency for patients at discharge during and immediately following the war, and they wanted to continue such efforts.

Occupational therapists tended to be divided over how involved they should become with the commercial side of their work. Their patients did, after all, produce large quantities of baskets, rugs and other woven products, metal products, jewelry, wooden toys, and myriad other useful and beautiful items with potential for sale. Debating the pros and the cons of the issue throughout the 1920s, they frequently asked themselves, "Should occupational therapy be concerned with the commercial value of its products?"[22]

They found no easy resolution to the problem, mainly because they too believed that economic independence, or at least productivity, was a necessary component of good health. Some occupational therapists, pushing for a modified commercialism, maintained, "The more valuable the product, the better the therapeutic effect."[23] Occupational therapists noticed that patients frequently became depressed and anxious when they were unable financially to take care of themselves or family members. Occupational therapists realized conversely that patients would likely benefit psychologically from producing salable products and realizing a profit. Thomas B. Kidner once pointed this out: "I am entirely aware of the therapeutic value to a patient of being able to produce a salable article, for I have known many patients, disheartened and unnerved for the future by a long illness, who have renewed their faith in themselves because of their having produced an article which some person was willing to buy for its intrinsic value."[24]

Nonetheless, Kidner warned against placing too much emphasis on the commercial value of craft products; after all, they had a very limited market in a society that increasingly valued efficient machine-made devices. To be safe, he and other occupational therapists firmly resisted commercialism by stressing the early stages of rehabilitation, which had to do with helping patients overcome the physical and psychological effects of illness. They widely distributed a set of principles that articulated the focus of their practice. In the principles they argued that the purpose of occupational therapy was to "arouse interest, courage and confidence; . . . to overcome disability; and to reestablish capacity for industrial . . . usefulness." In other words, occupational therapy prepared patients for what would come later—vocational training. Furthermore, the principles put the priority on care of patients by stating, "Quality and quantity of products may prove beneficial by satisfying and stimulating the patient but should always be kept secondary." According to the sixth principle, patients clearly came first: "The real product of occupational therapy and the only reliable measure of treatment is the effect upon the patient."[25]

Obviously, even in the 1920s the new profession of occupational therapy had to convince others of what its area of expertise encompassed. William Rush Dunton, Jr., and his colleagues on two association committees took up this problem.

## WILLIAM RUSH DUNTON, JR., AND THE COMMITTEE ON PUBLICITY AND PUBLICATION

From before World War I until after World War II, Dunton promoted occupational therapy through the written word. Before the founding of the National Society for the Promotion of Occupational Therapy in 1917 and until the society founded its own journal, Dunton published several articles about occupational therapy in the *Maryland Psychiatric Quarterly*, which he edited. In the years 1917–20 his own institution's press printed the association's proceedings, and occupational therapy patients at the institution bound the volumes.[26] In 1921, Dunton inaugurated the profession's first official organ, the *Archives of Occupational Therapy*, and edited it through 1923. He oversaw the renamed journal, *Occupational Therapy and Rehabilitation*, from 1924 to 1946, bringing his editorial contributions to over twenty-five years. All of this he did without remuneration. In addition, Dunton authored several books and nearly 100 articles on the subject of occupational therapy.[27] In one way or another, he used these many publications to publicize the profession's accomplishments, to provide a forum for an exchange of occupational therapy ideas, and to explain to outsiders what occupational therapy was all about.

Dunton worked indefatigably for the association. From its very founding he chaired the standing committee originally called the Committee on Finance, Publicity and Publication, later called simply the Committee on Publicity and Publication. In 1917 he sent announcements of the founding of the National Society for the Promotion of Occupational Therapy, with a photograph of the founders and, in some cases, copies of the papers read, to several professional periodicals, including the *Journal of the American Medical Association*, *Survey*, and *Modern Hospital*.[28] He and George Edward Barton sent similar materials to a number of newspapers, including the *Baltimore Sun*, the *Boston Transcript*, the *Chicago Sun*, and the *New York Times*, to name a few. Dunton, in his own words, made "every effort compatible with dignity . . . to bring the Society to the notices of the general public and those interested in occupational therapy."[29]

By 1921, Dunton had decided that the occupational therapy profession should have its own journal. He explained to the membership at the annual meeting, "Every specialty of medicine, excepting ours, has one or more periodicals devoted to its interests." Using the *Maryland Psychiatric Quarterly* to publicize occupational therapy news and accomplishments, he asserted, was no longer viable; it was "too much of an amateur periodical to meet our needs." He objected as well to printing association proceedings on an "amateur" basis. Dunton also thought that articles in *Modern Hospital* failed to meet the needs of the growing profession. Its editors rightfully had their own concerns about space and focus and therefore could not possibly publish all the literature that Dunton thought should be circulated. Dunton had sent ten papers from the fourth annual meeting to *Modern Hospital*; to his regret, only three appeared in print.[30]

Dunton negotiated with a Baltimore publishing house, and in February 1922 the first issue of *Archives of Occupational Therapy* appeared, with articles covering many of occupational therapy's most pressing contemporary concerns. About half of the articles were written by prestigious physicians such as Adolph Meyer, whose contribution was entitled "the Philosophy of Occupation Therapy." Several articles on education appeared, including "Training Aides for Mental Patients" by Eleanor Clarke Slagle; "The Training of the Occupational Aide" by John D. Adams, vice-president of the Massachusetts Association of Occupational Therapy; and "Scope of Occupational Therapy and Requirements for the Training of Occupational Aides" by Elliot G. Brackett, the orthopedic surgeon formerly associated with reconstruction. A few papers addressed care of patients with tuberculosis, including "The Trend of Occupational Therapy for the Tuberculous" by H. A. Pattison, president of the National Tuberculosis Association; and "Experience with Tuberculosis Patients" by Gertrude Sample, an occupational therapist. Also included were proceedings of the annual meeting, editorials, book reviews, abstracts, and a bibliography, all of which made the journal clearly professional in style and content.[31]

Dunton wanted the journal to serve "as an archives where those papers worthy of permanent preservation may be placed." By this he meant the professional papers and discussions that took place at annual meetings. He also wanted local occupational therapy professional societies to submit meritorious papers for publication. He discouraged members from sending in what he called "news of ephemeral moment," that is, reports on the current activities of various local institutions and societies. This material, he said, belonged in "journals of more general character, . . . [such as] *The Modern Hospital*."[32]

Costs and the preferences of subscribers and the editor shaped the journal in the next few years. Having stenographers capture every word at annual meetings and printing verbatim reports became financially prohibitive. *Archives* was far from self-supporting, especially because only about one-quarter of the active members of the association subscribed to it.[33] In late 1923, association members discussed incorporating into the dues a fee for a subscription to *Archives*, but the idea died without action. Raising annual dues from $2.00 to $3.00 was controversial enough that year; to add the cost of a subscription would have meant an additional $4.00 per person, far beyond the means of the average practitioner.[34]

In spite of these financial pressures, Dunton wanted to hold to his original concept of recording all the transactions of the association, partly for the sake of history but more importantly for the benefit of those unable to attend the annual meetings because of geographic constraints. Slagle, in her typically practical way, told Dunton that although he and the publisher did a fine job of recording all the details of meetings, she thought it was unnecessary. She wanted to see more practitioners attend meetings and otherwise participate more fully in the association. "Quite plainly," she told Dunton, it is "up to the occupational therapists to take on a little bit more responsibility relative to their own profession and not cast the burden upon the editor or the publishing firm."[35] Frustrated by what she perceived to be indifference to the association, she asked all the members present to take membership blanks back to their home institutions and personally assume responsibility for recruiting at least one new member for the following year.[36]

Slagle obviously thought that such a membership drive would automatically result in better support of the journal, but that was not the case. Dunton published an angry editorial the following year, admonishing the membership for its failure to subscribe to the journal. In 1923 he scolded, "227 of the subscribers of Volume I failed to renew for Volume II." The next year, 88 did not sign up again; and the following year, 110. This meant on the face of it that in 1925, only 340 of the association's 1,000 members were keeping up with their professional responsibilities. The reality, though, was even worse than that, Dunton explained. Only 120 subscriptions went to individuals; the rest belonged to libraries, hospitals, and schools.[37]

The fact that a mere 12 percent of association members found it imperative to subscribe to the journal surprised Dunton, who made assumptions about professional organizations according to his own experience as a physician. Occupational therapists, however, may have had different purposes in mind when they joined the association, job placement being among the most important. Obviously, only a few occupational therapists connected membership in the association with a subscription to the journal. Besides, an alternative existed that seemed not to cross Dunton's mind. Occupational therapists could read the issues in their libraries and institutions if they wanted to do so, without subscribing individually. Moreover, perhaps occupational therapists had less-formal means of communicating information among themselves.

Dunton's idea to combine membership in the national association with a subscription to the association's official journal became a reality in 1926, but not without administrative havoc and vocal opposition from the membership. Shortly after the 1925 meeting in Louisville, Kentucky, during which Dunton finally convinced those attending that the membership and subscription fees should be combined, the association entered into a contract with the Williams and Wilkins Publishing Company, pledging to pay for one annual subscription for every "sustaining" and "active" member in "good standing" as of January 1, 1926.

Slagle's office was inundated with complaints that first year, partly because some members resented the "increase of dues" imposed on them by the "officers" and also because the national office had difficulty providing the publisher with current addresses, resulting in some members not receiving their issues. To resolve the problem, President Thomas B. Kidner made a special trip to Baltimore for further discussions with the publisher, and special auditors were retained to bring the books up to date. The biggest problem to be resolved lay in the continuous failure of the rank-and-file to pay their membership fees on time. Without the payments the association could not maintain its financial obligation to the publisher. For example, in 1926 the association was scheduled to pay $1,750.00 to Williams and Wilkins; by September, it had paid only $1,141.50, leaving a balance of $608.50. Only 625 of 874 of the "members in good standing" had paid their dues for the year. Slagle scolded those who had not yet paid, saying that "if all members . . . had paid we should have $1650.00 in our treasury, which would have more than met every obligation of the association."[38]

In spite of all these problems, Dunton managed to keep the journal thriving. Moreover, his contributions as occupational therapy's publicizer went beyond the Committee on Publicity and Publication and the journal. Dunton led another AOTA committee that developed "an outline of lectures on occupational therapy to medical students and physicians."[39] The committee members realized that their own colleagues needed to be educated in the use of occupational therapy. G. Canby Robinson, a Vanderbilt University professor of medicine, thought it was just as important to teach "medical men . . . an intelligent conception of the methods, aims and possibilities of occupational therapy" as it was to "train occupational therapists to have an intelligent conception of the practice of medicine and of medical problems."[40]

The 1925 document that the committee produced offered a succinct overview of occupational therapy's growing relationships with different areas of medicine. The document defined occupational therapy, gave a history of the profession's development from ancient to contemporary times, explained occupational therapy's scope and application, laid out fifteen principles of occupational therapy, described different types of work and dosage, and then gave actual outlines of lectures in the specialty areas of general medicine and convalescence, surgery, tuberculosis, and mental illness.[41]

Curiously the document sped through all these topics quickly and superficially. Perhaps Dunton wanted only to pique the interest of physicians so that they would consider sending patients to the occupational therapy department, where the practitioner would take over. In an expanded version of this committee's work, a book specifically geared to physicians entitled *Prescribing Occupational Therapy*, Dunton explicitly stated that "brevity" was "purposely sought." He wanted merely to "present the subject so that it might be quickly apprehended by the busy physician or medical student." Going on the assumption that the readers were physician "specialists," "grounded" in their own branch, he wanted only to "correlate occupational therapy with [their] subject."[42]

## EVERETT S. ELWOOD AND THE PERILS OF PROFESSIONAL GROWTH

In 1926, at the tenth annual meeting of the association, Everett S. Elwood, representing the voice of physician-controlled organized medicine, spoke to the membership about the perils of professional growth and development. As managing director of the National Board of Medical Examiners, Elwood paternalistically advised the association on various means of "making certain that the back door is very carefully fastened against pretenders, that others do not crawl in under the fence and that those who are permitted to enter the front door have the proper credentials of admission." Medicine, he explained, had been "harassed by . . . various cults and quacks who . . . attempted to take advantage and capitalize on the great reputation" that the medical profession held. He pushed licensing as a legitimate and useful safeguard against quackery, a method successfully used by the medical profession. He also pledged support for development of a national examination for occupational therapists similar to the one that medical students had to take before they could obtain a license to practice. Further, Elwood urged university-affiliated training so that occupational therapy and medical students' paths would cross in teaching hospitals. Such contact, he argued, would ensure occupational therapy's status in medicine.[43]

In spite of occupational therapy's aim to establish itself in the medical world, the association's members resisted many of Elwood's suggestions. Licensing implied that physicians would take control of requirements for entry into the profession, and the occupational therapists did not want to lose that control. Rather than allow the state or the American Medical Association to license practitioners, the American Occupational Therapy Association intended to begin a system of registration, which it did set up by the end of the 1920s. The association resisted licensing until the 1970s.[44] Moreover, the notion of a national examination had already been considered by the association, and the issue had been resolved with the development of the minimum standards for training schools. Successful completion of a course of study in an endorsed school constituted proper preparation. Again, occupational therapy had created its own autonomous solution. Elwood's final suggestion, affiliation with the university, which often meant contact with medical schools, also went unconsidered. The independent schools held their ground for decades to come.

Indeed, occupational therapy held a precarious position in the world of medicine during the 1920s. Physicians could not control the new profession, yet many grew to depend on the services of occupational therapists. Usually physicians' acceptance of occupational therapy was based on its obvious utilitarian value. In 1925, B. W. Carr of the United States Veterans Bureau, whose usual work was to care for patients with tuberculosis, put it succinctly: "The patient is a unit of society, at present not only a non-producer, but an economic burden. Instead of an asset he has become a liability. Anything which will render him more contented in the hospital and will make it possible more quickly to return him to his work; anything which will make him a better citizen and of more value to himself, his family, and the community after his discharge should be given consideration. It has been found that occupational therapy, rightly used, is of material assistance in bringing about these desired results."[45]

Throughout the 1920s occupational therapists struggled to balance the profession's utilitarian and medical purposes.

Moreover, practitioners of the first generation strove to promote the service ideal that had been so prominent in women's reform work. The next section returns the focus to the world view of the practitioners of occupational therapy, most of whom were females. 🌿

## Notes

1. "Minutes of the Fifth Annual Meeting," *Archives of Occupational Therapy* 1 (1922): 232.

2. Ibid., 234, 160–61. In her comments to the membership Slagle did not specify whether she was talking about her work in the Illinois or New York State hospital system. She did say, however, that several hundred to twelve hundred patients were seen daily, all with prescriptions from physicians.

3. Mary M. Atwater, "Suggestion for a Classification of Occupations in Occupational Therapy," *Archives of Occupational Therapy* 1 (1922): 389.

4. "Minutes of the Fifth Annual Meeting," 232.

5. Herbert J. Hall died on February 19, 1923, of an unnamed long illness. He spent most of the last eight months of his life in the hospital. See Editorial, *Archives of Occupational Therapy* 2 (1923): 165–66.

6. "Fifth Annual Meeting of the National Society for the Promotion of Occupational Therapy," *Archives of Occupational Therapy* 1 (1922): 238–39.

7. "Round Table on Records Conducted by Horatio M. Pollock [*sic*]," *Archives of Occupational Therapy* 2 (1923): 217–18.

8. Horatio M. Pollack, "Outcome of Mental Diseases in the U.S.," *Mental Hygiene* 9 (1925): 783–804. In this article Pollack reported the results of his study of federal Census Bureau statistics as of January 1, 1923, of patients in residence in institutions for mental disease. The study included an analysis of first admissions, readmissions, discharges, and deaths. Other articles by Pollack include "Feebleminded in Institutions in the U.S.," *Mental Hygiene* 10 (1926): 804–10; "Frequency of Dementia Praecox in Relation to Sex, Age, Environment, Nativity, and Race," *Mental Hygiene* 11 (1926): 596–611; and "Progress and Present Status of Statistics in Mental Diseases," *Mental Hygiene* 11 (1927): 156–61.

9. Horatio M. Pollack, "Records and Statistics in Occupational Therapy," *Mental Hygiene* 5 (1921): 566–73.

10. Horatio M. Pollack, "Organization of Occupational Therapy in a State Hospital," *Mental Hygiene* 7 (1923): 149–53.

11. Horatio M. Pollack, "Six 'Musts' for Occupational Therapy," *Modern Hospital* 16 (1921): 169.

12. Pollack, "Organization of Occupational Therapy," 151–52.

13. G. L. Bellis, "Occupational Therapy in the Sanatorium Treatment of the Tuberculous," *Archives of Occupational Therapy* 3 (1924): 363–66.

14. "Report of the Committee on Research and Efficiency," in *Proceedings of the Fourth Annual Meeting of the National Society for the Promotion of Occupational Therapy* (Towson, Md.: NSPOT, 1920), 5–9.

15. Thomas B. Kidner, "Work for the Tuberculous during and after the Cure," pt. 2, *Archives of Occupational Therapy* 3 (1924): 169–93.

16. Thomas B. Kidner served as the institutional secretary of the National Tuberculosis Association in the early 1920s, working with the Institutional Construction Advisory Service. Some of his work was published in *American Architect* and *Modern Hospital*. See, for example, "Accommodation for Occupational Therapy in Federal Tuberculosis Sanatoriums," *Modern Hospital* 18 (1922): 292–94; and "Planning for Occupational Therapy," *Modern Hospital* 21 (1923): 414–28, which included many architectural drawings of occupational therapy departments in United States and Canadian hospitals.

17. Kidner, "Planning for Occupational Therapy," 418–19.

18. As quoted in Thomas B. Kidner, "Work for the Tuberculous during and after the Cure," pt. 1, *Archives of Occupational Therapy* 1 (1922): 375.

19. As quoted in Glenn Gritzer and Arnold Arluke, *The Making of Rehabilitation* (Berkeley: University of California Press, 1985), 78–79.

20. Following is a small sample of articles in which occupational therapists and their supporters argued for medical supervision in the care of patients with tuberculosis: H. A. Pattison, "The Trend of Occupational Therapy for the Tuberculous," *Archives of Occupational Therapy* 1 (1922): 19–24; Martin F. Sloan, "Occupational Therapy as Applied at Eudowood Sanatorium," *Archives of Occupational Therapy* 1 (1922): 121–29; Ruth B. Harter, "Organizing Occupation Therapy in New York County Hospitals," *Archives of Occupational Therapy* 1 (1922): 201–5; and Gertrude Sample, "Experience with Tuberculous Patients," *Archives of Occupational Therapy* 1 (1922): 205–13.

21. Kidner, "Work for the Tuberculous," pt. 1, 363–76.

22. A small sample of articles focusing on this debate follows: "Should Occupational Therapy Be Commercialized?" editorial, *Modern Hospital* 18 (1922): 294; "Commercialism," editorial, *Modern Hospital* 18 (1922): 374; William H. Livingston, "Useful Occupational Therapy vs. Useless Occupational Therapy," *Modern Hospital* 21 (1923): 210–12; Blanche B. McNew, "'Useless' versus Useful Occupational Therapy, *Modern Hospital* 21 (1923): 656–58; Susan C. Johnson, "Occupational Therapy and Post-Hospital Employment," *Modern Hospital* 22 (1924): 196–98; Ernest P. Boas, "In Defense of the Secondary Value of Occupational Therapy Work," *Modern Hospital* 22 (1924): 432; Thomas B. Kidner, "Therapeutic versus Selling Value of Occupational Therapy Work," *Modern Hospital* 23 (1924): 96–98; and Boston School of Occupational Therapy, "Outline of District and Curative Work Shop Department," *Modern Hospital* 23 (1924): 276–80, especially the sections titled "Product

Secondary to Curative Results" and "Aims Simply to Hasten Recovery."

23. "Commercialism," 374.

24. Boas, "In Defense of the Secondary Value"; Kidner, "Therapeutic versus Selling Value," 97.

25. "The Principles of Occupational Therapy," listed at the opening of this chapter, began to appear in various forms in many different publications beginning in 1918 when William R. Dunton presented a list at the Second Annual Meeting of the National Society for the Promotion of Occupational Therapy. For a longer version, which includes fourteen principles, see William R. Dunton, *Prescribing Occupational Therapy* (Springfield, Ill.: Charles C Thomas, 1928), 12–15.

26. On the back of the title page of the proceedings of the annual meeting of the National Society for the Promotion of Occupational Therapy for 1917 is this announcement: "The minutes of the meeting were printed by the Spring Grove Hospital Press and the remainder by the Sheppard Hospital Press. Bound by Sheppard Hospital Press all as a part of occupational therapy." A slightly modified statement appears in the 1918 and 1919 proceedings: "This book was printed and bound by patients at the Sheppard and Enoch Pratt Hospital as a form of occupational therapy." In the 1920 proceedings, the message is, "This book was printed and bound by patients at the Spring Grove State Hospital and the Sheppard and Enoch Pratt Hospital as a form of occupational therapy."

27. Robert K. Bing, "William Rush Dunton, Jr.—American Psychiatrist: A Study in Self" (Ed.D. diss., University of Maryland, 1961), chaps. 6, 7. Bing also points out that Dunton was affiliated with the *American Journal of Psychiatry* in various capacities from 1927 until the late 1950s.

28. "Report of the Committee on Finance, Publicity and Publication," in *Proceedings of the First Annual Meeting of the National Society for the Promotion of Occupational Therapy* (Towson, Md.: NSPOT, 1917), 29–31.

29. Ibid., 29–30.

30. "Report of the Committee on Finance, Publicity and Publication," *Archives of Occupational Therapy* 1 (1922): 64–66; see also the discussion following the report, 66–71.

31. See Contents, *Archives of Occupational Therapy* 1 (1922): iii–xviii.

32. Editorial, *Archives of Occupational Therapy* 1 (1922): 87–88.

33. Editorial, *Archives of Occupational Therapy* 3 (1924): 333–36.

34. "The Seventh Annual Meeting of the American Occupational Therapy Association," *Archives of Occupational Therapy* 3 (1924): 68–73.

35. Editorial, *Archives of Occupational Therapy* 3 (1924): 335.

36. "The Seventh Annual Meeting of AOTA," 72.

37. Editorial, *Archives of Occupational Therapy* 4 (1925): 391–93.

38. "Report of the Secretary-Treasurer, Year Ending September 15, 1926," *Occupational Therapy and Rehabilitation* 6 (1926): 451–63.

39. John D. Adams, B. W. Carr, G. Canby Robinson, and William R. Dunton, "An Outline of Lectures on Occupational Therapy to Medical Students and Physicians," *Occupational Therapy and Rehabilitation* 4 (1925): 277–92.

40. G. Canby Robinson, "The Relation of Occupational Therapy and Medicine," *Occupational Therapy and Rehabilitation* 4 (1925): 2–3.

41. Adams et al., "An Outline."

42. Dunton, *Prescribing Occupational Therapy*, v–vi.

43. Everett S. Elwood, "The National Board of Medical Examiners and Medical Education, and the Possible Effect of the Board's Program on the Spread of Occupational Therapy," *Occupational Therapy and Rehabilitation* 6 (1927): 341–47.

44. Gritzer and Arluke, *The Making*, 78–81.

45. B. W. Carr, "A Progressive Program of Occupational Therapy for Tuberculous Patients," *Occupational Therapy and Rehabilitation* 5 (1926): 175–85.

# PART IV

### ❦ ❦ ❦

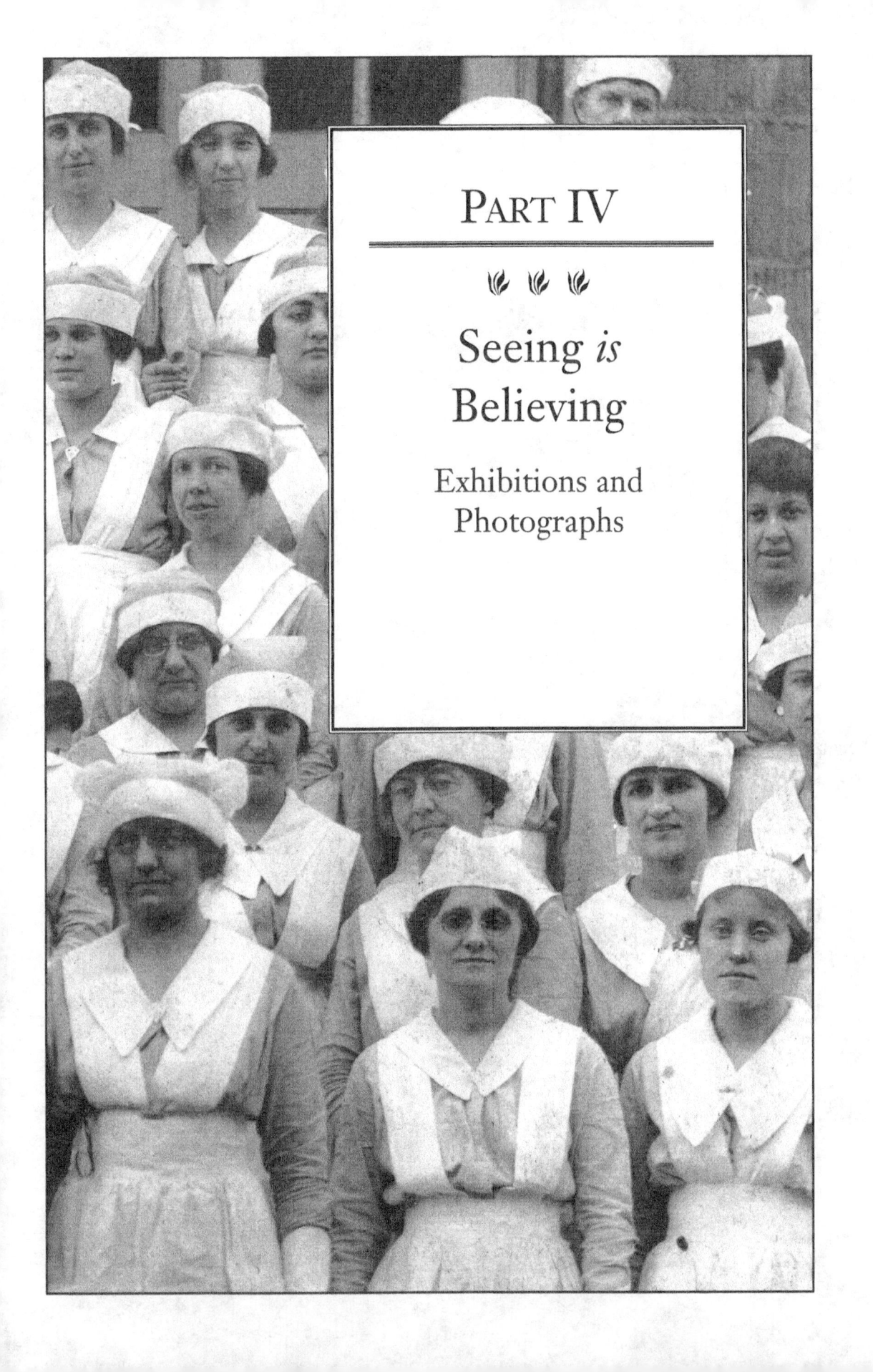

# Seeing *is* Believing

Exhibitions and Photographs

In 1937 in an Atlantic City hotel, 324 guests paid tribute to Eleanor Clarke Slagle at an American Occupational Therapy Association testimonial dinner. On the eve of Slagle's retirement from professional life, several speakers traced her many contributions to building the profession of occupational therapy and its national association. Fittingly two of the evening's speakers emphasized issues close to Slagle's heart. Adolph Meyer traced her important work in mental hygiene, saying that she had helped turn "psychology from esoteric contemplation into the service of actual life."[1] First Lady Eleanor Roosevelt, an activist in women's reform work in her own right, stressed Slagle's commitment to helping "those fighting their way back to health by way of the occupational therapy route."[2] Slagle certainly ended her occupational therapy career in a dignified but bright blaze of glory.

By the time that Slagle retired from occupational therapy, she and other members of the founding generation had established the profession's medical identity. They left another legacy as well. The vast majority of practitioners, like Slagle, found that they continued to dwell in two worlds, medicine and the culture of women's reform. They straddled these worlds in part because the work that they were doing did not fit comfortably into the world of scientific medicine. Their actual practice focused on attracting patients' attention to craft work, teaching patients the skills necessary to conduct such work, and supervising patients' progress through such activities. Craft work made it difficult for practitioners to demonstrate tangible improvement in patients, at least by the standards of scientific medicine. Rather than struggle to find methods of producing "objective" evidence, however, first-generation occupational therapists persisted in embracing the experiential and practical traditions begun in the Hull House Labor Museum decades before.

Still leaning on the methods and the philosophies of early-twentieth-century teaching and arts and crafts, occupational therapists gave both medical colleagues and women's reform constituents opportunities to make their own observations about patients' progress. Occupational therapists accomplished this by regularly and formally exhibiting patient-made craft products in hospitals, at school fund-raising events, and at national association meetings. Slagle, for example, showed a delighted Eleanor Roosevelt what wonderful work recovering patients could accomplish by guiding her through the exhibition held during the 1937 annual meeting (see photograph 10).

Part IV:
Seeing is Believing

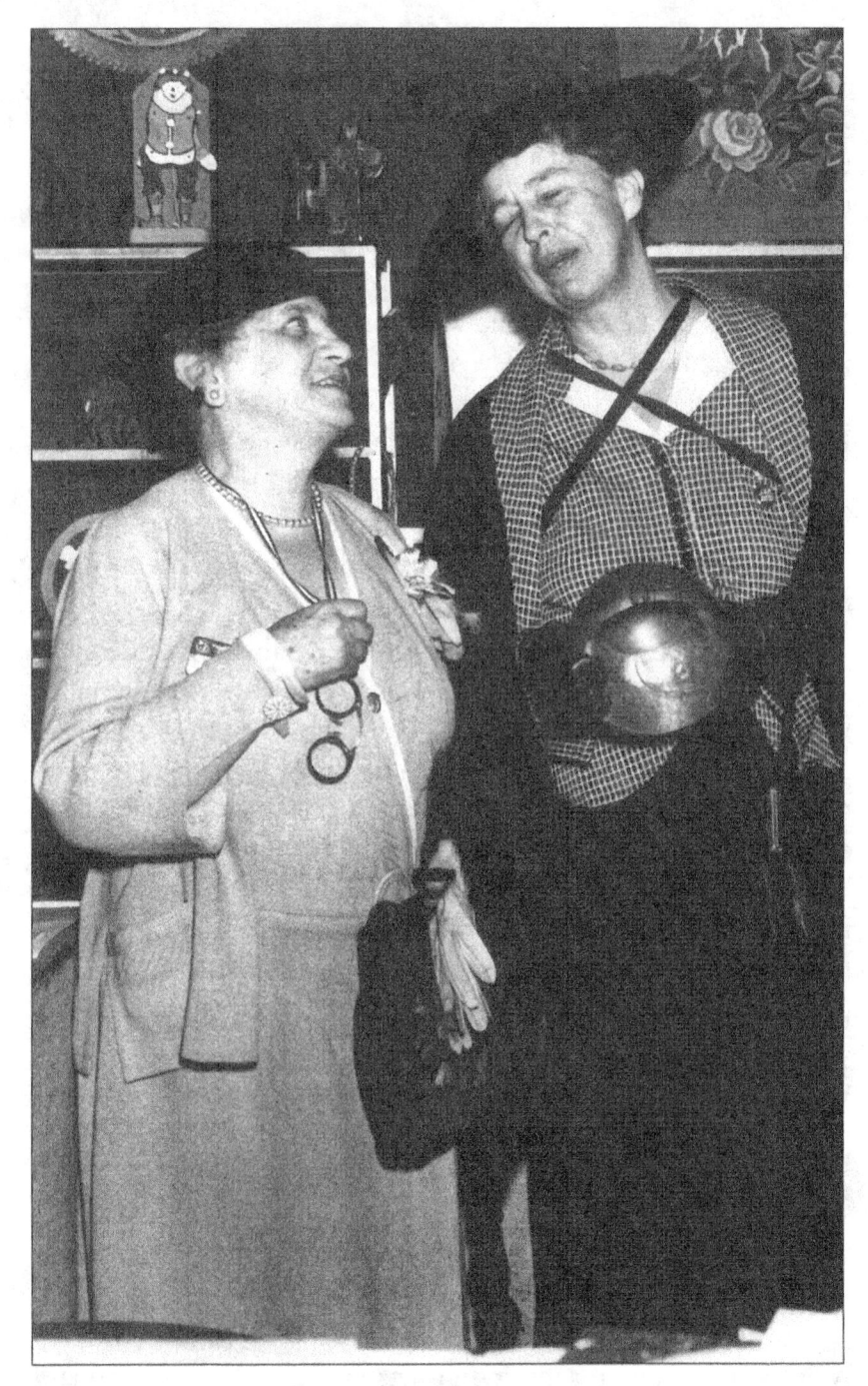

**Photograph 10:** Eleanor Clarke Slagle and Eleanor Roosevelt at the 1937 Annual Meeting of the AOTA. (John Davenport Clarke Papers, New York State Historical Association, Cooperstown)

Typically the annual meeting exhibitions contained a variety of patient-made products from institutions all over the country. In addition to displaying craft products, exhibitions often included photographs depicting patients at work and written case histories of patients. Fifty-one institutions contributed displays to the exhibition that accompanied the 1923 annual meeting in Milwaukee. Exhibitors asserted that the patient-made articles on display showed "therapeutic value." Half the exhibitors attached what they called "the history of the patient," otherwise called "series of charts," as a way of quantifying patients' progress and productivity, which they interpreted as meaning good health.[3] Sometimes photographs depicted practitioners closely supervising patients, underscoring the importance of the occupational therapist's role in managing individual patients' activity.

Given that craft work bonded patients and practitioners, it is not surprising that occupational therapists persistently used the finished products—the crafts—as a means of measuring and demonstrating patients' progress. This practice was of course slightly problematic because in certain circles occupational therapists had to deemphasize the objects that patients made. The problem of commercialism frequently compelled them to assert, "The real product of occupational therapy and the only reliable measure of treatment is the effect upon the patient."[4] Yet even though they dared not overemphasize to their medical constituency the importance of the craft product, first-generation occupational therapists deeply believed that if they persuaded patients to participate in craft activity, and pressed patients to complete a tangible object in the process, they contributed to the healing of patients.

Occupational therapists conducted exhibitions for several reasons. Hospital displays of patients' products helped in a practical way to attract physicians and patients to the occupational therapy department. Actually seeing interesting and useful items may have persuaded many skeptics to try the department's services. Occupational therapists also geared presentations to their female lay constituency—members of women's clubs and charity organizations—who often provided the raw materials for crafts and later disposed of finished products at fund-raising sales. Thus the exhibitions reinforced links to lay women, on whom the occupational therapists still depended for financial and moral support. Exhibitions conducted at meetings provided the additional function of giving practitioners a means of exchanging information about techniques. "Gaining new ideas" at exhibits was nearly as important as showing "the public that occupational therapy [meant] something far more than mere recreational handwork," according to the Exhibition Committee of the 1923 annual meeting.[5] Thus exhibitions became a crucial form of communication among practitioners as well as an effective public relations strategy, differing substantially from the written word with all its limitations.

First-generation occupational therapists left a remarkable photographic record to document their activities and their patients' work. Virtually every depository of occupational therapy historical materials contains numerous photographs of patient-made products in exhibition. "Reading" these photographic documents helps one understand the institutionalization of exhibitions in occupational therapy's history and the extent to which practitioners used patients' engagement in activity as a means of validating successful practice.

What follows is an analysis of exemplary photographs from hospital and school historical collections and from printed sources. These photographs, which vividly depict the experiences of first-generation occupational therapists, provide visual evidence of many changes that occurred during the profession's formative years. The photographs represent the three phases of occupational therapy history delineated in this book: the preprofessional/prewar years in the early 1910s, when practitioners primarily identified with the arts and crafts movement and women's altruistic reform work; the patriotic World War I period, when volunteers were swept up in a process that turned occupational therapy in the direction of a profession; and the 1920s, when occupational therapy took on its medical identity. The photographs range in subject matter: some depict patients and practitioners at work; others display of craft work; still others illustrate students in training. They were taken with deliberate purposes in mind: they project powerful images and messages, different than but just as meaningful as words. Overwhelmingly the photographs depict the ideas that work is a necessary means of achieving good health and that occupational therapists create the atmosphere in which the nexus between work and health occurs.

### THE PREWAR ERA (PHOTOGRAPHS 11–14)

In the prewar era (photographs 11–14), women took domestic activities such as cloth production and basket weaving to institutional settings such as tuberculosis and children's hospitals. They did so in the tradition of women's altruistic work with deprived or dependent populations, and as arts and crafts enthusiasts.

Photographs 11–13 were published in a series of books by Herbert James Hall and his colleague Mertice M. C. Buck.

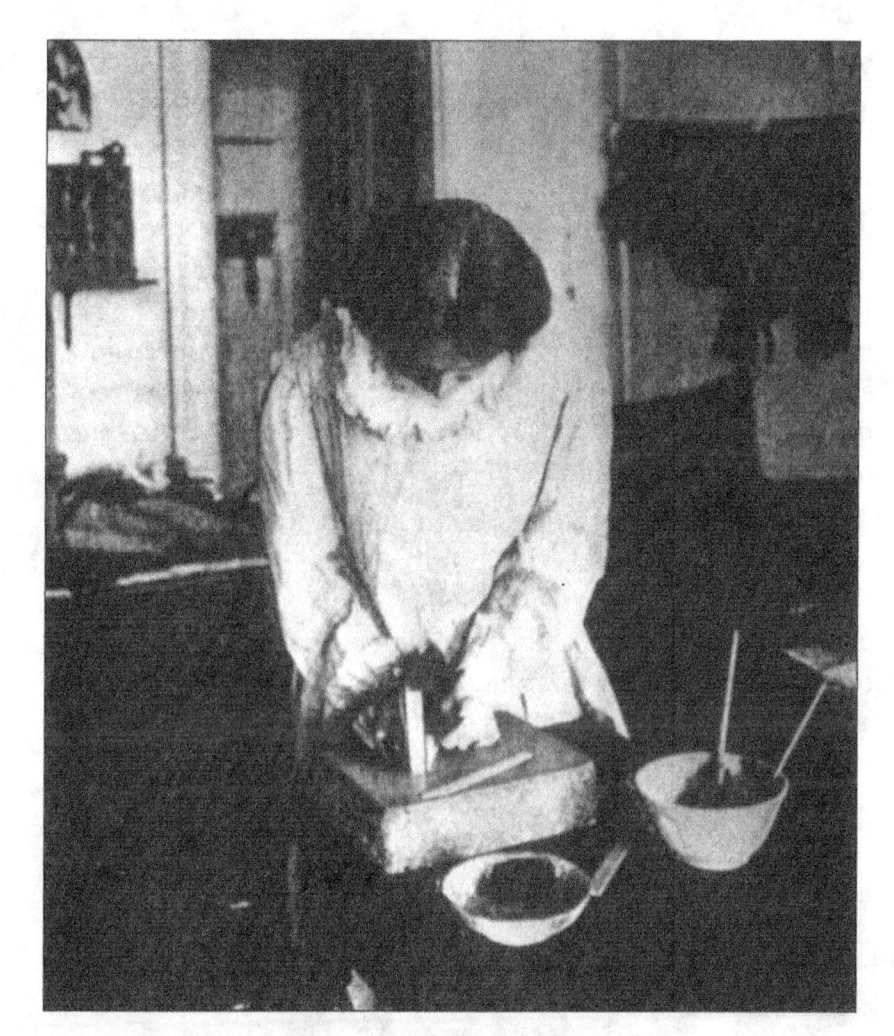

*Exhibitions and Photographs*

**Photograph 11:** Covering a full-bound book. (Hall and Buck, *Handicrafts for the Handicapped*, p. 108)

Dressed in a craftswoman's apron, the woman in photograph 11 devotes all her attention to bookbinding, a craft that was extremely popular and readily affordable in the early twentieth century. Some arts and crafts enthusiasts wanted to preserve the tradition of medieval bookbinding; others simply wanted to rebind old books or make portfolios and guest books. Participating in the amateur photography craze of the early twentieth century, still others made albums in which they could place photographs taken by "the family kodak [*sic*] fiend."[6]

Set in a room that looks like a shop, the photograph shows a bookbinder at work. On the worktable are several tools of the trade, including glue pots, sticks and brushes for mixing and application, and measuring instruments. A sewing frame and tapes, needed to put pages of a book together, stand ready behind her. A supply of leather, the raw material for covering books, hangs on the rack against the wall on the right. As well as tools and works-in-progress, there is a shelf of books already beautifully bound.

Although bookbinding is depicted in the photograph as individual work, many occupational therapy advocates recommended it as an excellent industry for workers with disabilities. Hall, for example, described a Scandinavian "cooperative industry" in schools for persons with physical disabilities, where government reports were both printed and bound under large contracts.[7] In the 1910s, William R. Dunton's patients printed and bound books in shops at the Sheppard-Pratt Hospital.

Arts and crafts enthusiasts and occupational therapists alike were fascinated with the loom, "a machine in which yarn or thread is woven into a fabric by the crossing of threads called chain or warp, running lengthwise with others called weft, woof or filling."[8] Typically the frame of a loom was made of wood and measured approximately 5 feet high, 5 feet wide, and 6 feet long. With very old looms, weavers made fabric by darning or

**Photograph 12:** A light weight loom. (Hall and Buck, *Handicrafts for the Handicapped*, p. 80)

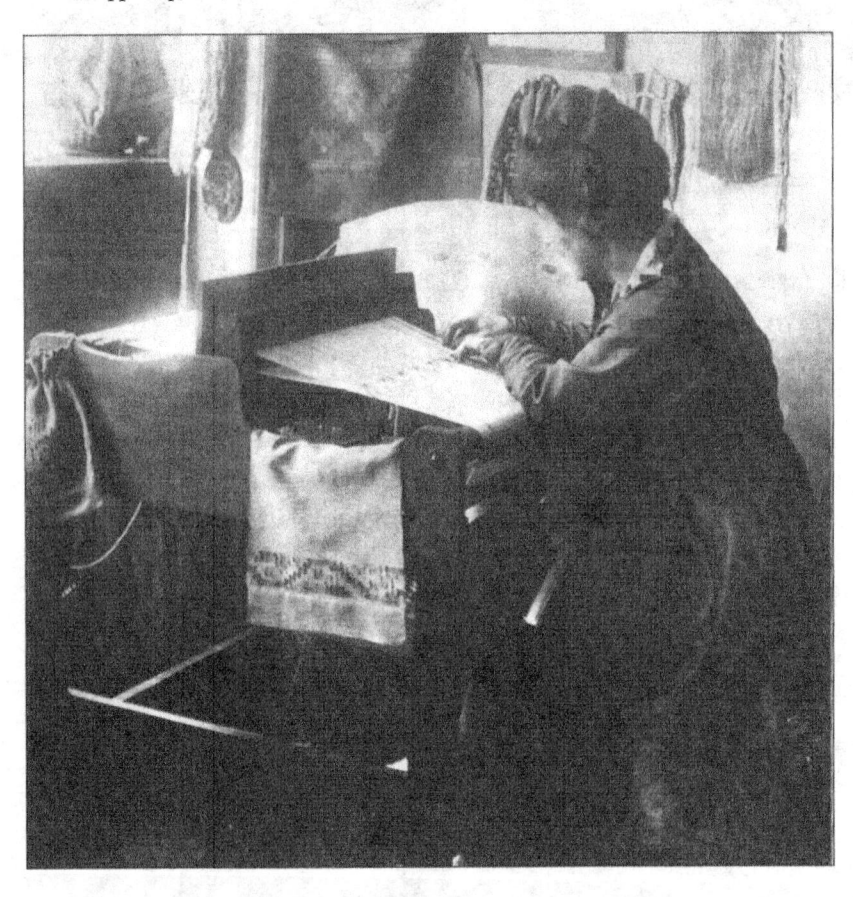

passing a needle or a shuttle over one thread and under another. By the colonial period a pedal-driven shedding method that mechanically arranged the position of alternate threads was common. Often schools or hospitals hired a well-experienced weaver to set up the looms and put on the warps as needed because these processes required considerable skill.

Using large looms, early-twentieth-century weavers—whether they were arts and crafts enthusiasts or occupational therapy patients—made rag rugs or denim, chintz, or flannel fabrics that could be used as bedspreads, curtains, blankets, or other such objects. The small, lightweight loom depicted in photograph 12, which could be purchased already threaded, was ideal for producing smaller objects such as bags, place mats, pillow covers, hatbands, and decorative patterned pieces.[9]

Photograph 12 shows a female weaver near a window, the light from which idealizes the work she does by forming a halo around the loom. Although the woman is turned away from the camera, the many beautiful patterned objects that she has produced with her loom face the camera for all to see. Dressed in a matronly fashion and working in what appears to be a tiny corner of her home, the woman evokes early-twentieth-century notions of femininity and domesticity.

Before World War I, occupations workers toiled mainly in tuberculosis and mental hospitals, and on a smaller scale, with patients who were physically disabled or visually impaired. As physicians became more involved in chronic disease and orthopedics, they opened specialized clinics and hospitals for their patients, and occupations workers flocked to these institutions for employment. Especially when children with disabilities needed assistance, participating in their care seemed natural because tending to children had long been women's purview.

In photograph 13, taken at the Hospital for Ruptured and Crippled in New York City, two women supervise a neat row of children with disabilities, in a large room filled with light from overhead windows. The children appear to be cared for according to middle-class standards. Outfitted impeccably, the girls wear dresses and hair bows, and the boy sports a fine shirt and pants. The nurse, clad in a uniform, projects an image of gentleness, overseeing the patients as a mother would her own children. The other woman has the technical and personal skills needed to encourage young sick children to participate in making decorative boxes. Crutches, a wheelchair, and leg braces are

*Part IV: Seeing is Believing*

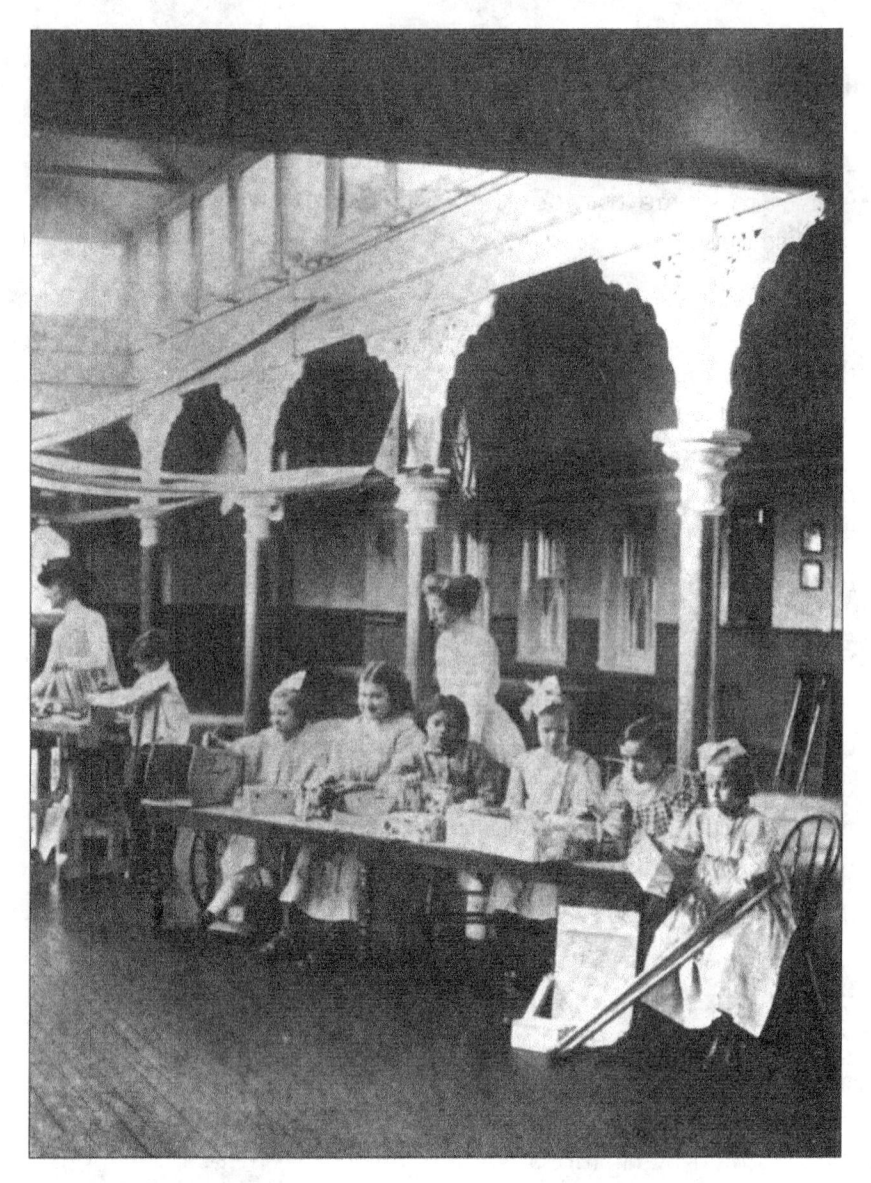

**Photograph 13:** Occupation room at the Hospital for Ruptured and Crippled in New York City. (Hall and Buck, *The Work of Our Hands*, p. 182)

not hidden from the camera, sending the message that in spite of disability, the children are capable of working independently on projects.

The children's work is differentiated by gender. The girls, all at one table, are finishing boxes by decoratively papering or painting them. The boy, at a different table, constructs boxes with tools such as a hammer, a saw, and a vise. The photograph gives a mixed message: it reinforces early-twentieth-century sex roles by saying that boys do carpentry while girls decorate, yet it shows a woman teaching what is traditionally a man's occupation, carpentry. The viewer overlooks the paradox because teaching is considered a woman's vocation and because the students are children and they are ill.

The leaders of the Arequipa Sanatorium in Fairfax, California, like the leaders of most hospitals and sanatoriums, had many photographs taken for their institution's annual reports and other public relations pieces. Arguing that persons with tuberculosis had to be removed from the unhealthful city environment, the leaders touted the sanatorium's modern facilities, which were located in the pristine setting of Marin County

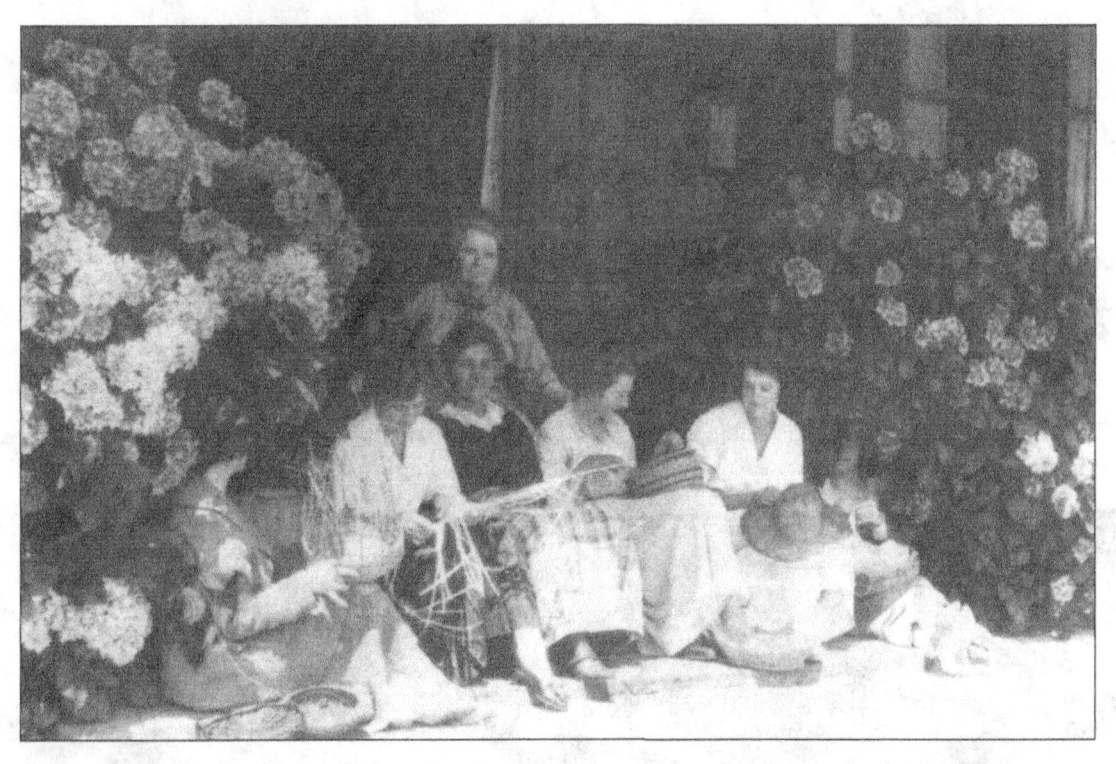

**Photograph 14:** Occupational therapy activities at Arequipa Sanatorium, Marin County, California. (AOTA Archives)

in the 1910s. Philip King Brown wanted everyone to know that the rural sanatorium saved his urban, female, working-class patients from the physical and moral ravages of tuberculosis.

In photograph 14, several women work on baskets, shown in several stages of completion. Seated on the front porch steps of the main building at the Arequipa Sanatorium, the women are nestled between blooming hydrangea shrubs. The healing sun shines on the women, who seem to be enjoying one another's company as well as the work that they are doing collectively. One woman, who appears to be the institution's matron, affectionately touches a patient on the shoulder. Such a gesture, and the front porch setting, suggest a personal or family relationship between the matron and the patients that is reminiscent of typical nineteenth-century hospitals. In fighting the dreaded disease tuberculosis, Arequipa Sanatorium personnel seemed to reject twentieth-century professional standards of objective relations between patient and practitioner. Practitioners would be much more conscious about projecting professional images by World War I.

## WARTIME (PHOTOGRAPHS 15–19)

In wartime (photographs 15–19), the reconstruction aides became invaluable members of the war effort, and worked in army hospitals at home and abroad. The following photographs highlight the variety of settings and activities in which they were involved.

**Photograph 15:** Reconstruction aide Lena Hitchcock with a patient with gunshot wounds in both legs, Chateauroux, France. (National Library of Medicine)

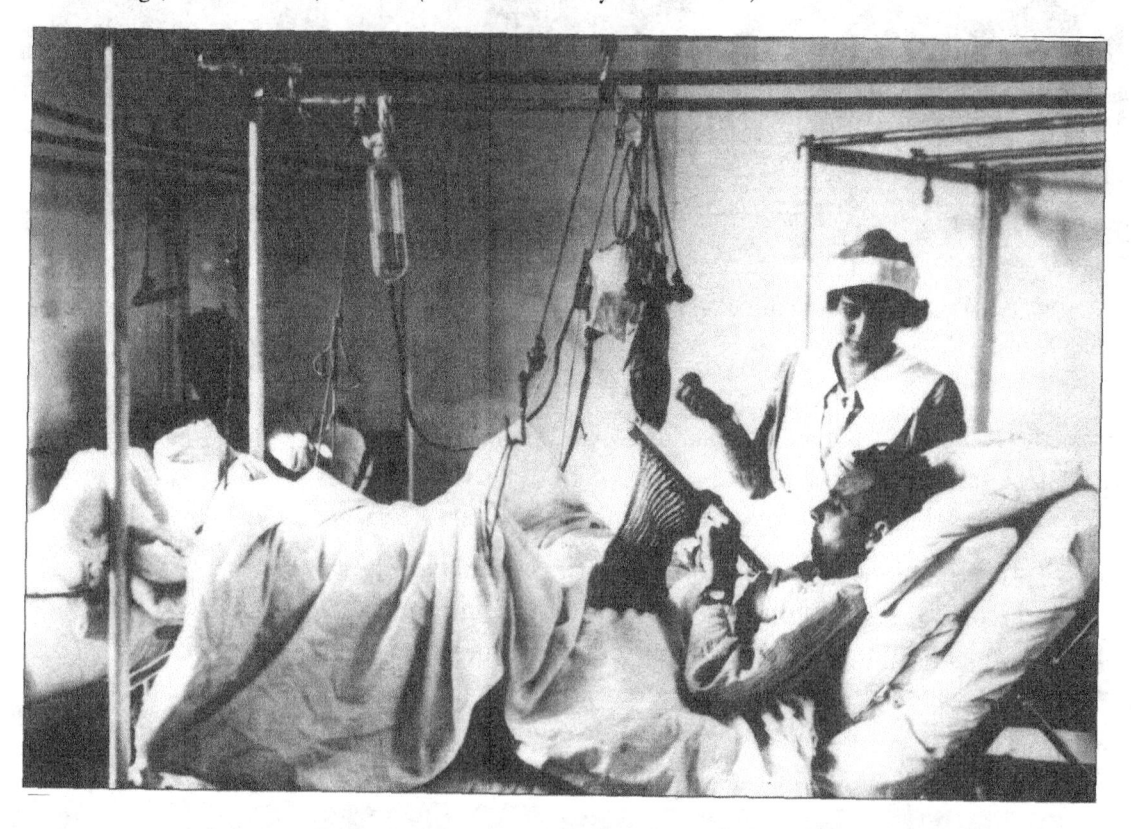

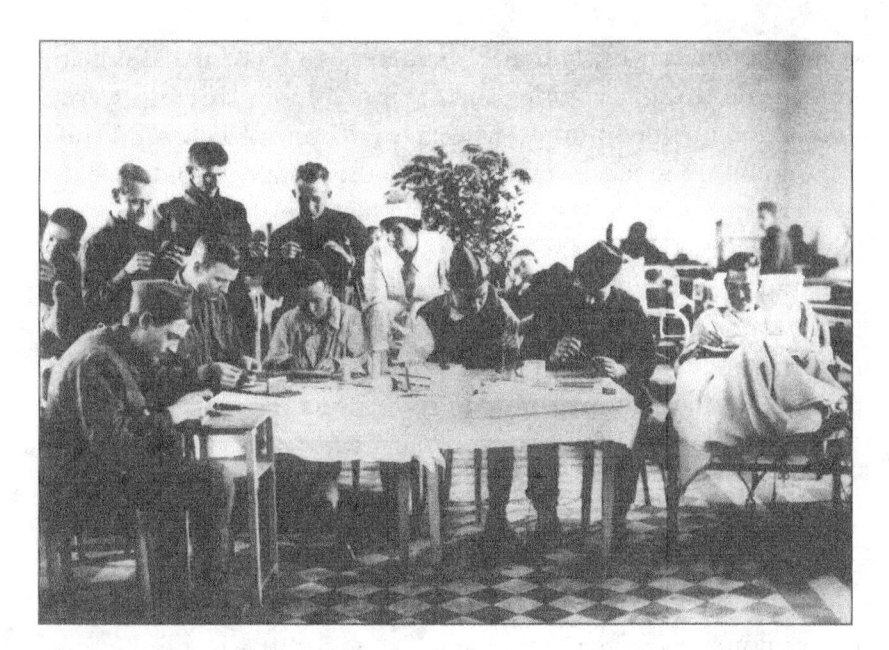

**Photograph 16:** Class in occupational therapy, Chateauroux, France. (National Library of Medicine)

In photographs 15 and 16, reconstruction aide Lena Hitchcock treats patients at Base 9, Chateauroux, France. Hitchcock was among the first reconstruction aides ordered overseas. They landed in France on August 11, 1918, and stayed until May 11, 1919. This original group included thirteen occupational therapists and fourteen physical therapists. Led by Susan Hiels from Boston, who had trained under Dr. Joel E. Goldthwait (by then in charge of Orthopedic Surgery in France), the occupational therapy reconstruction aides consciously strove to establish their profession as legitimate. They faced very difficult circumstances in France. Their tools and materials had been lost in transit, and because the government provided no money for materials, they were forced to beg and borrow in order to get started. According to Hitchcock, the reconstruction aides had tools "copied in the blacksmith shop, begged others from the Engineers and Aviation Camp nearby, and out of our own pockets bought the necessary things and materials." In spite of these obstacles this first group succeeded in convincing the chief surgeon of the American Expeditionary Forces, General Ireland, that the work that they were doing "was of a very high order" both "curatively and by way of morale." General Ireland cabled home for additional reconstruction aides, who served at Base 9, Chateauroux, and then at Base 114 in Beau Desert, near Bordeaux, and Base 8, Savenay, near Britanny.[10]

In photograph 15, Hitchcock supervises a weaving patient at the bedside. Light activities such as small-loom weaving were often recommended in the early stages of convalescence. In the photograph, Hitchcock stands close to the wounded soldier, but she does not touch him, nor does she make eye contact as she gives directions about the work he is doing. Every reconstruction aide knew instinctively that a patient could not be "ordered to do occupational work"; rather, he should be "induced to do so through the [individual] interest taken in him by the aides."[11] This photograph shows how the reconstruction aide took personal interest in a patient without being personal.

In photograph 16, Hitchcock supervises a class of patients in various stages of convalescence. Of particular interest is the way in which Hitchcock and the patients concentrate on the work that they are doing. This image suggests to the viewer that anyone, even a person who is sickly or disabled, can become useful, given the right circumstances. Clad in her blue uniform, Hitchcock shows that viewer that patriotic duty drew her to "do her bit for the boys."

In photograph 17 the reconstruction aide, who may be an occupational therapist or a physical therapist, demonstrates a

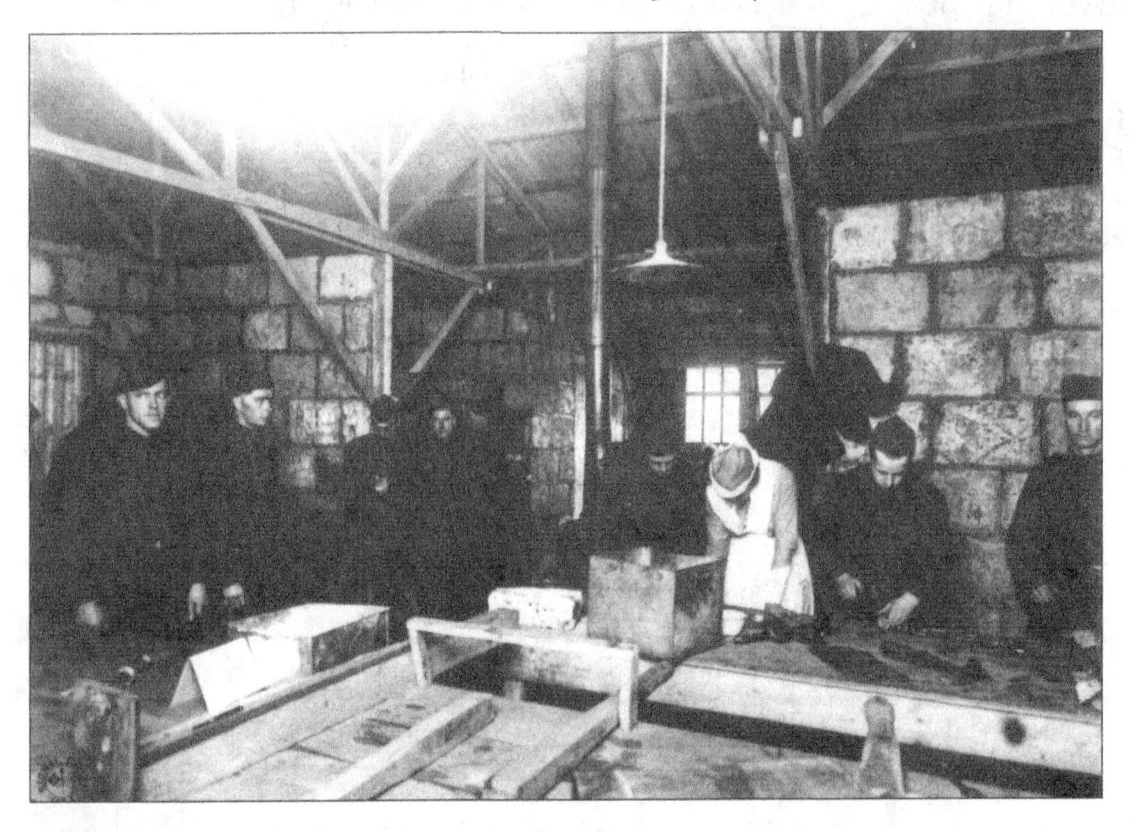

**Photograph 17:** General workshop, occupation building, Savenay, Loire Inferieure, France.

procedure to a class of wounded convalescing soldiers in a makeshift workshop. Identifying with middle-class values about productive work and good citizenship, female reconstruction aides participated in reaching the goals of the larger reconstruction movement. They helped lead soldiers back to a socially useful role in postwar American society.

In photographs 18 and 19, soldiers in various stages of convalescence are making jewelry in a stateside hospital. The men are not only recovering from their wounds, but are also learning new vocational skills that will provide them with economic independence when they are discharged from the armed services. The close-up image of the soldier in photograph 19 emphasizes that even men with serious injuries can be made productive again.

**Photograph 18:** Group craft activities in the workshop, U.S.A. General Hospital No. 36, Detroit, Michigan. (National Library of Medicine)

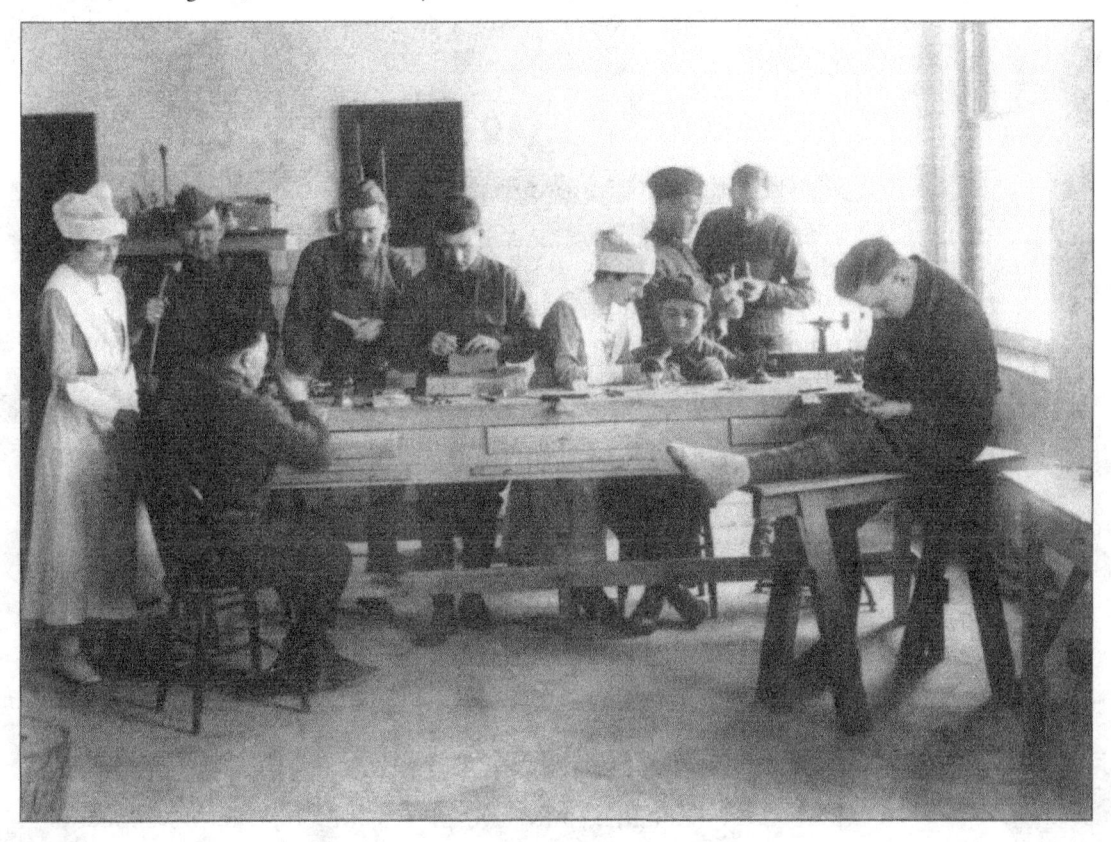

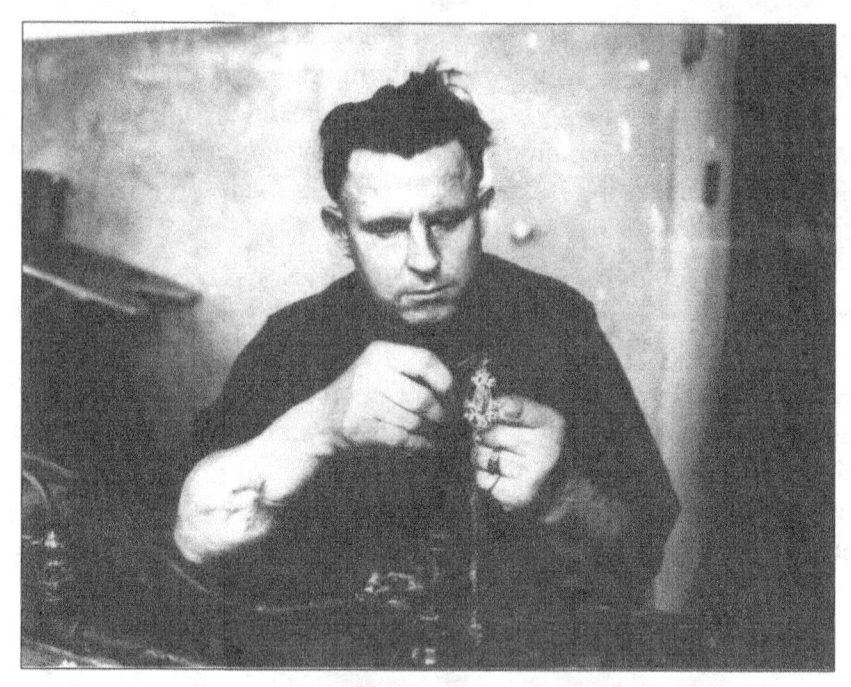

**Photograph 19:** Patient making jewelry to regain finger motion and dexterity following forearm injury, U.S.A. General Hospital No. 36, Detroit, Michigan. (National Library of Medicine)

## THE POSTWAR PERIOD (PHOTOGRAPHS 20–24)

After the war (photographs 20–24), many reconstruction aides continued to claim the professional identity of occupational therapist. They took jobs in a variety of institutions that delivered occupational therapy services, including hospitals and rehabilitation centers, often called "sheltered workshops." Many served as mentors to newcomers in the field, frequently in educational and clinical settings. Usually these institutions were financed by women's charity networks. Photograph 20 shows products of the 1920–21 class of students at the St. Louis School of Occupational Therapy, all of whom received training in several crafts. The sign above the fireplace mantel says that the crafts that are taught include design, basketry, beadwork, metal work, weaving, pottery, bookbinding, modeling, leather work, toy making, wood carving, printing, woodworking, and stenciling.

As well as learning craft skills, occupational therapy students were socialized into the profession. Instructors expected students to display certain personality traits and habits that they saw as fitting for professional women. For example, instructors at the St. Louis School of Occupational Therapy looked for qualities such as adaptability, resourcefulness, intelligence (the ability to understand new ideas or instructions), judgment and common sense (the ability to think clearly and arrive at logical conclusions), tact (the faculty of being considerate and sensible in dealing with others), initiative (the trait of beginning needed work or taking appropriate action on one's own responsibility), punctuality, neatness and personal appearance, dependability, and loyalty.[12] These were the very traits that occupational therapists hoped to instill in patients.

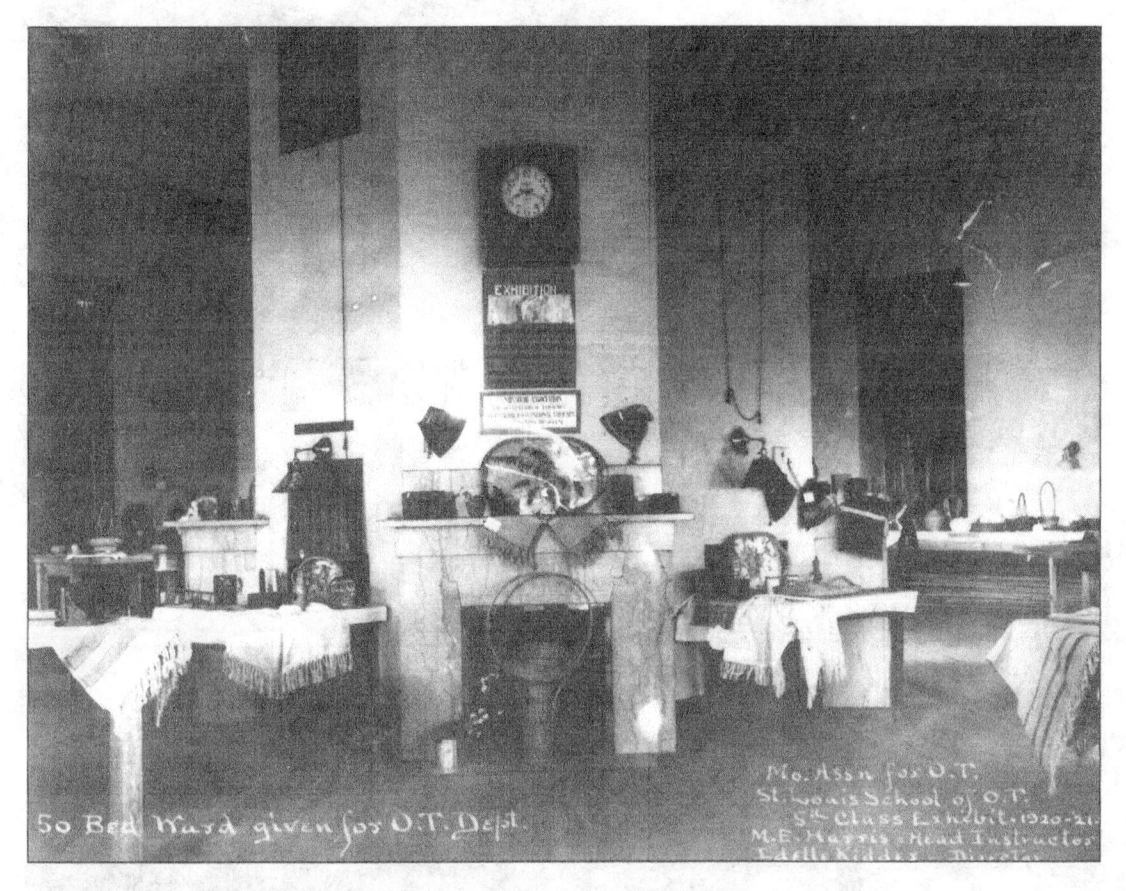

**Photograph 20:** St. Louis School of Occupational Therapy Workshop. (Historical files, St. Louis School of Occupational Therapy photograph collection)

In photograph 21 an occupational therapist, in uniform, is showing patient-made products to a woman dressed in a coat. The setting is the Robert Koch Hospital for tuberculosis care, in St. Louis, Missouri. One woman is a professional, the other an interested citizen who will support the work of patients with tuberculosis by buying products that they have made.

Photograph 22, also taken at the Robert Koch Hospital, depicts an occupational therapist overseeing the weaving work of three patients, who are outside even though it is winter.

Part IV: Seeing is Believing

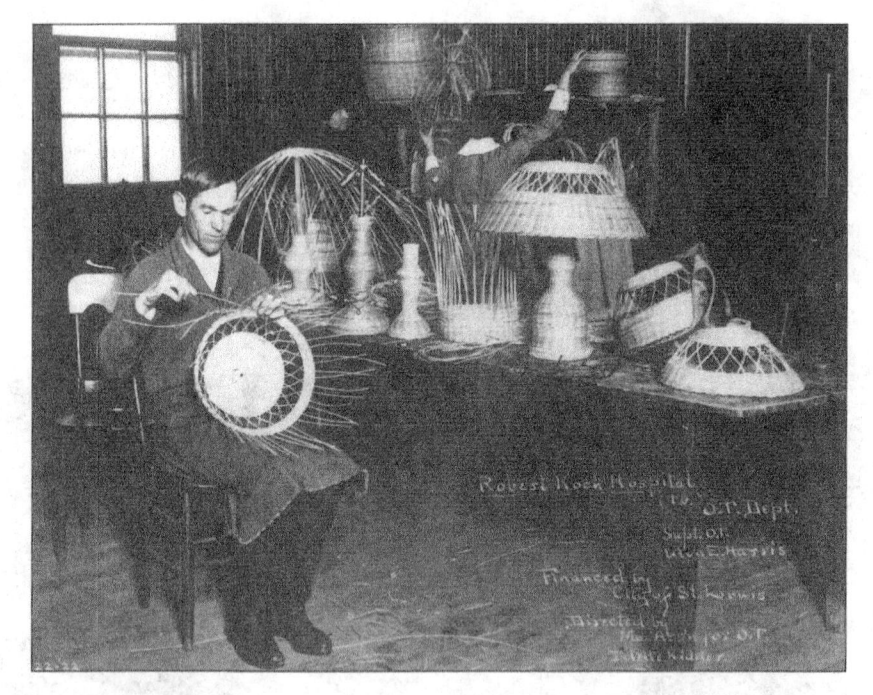

**Photograph 21:** Occupational therapy department, Robert Koch Hospital. (Historical files, St. Louis School of Occupational Therapy photograph collection)

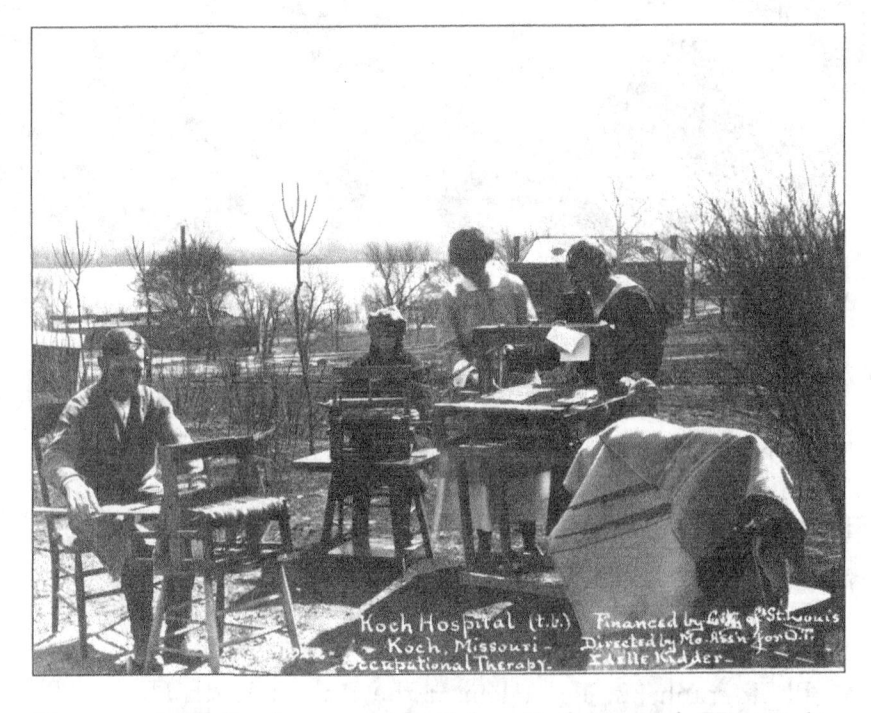

**Photograph 22:** Outdoors weaving, Robert Koch Hospital. (Historical files, St. Louis School of Occupational Therapy photograph collection)

Early-twentieth-century medical practice called for patients with tuberculosis to receive plenty of fresh air and sunshine in order to get well. Supervised work, in the view of occupational therapists, enhanced such practice. The photograph shows not only patients at work, but also beautiful finished products. There is an absence of division of labor by gender; weaving was appropriate for male or female patients.

**Photograph 23:** Curative workshop, U.S. Veterans Hospital, Maywood, Illinois, 1924. (AOTA Archives)

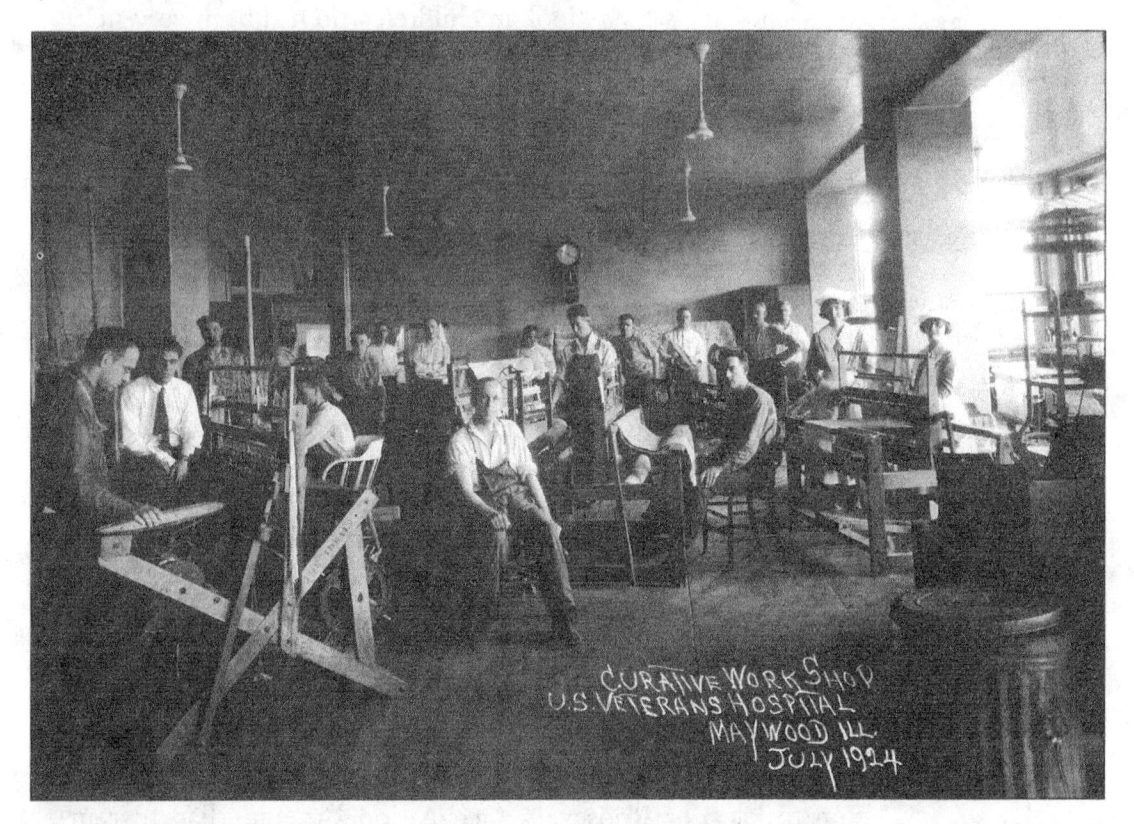

Photograph 23, taken in the curative workshop at the United States Veterans Hospital in Maywood, Illinois, is interesting because it is unlike most other occupational therapy photographs. Instead of presenting patients hard at work, it shows them looking at the camera. Rather than representing occupational therapists in a supervisory role, it displays them standing passively near the window, not among the patients. Only two patients (on the left) are actually working; one is weaving, the other making a basket. A man in a shirt and tie seems to be advising them. He is probably a physician, the person most obviously in charge in this setting.

Although some reconstruction aides continued to work as occupational therapists long after the war, others eventually "gave in and got married," as Anna Wheelright Codman did after seven years of practice. Codman continued to apply the world view and the skills that she had acquired during her years as a reconstruction aide, however. Her role as housewife and mother of two children precluded her working in a professional capacity, but she still taught what she had learned in occupational therapy to others. As she raised her two children, she volunteered at the Red Cross, the Girl Scouts summer camp, and on Children's Island in Massachusetts, which "took in children who had been very sick." In these settings, in her own words, she applied "extensions of O.T.'s way of looking at the world," which for her mainly meant service to others.[13] This value was shared by many other occupational therapists of the first generation.

## The Legacy of the First Generation

Eleanor Clarke Slagle's retirement in 1937 represented much more than the experience of one person. Her career, which began at Hull House in the first decade of the twentieth century, spanned a period in which a generation of American women first participated in professional work. Moreover, she embodied the combination of women's reform and scientific values and ideas that set occupational therapy on its professional trajectory. An influential person, Slagle largely shaped the profession of occupational therapy, helping to keep in balance its many disciplinary aspects internally while skillfully fixing connections to outside supporters.

As Slagle left occupational therapy in 1937, she pointed the way for the next generation in her brief but significant connection to Eleanor Roosevelt. Occupational therapy had to reinforce and build on its connections with state and federal governments in order to continue its growth and development. Legislation such as the National Emergency Act of the 1930s, the World War II Disabled Veterans Rehabilitation Act of 1943, and the Vocational Rehabilitation Act Amendments of 1943 and 1954 would continue to shape the opportunities for practice in occupational therapy.

This book has contended that the founding generation of occupational therapists observed a gender-defined division of labor. The men conducted the work necessary to broadcast and strengthen the relationships between occupational therapy and various medical specialties. The women concentrated on the internal workings of the profession by building and developing

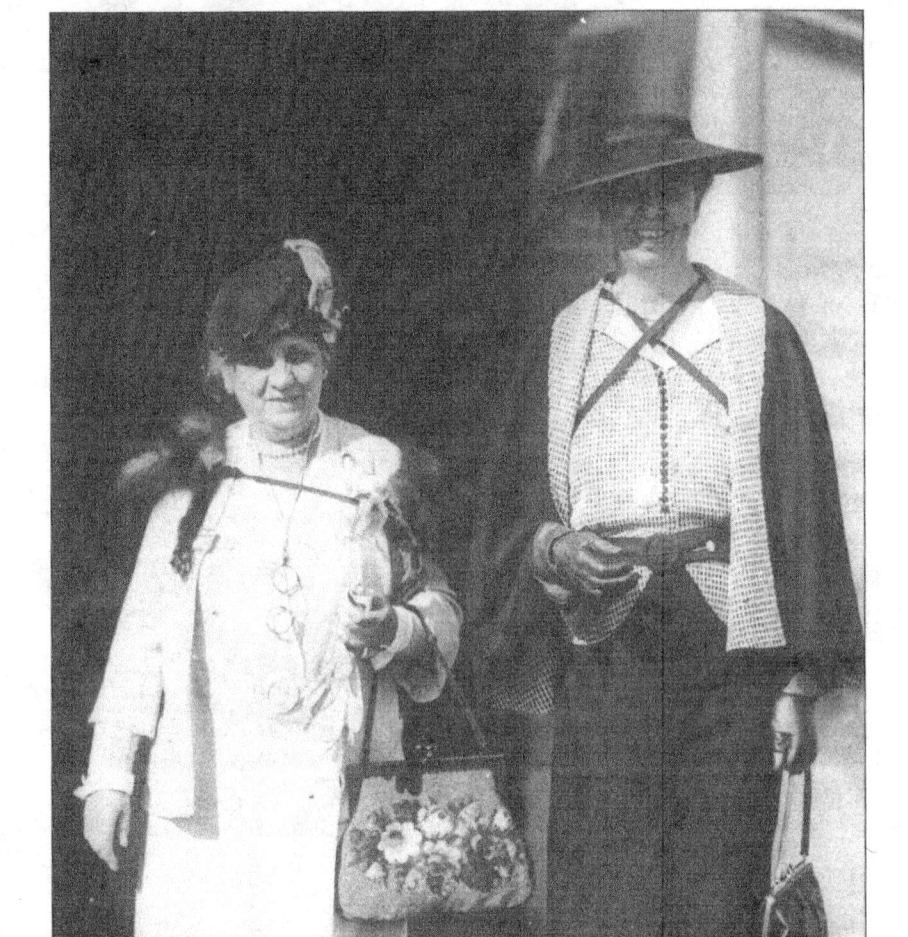

*Exhibitions and Photographs*

**Photograph 24:** Eleanor Clarke Slagle and Eleanor Roosevelt at the 1937 Annual Meeting of the AOTA. (John Davenport Clarke Papers, New York State Historical Association, Cooperstown)

teaching and practice institutions and by socializing newcomers to the field—all while struggling to find their own identity as professionals.

The experience of the second generation of occupational therapists differed greatly from that of the first generation. As women trained in the 1920s by the first generation took leadership roles in occupational therapy institutions during the 1930s, they had to learn to negotiate with a medical world that held more and more power over hospital policy. They also had to fight for the profession's integrity when physical medicine rose in stature and threatened to merge occupational therapy into physical therapy. They would serve in the military during World War II, bringing home experiences that needed to be analyzed differently from those of World War I. After World War II, female practitioners took over the leadership positions in the American Occupational Therapy Association previously held by male physicians, blurring the gender-defined division of labor observed by the first generation.

At the same time, the second generation of occupational therapists had certain values and orientations in common with their predecessors. They used crafts in therapy, and they maintained relationships with women's clubs and reform organizations. Most important, they experienced the culture of a profession dominated by women. Further scholarly work may reveal how the traditions laid down by the first generation evolved as women's status and position in American society changed over time. 🍃

## Notes

1. Adolph Meyer, "Address in Honor of Eleanor Clarke Slagle," *Occupational Therapy in Mental Health* 5 (1985): 111.

2. As quoted in newspaper clipping, Charlotte Johnson, "I Cover the Beachfront: First Lady Here; Escapes Crowds; Simplicity Striking," scrapbook, John Davenport Clarke Papers, New York State Historical Association, Cooperstown. For background on Eleanor Roosevelt's long and distinguished work in women's reform, see Blanche Wiesen Cook, *Eleanor Roosevelt* (New York: Viking, 1992).

3. "Fifty-one Institutions Display Work at Occupational Therapy Exhibit," *Modern Hospital* 21 (1923): 652–54.

4. William R. Dunton, "Principles of Occupational Therapy," in Proceedings of the Second Annual Meeting of the National Society for the Promotion of Occupational Therapy (Towson, Md.: NSPOT, 1918), 26–30.

5. "Fifty-one Institutions," 654.

6. Herbert J. Hall and Mertice M. C. Buck, Handicrafts for the Handicapped (New York: Moffat, Yard and Company, 1916), 83–85.

7. Ibid., 84.

8. Ibid., 62.

9. Ibid., 7.

10. Laura Brackett Hoppin, ed., *History of the World War Reconstruction Aides* (Millbrook, N.Y.: William Tyldsley, 1933), 50–51.

11. Manuscript B-122, exhibit "B," U.S. Army General Hospital 6, Observations and Suggestions by the Chief Educational Officer, p. 10; History of Medicine Division, National Library of Medicine, Bethesda, Maryland; manuscript B-122, exhibit "N," U.S. Army General Hospital 6, Cases, History of Medicine Division, National Library of Medicine.

12. "Reports of Practice Training of the St. Louis School of Occupational Therapy," mss., 1923–26, Papers of the St. Louis School of Occupational Therapy, School of Medicine Library, Washington University, St. Louis, Missouri.

13. Anna Wheelright Codman, interview by Nedra Gillette, 6 August 1986, Oral History Collection, American Occupational Therapy Foundation, Bethesda, Maryland.

# Index

## A

Activity treatment, pre-20th century, 19–22
Adams Nervine Asylum, Tracy, Susan E., 73–79
Addams, Jane, 37–41
Allen, Jenny Kaye, 211
Alternative medicine, 5
Altruism, 77–78, 83, 132–133
Amar, Jules, 152
American Expeditionary Forces, 164–165
    reconstruction aide, 164–165
American Federal Board for Vocational Education. *See* Federal Board for Vocational Education
American Occupational Therapy Association, 212. *See also* National Society for the Promotion of Occupational Therapy
    Barton, George Edward, 174–175
    Committee on Admissions and Positions
        Davis, Elizabeth Upham, 218–220
        education reform, 218–220
        Johnson, Susan Cox, 218–220
    Committee on Publicity and Publication, Dunton, William Rush, Jr., 245–250
    East Coast bias, 216–217
    foundation, 174
    Johnson, Susan Cox, 175
    Kidner, Thomas B., 174–175
    leadership, 15
    member services, 216
    minimum training standards, 223–226
    regional rivalry, 216–218
    Slagle, Eleanor Clarke, 176–177
    Wade, Beatrice, 211–212
Annual meeting exhibitions, 261, 262–263

*Archives of Occupational Therapy,* 174, 246
    founding, 247
    purposes, 247–248
    subscriptions to, 248–249
Arequipa Sanatorium, Brown, Philip King, 125, 128–129
Arts and crafts movement, 39, 93
Asclepiades, 19
Atwater, Mary M., 236
Autonomy, 83

## B

Barton, George Edward, 116–125, 120
    American Occupational Therapy Association, 174–175
    Consolation House, 117–119
    Dunton, William R., 120–122, 123
    early life, 116–117
    efficiency, 119
    hospital, 119–120
    illness, 117
    National Society for the Promotion of Occupational Therapy, 116, 122–123
Basketmaking, 264, 269–270, 274, 277
Beers, Clifford W., 119–120
Bing, Robert K., 16
Bookbinding, 265–266
Boston School of Occupational Therapy, 96
Boxmaking, 267–268
Brackett, Elliot G., 152–153
Brackett, Minnie, 181
Brown, Philip King
    Arequipa Sanatorium, 125, 128–129
    early life, 126
    medical credentials, 126
Brush, Edward N., Sheppard-Pratt Hospital, 55–56, 62–63

Buck, Mertice M.C., 99
Byrdcliffe School, 222

## C

Carpentry shop, 268–269
Celsus, 19
Charity network, 15, 185–186, 214–215
Cheer-up worker, 156
Chicago School of Civics and Philanthropy, 35
    Slagle, Eleanor Clarke, 45, 46
Children's Bureau, 38
Children's work, 267–269
Christian Science, 105, 106
Chronic physical illness, 115
City politics, Hull House, 38
College education, 37
Collins, Evelyn Lawrence
    remuneration, 132–133
    Teachers College, 130, 131–133
    volunteer charity work, 132
Consolation House, Barton, George Edward, 117–119
Contagious disease, 188
Course in curative occupations, 42
Craft work, 39
Credentials, 7, 250
Cult of true womanhood, 35–36
Cultural diversity, 5–6
Cultural synthesis, 5
Curative workshop, 277

## D

Davis, Elizabeth Upham, Committee on Admissions and Positions, 218–220
Devereux Workshops
    Hall, Herbert J., 96–101
    Luther, Jessie, 96
Dunton, William Rush, 99
    Barton, George Edward, 120–122, 123

Dunton, William Rush, Jr., 16, 53
    Committee on Publicity and Publication, 245–250
    early life, 53–54
    education, 54–55, 56
    National Society for the Promotion of Occupational Therapy, 122–123
    in professionalizing occupational therapy, 53
    Sheppard-Pratt Hospital, 54, 57, 62–63
    Slagle, Eleanor Clark, professional relationship, 61–62

## E

Education, of women, 36–37
Education reform
    beginnings, 218–222
    Committee on Admissions and Positions, 218–220
Elwood, Everett S., 250–252
Emmanuelism, 103, 105–107
    Hall, Herbert J., 106–107
Equivalents, 101–102
Experiment Station for the Study of Invalid Occupations
    resource center, 80
    Tracy, Susan E., 79–80
    training, 80–81

## F

Family responsibilities, 190
Fatigue, 98, 119
Fechner, Gustav, 104
Federal Board for Vocational Education, 153–154
Federal Board for Vocational Education, Upham, Elizabeth Greene, 158, 184
Follett, Mary Parker, 3
Freudianism, 62, 63
    Hall, Herbert J., 106–107
Frustration, 98
Fuller, Daniel H., 73, 75, 79, 99
Fundamentalism, 5

## G

Gender role, 14–15, 35–36, 73, 83–84, 157, 189–190, 278–280

General Federation of Women's Clubs, 214–215

Goldthwait, Jessie, 181

Goldthwait, Joel E., 94, 96, 152

Goodman, Hilda B., Milwaukee-Downer College, 184

## H

Habit training, 45, 104

Hall, Herbert J., 74, 75, 84–85, 93, 235, 238–239
- criticism, 84
- Devereux Workshops, 96–101
- early life, 95–96
- education, 95
- Emmanuelism, 106–107
- equivalents, 101–102
- Freudianism, 106–107
- immunities, 102
- Marblehead workshops, 93, 94
- National Society for the Promotion of Occupational Therapy, 176
- patient socioeconomic backgrounds, 99–100
- recordkeeping, 238
- substitutions, 102

Health care, 6

Henry Phipps Psychiatric Clinic, Meyer, Adolph, 58

Henry Street Settlement, 130, 131

Hitchcock, Mrs. Ripley, 178–179

Holistic medicine, 13

Horner, Rachel, Muirdale Hospital, 183

Hospital
- Barton, George Edward, 119–120
- early craft work, 60–61
- establishment, 20
- reform, 21

Hull House, 37–42
- city politics, 38
- in contemporary social movements, 39
- educational activities, 40–41
- female patrons, 38–39
- founding, 37
- industrialization, 39–40
- objectives, 37
- projects, 38

Hull House Labor Museum, 40–41

## I

Immunities, 102

Independence, 83

Industrialization, Hull House, 39–40

## J

Jewelry making, 273, 274

Johnson, Susan Cox, 17, 129, 130–134, 162, 163, 182, 221
- American Occupational Therapy Association, 175
- Blackwell's Island Hospital, 130
- Committee on Admissions and Positions, 218–220
- National Society for the Promotion of Occupational Therapy, 122–123
- patients' productivity, 130–131
- programs, 130
- Teachers College, 133
- training, 133

Junior League, 215

## K

Kidner, Thomas B., 242–243
- American Occupational Therapy Association, 174–175
- National Society for the Promotion of Occupational Therapy, 122, 123–124

Kirkbride, Thomas Story, 21

## L

Lathrop, Julia, 41–42

Licensing, 250–251
Licht, Sidney, 16
Loom, 266–267
Luther, Jessie, 94
    Devereux Workshops, 96

## M

Management consultant, 3
Mansfield, Helen, War Service Classes for Training Reconstruction Aides in Occupational Therapy, 177
Marblehead workshops, Hall, Herbert J., 93, 94
Massachusetts General Hospital, 177
McComb, Samuel, 105
McMurtrie, Douglas C., 153–154
Mental hygiene movement, 35, 120, 240–241
    Slagle, Eleanor Clarke, 45
Mentoring
    professional culture, 212–218
    Slagle, Eleanor Clarke, 213
Meyer, Adolph, 74–75
    Henry Phipps Psychiatric Clinic, 58
    Sheppard-Pratt Hospital, 58–59
Millenium, 3–5
Milwaukee-Downer College
    Goodman, Hilda B., 184
    philanthropic organization support, 185–186
    Sabin, Ellen, 183, 184
    Upham, Elizabeth Greene, 182–185
*A Mind That Found Itself*, 120
Mitchell, S. Weir, 104
Morrison, Mrs. Horace, 181
Muirdale Hospital, Horner, Rachel, 183

## N

National register of qualified practitioners, 226

National Society for the Promotion of Occupational Therapy, 174–177, 175–176. *See also* American Occupational Therapy Association
    Barton, George Edward, 116, 122–123
    conferences, 174
    Dunton, William Rush, Jr., 122–123
    foundation of, 81–82
    founders, 122
    Hall, Herbert J., 176
    Johnson, Susan C., 122–123
    Kidner, Thomas B., 122–123, 123–124
    name change, 174
    presidency, 174
    Slagle, Eleanor Clarke, 122–123, 175–176
    Tracy, Susan E., 81, 122–123
Networking
    professional culture, 212–218
    Slagle, Eleanor Clarke, 215–216
Neurasthenia, 73–74, 98
New Age, 4–5
New woman, 189–190
New York War Service Classes for Training Reconstruction Aides in Occupational Therapy, 222
Nursing
    occupational therapy, interrelationship, 81–82
    Tracy, Susan E., 76
Nutting, Adelaide, 71

## O

Obedience, 78–79
Occupational therapist, family responsibilities, 190
Occupational therapy
    antimodernist movement, 116
    charity organization support, 15, 38–39, 132, 185–186, 214–215
    craft work, 41
    crafts selection, 98
    credentials, 17, 250
    current issues, 6–7
    defined, 13

Occupational therapy *(cont.)*
   experiential learning, 41
   first generation legacy, 278–280
   funding, 242–243
   gender-defined division of labor, 278
   gender-defined framework of organization, 73
   historical materials, 16
   ideals, 7–9
   ideology, 116
   implicit elitism, 187–188
   inspiration for, 77–78
   medical identity, 235–236
   medical legitimacy, 237–238
   medical model of, 212
   midwestern practitioners, 212
   moral therapy regimens, 98
   networking, 173
   nursing
      interrelationship, 188, 221
   nursing, interrelationship, 81–82
   organizational strategies, 181
   principles, 98, 235
   problem of commercialism, 244–245
   profession status evaluation, 219–220
   promotion, 173, 181
   reasons for vocation, 77–78
   reconstruction, 159
   reconstruction aide, 159
   selection, 173
   theoretical basis, 61, 62
   therapeutic world view, 116
   training, 177
   volunteer service, 162
   western practitioners, 212
   women's organization support, 185–186
   women's values, 15
*Occupational Therapy: A Manual for Nurses*, 62
*Occupational Therapy and Rehabilitation*, 243, 246
Orthopedics, 152–153
*O.T.: A New Profession*, 101

## P

Philadelphia School of Occupational Therapy, 82
Philanthropic organization, 15, 38–39, 132, 185–186, 214–215
Phipps Clinic, Slagle, Eleanor Clarke, 45–46
Physical therapy, 160
Physicians' prescription, 235, 236, 243
Pinel, Philippe, 20
Politically active family, 187
Pollack, Horatio M., 239–241
   recordkeeping, 239
Pratt, Joseph H., 104–105
*Prescribing Occupational Therapy*, 250
Professional culture
   mentoring, 212–218
   networking, 212–218
   recruitment, 212–218
Professionalism, 206
   cultural context, 16
   documentation, 17
   ideological context, 16
   Tracy, Susan E., 72–73, 77
Psychiatric care, 53, 57, 188–189
Psychobiology, 58
Psychology, 103
Public service, 187

## R

Reconstruction aide, 19, 20, 21, 82, 157–166, 270, 274, 278
   accomplishments, 165
   American Expeditionary Forces, 164–165
   authority over, 161
   career tracks, 189–192
   characteristics, 161
   effects, 173
   occupational therapy, 159
   placement, 163
   recruitment, 157–158, 160
   training, 160
   types, 160
   Upham, Elizabeth Greene, 158

## Index

Reconstruction aide *(cont.)*
   *vs.* hospitals, 173
   *vs.* occupational therapy, 205–206

Reconstruction movement, 151
   authority in, 153–154
   European model of reconstruction, 157
   gender-defined division of labor, 157
   occupational therapy, 159
   recruitment, 157–158

Recruitment
   professional culture, 212–218
   Slagle, Eleanor Clarke, 214–215

Red Cross Institute for Crippled and Disabled Men, 153–154

Reeducation, 151, 152

Reform, 35–36, 37, 39, 261

Rehabilitation, World War I, 151–166
   Canada's system, 152

Reil, Johann Christian, 20

Remuneration, Collins, Evelyn Lawrence, 132–133

Rest cure, 74, 104
   critique, 74

Revivalism, 5

Roosevelt, Eleanor, Slagle, Eleanor Clarke, 261, 262, 278, 279

### S

Sabin, Ellen, Milwaukee-Downer College, 183, 184

Salmon, Thomas W., 155

Sanderson, Marguerite, 158–159, 161

Scattergood, Thomas, 21

Scientific medicine, 13

Self-absorption, 98

Self-sacrifice, 78–79

Service to society, 77–78, 132–133

Settlement house movement, 37–42

Sheppard-Pratt Hospital
   Brush, Edward N., 55–56, 62–63
   development of, 57–61
   Dunton, William Rush, Jr., 54, 57, 62–63
   early crafts, 59
   Meyer, Adolph, 58–59
   records, 59–60

Shut-In Society, 132

Slagle, Eleanor Clarke, 17, 35–37, 162, 235
   American Occupational Therapy Association, 176–177
   Chicago School of Civics and Philanthropy, 45, 46
   early life, 42–43
   education, 35, 43, 45, 175
   Experimental Station, 46
   family gender roles, 43
   family health history, 44–45
   family life, 191
   legacy, 278
   marriage, 43
   membership drive, 248
   mental hygiene movement, 45
   mentoring, 213
   National Society for the Promotion of Occupational Therapy, 122–123, 175–176
   networking, 215–216
   Phipps Clinic, 45–46
   professional persona, 175–176
   recruitment, 214–215
   Roosevelt, Eleanor, 261, 262, 278, 279
   testimonial dinner, 261
   work experience, 175

Slagle, Eleanor Clarke, Dunton, William Rush, Jr., professional relationship, 61–62

Smith, Mrs. Charles Sprague, 178

Smith-Sears Act, 154

Soldiers (Veterans) Rehabilitation Act, 154, 158

Starr, Ellen Gates, 37, 39, 40

Substitutions, 102

Suffrage, 187

Sullivan, Mrs. Cornelius J., 178

## T

Taylor, Frederick W., 151–152
Taylor, Graham, 42
Teachers College, 177, 219–221
- Collins, Evelyn Lawrence, 130, 131–133
- Johnson, Susan Cox, 133

Tracy, Susan E., 17, 71
- Adams Nervine Asylum, 73–79
- early life, 71
- education, 76
- as educator, 71
- Experiment Station for the Study of Invalid Occupations, 79–80
- female model, 83–84
- home-based care, 71
- mythologizing, 76–77
- and national organization, 71
- National Society for the Promotion of Occupational Therapy, 81, 122–123
- nursing, 76
- private-duty nursing, 75
- professionalism, 72–73, 77

Training, 181–182
- competition, 184
- educational reform, 218–222
  - Committee on Admissions and Positions, 218–220
- Experiment Station for the Study of Invalid Occupations, 80–81
- Johnson, Susan Cox, 133
- minimum standards, 223–226

"True" womanhood, 35–36
Tuberculosis, 125–129, 241, 242, 243, 264, 267, 269–270, 275, 277
Tuke, William, 20, 56, 57

## U

Upham, Elizabeth Greene, 158, 161, 162, 182
- early life, 182–183
- family life, 190
- Federal Board for Vocational Education, 158, 184

Upham, Elizabeth Greene (cont.)
- Milwaukee-Downer College, 182–185
- reconstruction aide, 158

## V

Volunteer service, 38–39, 132, 214–215, 236
- occupational therapy, 162
- *vs.* professional types, 162

## W

Wade, Beatrice
- American Occupational Therapy Association, 211–212
- family life, 191

Wadsworth, Martha, 161–162, 177
War Risk Insurance Act, 158
War Service Classes for Training Reconstruction Aides in Occupational Therapy, 177–182
- classes, 179
- founders, 177–179
- Mansfield, Helen, 177
- placement, 179–180
- student background, 179
- Surgeon General's Office, 177, 179

Weaving, 274–275, 277
Wembridge, Eleanor Rowland, 165
Wigglesworth, Ruth, 223
Williams, Frankwood E., 163–164
Women professional
- cultural context, 16
- documentation, 17
- ideological context, 16

Women's club, 214
Women's philanthropic support, 38–39, 132, 185–186
Women's role, 14–15, 35–36, 73, 83–84, 157, 189–190, 280
Women's role, altruistic lady *vs.* independent professional, 83
Women's suffrage movement, 187
Worcester, Elwood, 103–105, 117
*The Work of Our Hands*, 99–100

Workshop, 272, 273, 274, 275, 277

World War I, 130, 134, 145–146, 264, 270–274. *See also* Reconstruction aide; Reconstruction movement
    Creed of the Disabled, 155
    psychological aspects, 155–156
    rehabilitation, 151–166
        Canada's system, 152
    wartime reconstruction movement, 151–152
    women's role in reconstruction, 155

World War Reconstruction Aides Association, 191

Wundt, Wilhelm, 103–104

Wyman, Rufus, 21

# Y

York Retreat, 56, 57